An Atlas of
LASER OPERATIVE
LAPAROSCOPY AND
HYSTEROSCOPY

THE ENCYCLOPEDIA OF VISUAL MEDICINE SERIES

An Atlas of
LASER OPERATIVE LAPAROSCOPY AND HYSTEROSCOPY

J. Donnez and M. Nisolle

Catholic University of Louvain
Brussels, Belgium

With a foreword by
Alan H. DeCherney
Tufts University School of Medicine
Boston, Massachusetts, USA

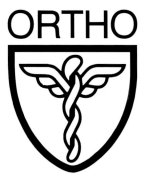

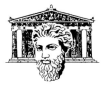

The Parthenon Publishing Group
International Publishers in Medicine, Science & Technology

NEW YORK   LONDON

Published in the USA by
The Parthenon Publishing Group Inc.
One Blue Hill Plaza, PO Box 1564, Pearl River, New York 10965, USA

Published in the UK by
The Parthenon Publishing Group Limited
Casterton Hall, Carnforth, Lancs, LA6 2LA, UK

Library of Congress Cataloging-in-Publication Data
Donnez. J.
   An atlas of laser operative laparoscopy and hysteroscopy /
J. Donnez and M. Nisolle: with a special introduction by Alan DeCherney.
       p.   cm. – (Encyclopedia of visual medicine series)
   Includes bibliographical references and index.
   ISBN 1-85070-464-3
   1. Generative organs, Female – Endoscopic surgery – Atlases.
2. Laser endoscopy – Atlases. I. Nisolle, M. II. Title.
III. Title: Laser operative laparoscopy and hysteroscopy. IV. Series.
   [DNLM: 1. Genital Diseases, Female – surgery –atlases. 2. Surgery,
Laparoscopic – methods – atlases. 3. Hysteroscopy – methods – atlases.
4. Laser Surgery – methods – atlases. WP 17 D686a 1994]
RG104.7.D66 1994
618.1'059 – dc20
DNLM/DLC
for Library of Congress   94-13476
                                                    CIP

British Library Cataloguing-in-Publication Data
Atlas of Laser Operative Laparoscopy and
Hysteroscopy. – (Encyclopedia of Visual Medicine Series)
   I. Donnez, J. II. Nisolle, M. III. Series
   618.107545
   ISBN 1-85070-464-3

Composition by Ryburn Publishing Services, Keele University, UK
Color reproduction by Colorplan, Leeds, UK
Printed and bound in Spain by T.G. Hostench, S.A.

Contents

List of principal contributors

S. Bassil
Department of Gynecology
Catholic University of Louvain
Cliniques Universitaires St Luc
Avenue Hippocrate 10
B-1200 Brussels
Belgium

M. Canis
Gynécologie-Obstétrique-Reproduction Humaine
Polyclinique Hôtel-Dieu
13, Boulevard Charles de Gaulle
F 63033 Clermont-Ferrand Cedex
France

A.H. DeCherney
Department of Obstetrics and Gynecology
Tufts University School of Medicine
Boston
Massachusetts
USA

J. Donnez
Department of Gynecology
Infertility Research Unit
Catholic University of Louvain
Cliniques Universitaires St Luc
Avenue Hippocrate 10
B-1200 Brussels
Belgium

J.B. Dubuisson
Service de Gynécologie Obstétrique II
Maternité Baudelocque
123 Bd Port Royal
75014 Paris
France

S. Gordts
Department of Gynecology
Catholic University of Louvain
Cliniques Universitaires St Luc
Avenue Hippocrate 10
B-1200 Brussels
Belgium

G. Mage
Gynécologie-Obstétrique-Reproduction Humaine
Polyclinique Hôtel-Dieu
13, Boulevard Charles de Gaulle
F 63033 Clermont-Ferrand Cedex
France

D.C. Martin
Baptist Memorial Hospital
University of Tennessee
Memphis
Tennesee
USA

C. Nezhat
Department of Obstetrics and Gynecology
Mercer University School of Medicine
Macon
Georgia
USA

M. Nisolle
Department of Gynecology
Infertility Research Unit
Catholic University of Louvain
Cliniques Universitaires St Luc
Avenue Hippocrate 10
B-1200 Brussels
Belgium

H. Reich
Wyoming Valley GYN/OB Associates
48 Pierce Street
Kingston
Pennsylvania
USA

R. Sinai
Sharplan Laser Industries
Tel Aviv
Israel

C.J.G. Sutton
Department of Gynecology
Royal Surrey County Hospital
Guildford
Surrey
UK

Y. Tadir
Beckman Laser Institute and Medical Clinic
Department of Surgery
University of California, Irvine
1002 Health Science Rd
Irvine, CA 92715
USA

M.J. Van Boven
Department of Anesthesiology
Catholic University of Louvain
Cliniques Universitaires St Luc
Avenue Hippocrate 10
B-1200 Brussels
Belgium

L. Van Obbergh
Department of Anesthesiology
Catholic University of Louvain
Cliniques Universitaires St Luc
Avenue Hippocrate 10
B-1200 Brussels
Belgium

Foreword

Professor Donnez and Dr Nisolle have written a classic, *An Atlas of Laser Operative Laparoscopy and Hysteroscopy*. Its major attributes are, first, it is state of the art; second, it is a superb atlas; and, third, it is a text filled with theory, understanding and wisdom. The illustrations are excellent and serve as guidelines for this specific genre of surgery.

In the last decade, there has been a burgeoning of information, innovative techniques and new technology in regards to endoscopic surgery. The introduction of the laser and the renaissance in electric power to carry out complicated surgical techniques through the endoscope have come to the fore in regards to what is done.

In most institutions, gynecological services and gynecology itself have changed dramatically, based on these new surgical techniques and approaches. The number of inpatient procedures has, in general, declined dramatically, and they have been replaced by newer techniques which can be performed in an outpatient setting such that the patient may go home the same day. Two examples come immediately to mind. The first is laparoscopically assisted vaginal hysterectomy. This procedure has revolutionized hysterectomy because not only do patients who undergo an endoscopically assisted procedure recuperate more rapidly, allowing them to go home earlier from the hospital, but the lessons learned have been applied to classically performed hysterectomies as well. The second example is the management of ovarian cysts which has a varied past, from medical treatment to observation to laparotomy. Now, with the advent of a laparoscopic alternative and the ability preoperatively to diagnose the presence of malignancy with fair accuracy, the majority of ovarian cysts are being treated in this fashion.

The history of laparoscopic surgery is perhaps best illustrated through ectopic pregnancy. For years it was controversial to perform linear salpingostomies through the endoscope, and in fact, as with most new ideas, it is one that required tremendous marketing in order to incorporate it into the armamentarium of the surgeon. Now, in some instances, it is considered less than optimal care to remove an ectopic pregnancy by means other than endoscopic. In fact, there are some pioneering researchers evaluating laparoscopic techniques as applied to carcinoma.

Hysteroscopy has an even more interesting past than laparoscopy in regards to gynecology. Hysteroscopy as a diagnostic technique remained only a possibility for many years, and it was only when surgery became possible that it took on added perspective and importance. This is best exemplified by the treatment of Müllerian fusion defects. For years these were treated with abdominal metroplasty. These procedures (Thompkins and Jones) have been totally replaced by an endoscopic approach.

Classic textbooks are therefore needed in order for the operating surgeon to learn and carry out these new tasks, and Professor Donnez and Dr Nisolle have provided us with just such a resource. As with any new 'science', principles must be laid down, pioneering approaches must be tried, and we must re-evaluate what we already know. To paraphrase the Queen of Hearts in Alice in Wonderland, When everyone is so sure it's the truth, it probably is not the truth.

This book is written by just a few authors, all with international reputations for excellence and innovation. Basic principles such as laser physics are extremely well explained and illustrated. The pathogenesis of the disease processes which we treat through an endoscopic approach are likewise handled. And, most importantly, the techniques are well described in that, not only does this serve as a reference book, but also as a manual for procedure.

Complications have long been a neglected area in endoscopic surgery. It began as a field of 'show and tell', and people were mainly interested in what could be done. What Professor Donnez and Dr Nisolle have contributed with this textbook is a large compendium on complications: identification, diagnosis, treatment and prevention. This I believe is the most significant portion of the book because this topic has been heretofore neglected. Any surgical field has complications. It is our obligation to present them so that others can benefit from past experience.

The future of gynecological surgery is clearly founded upon endoscopy and I feel that this book is the 'TeLind', that standard textbook of surgery that has become legendary, of the future.

Alan H. DeCherney
Louis E. Phaneuf Professor and Chairman
Department of Obstetrics and Gynecology
Tufts University School of Medicine
Boston, Massachusetts, USA

Laser physics and laser instrumentation

R. Sinai

INTRODUCTION

The utilization of the laser in advanced modern surgery owes its wide dissemination to the fact that lasers, commonly used in industrial, military, commercial or scientific applications, interact with biological tissue in such a way that localized and precisely controlled alterations of the cellular structure are effected irreversibly.

In the hands of the skilled surgeon, the laser becomes an instrument capable of inducing desired therapeutic effects, far beyond the scope of conventional surgical tools such as cold knives or electrocautery probes. The laser enables the surgeon to utilize a variety of operational modalities for the treatment of diseased tissue. Precise incisions can be performed, lesions extending over large areas can be vaporized, and voluminous lesions can be debulked and destroyed by ablation or necrotization. Very often, it is possible to target the therapeutic energy selectively at cells characterized by a well-defined property (e.g. color), implementing the selectivity of the interaction process between the laser and the tissue.

Laser energy can be delivered to tissue in a variety of ways: by contact or from a distance, in conjunction with an operative microscope, through an endoscope, or with the aid of freehand tools.

Finally, laser treatments provide significant advantages, unmatched by competitive techniques: in the majority of cases the operation is largely hemostatic. Thus, the surgeon enjoys the convenience of a dry and clear field, even when operating in an environment of high vascularity. Moreover, contamination of adjacent areas is considerably reduced because of the sealing of blood and lymph vessels. The extent of injury to surrounding tissue is, to a high degree, controllable. Consequently, the risk of postoperative pain, complications or irreversible damage is diminished considerably. In some cases, the recurrence rate of the disease also appears to be reduced. The laser enables the surgeon to reach anatomical structures whose size or location render them inaccessible to any other known surgical instrument.

The reasons for this impressive procedural variety and wealth of benefits lie in the particular properties of the laser as a special source of energy. In order to achieve the best clinical use with this surgical tool, it is necessary to understand what a laser is, how it operates, and how the parameters that govern its operation can be controlled by the surgeon.

WHAT IS A LASER?

Light as a wave phenomenon

The laser is merely a beam of ordinary light radiation. Visible light, which is a day-to-day experience in our natural environment, represents only one facet of a much broader physical phenomenon known as electromagnetic radiation.

Classical physics regards electromagnetic radiation as a wave phenomenon, much like the waves generated by throwing a stone into a pond or the audible sound waves emitted by a tuning fork (Figure 1). A wave-type phenomenon is manifested by periodic vibrations of physical quantities, such as the height of the pond surface, the air pressure or the electromagnetic field. These undergo a cyclical change in magnitude – the cycle repeating itself, in principle, over an indefinite period of time. In the case of the pond, the surface at each specific location is displaced and elevated above its rest value to a certain maximum displacement – the crest of the wave. Subsequently, the pond surface sags under gravity and a trough is created at the same location, below the same rest value. The downward displacement is equal to the displacement of the crest. The cycle repeats itself, and were it not for the dissipative forces which ultimately return the pond to the rest position, the oscillation would continue *ad infinitum*. Moreover, as a result of the temporal oscillations occurring at one particular location, adjacent areas are also set in motion and the wave propagates over the pond surface, away from the origin of disturbance, creating a sequence of crests and troughs which propagate as spatial oscillations.

A similar phenomenon occurs in the case of sound waves: the crests and troughs of the pond waves are substituted by alternate compressions and rarifications of the gas (air) through which the sound propagates.

The quantity that vibrates in the case of electromagnetic waves is an electrical field (always paired with a concurrent magnetic field to which it is related by a well-defined mathematical relation).

Four basic parameters describe the wave phenomenon:

(1) The magnitude of the displacement represents the intensity of the wave and is a direct outcome of the energy invested in its generation (the impact of the stone on the surface of the pond). This is the *amplitude* (A) of the wave (Figure 1).

(2) The *wavelength* (λ) is the distance between two successive crests or troughs (Figure 1). The unit of measurement is:

$$1 \text{ nm} = \frac{1 \text{ mm}}{1\,000\,000} \quad \text{or} \quad 1 \text{ μm} = \frac{1 \text{ mm}}{1000}$$

(Obviously, 1 μm = 1000 nm.)

(3) The *speed* of propagation (c), is measured in cm/s.

(4) The *frequency* (f) is measured in Hertz (cycles/s) and represents the number of vibrations per second, occurring at a given spatial location. In the case of sound waves, the frequency translates into the pitch of the sound.

Wavelength (λ), speed of propagation (c), and frequency (f) are related by:

$$\lambda f = c$$

In the case of electromagnetic waves, the speed of propagation in the void is a universal constant, namely the speed of light:

$$c = 300\,000 \text{ km/s}$$

Consequently, the higher the frequency, the shorter the wavelength.

The electromagnetic spectrum

Electromagnetic radiation of different wavelengths is manifested in diverse physical phenomena:

(1) The wavelength of ordinary radio waves ranges from approximately 1000 m (AM radio waves, hundreds of kHz in frequency) to 1 m (FM radio waves, hundreds of MHz in frequency).

(2) Radar occupies the range of cm waves (frequency in GHz) in the electromagnetic spectrum.

(3) Microwaves or mm waves used in consumer products feature frequencies up to 100 GHz.

(4) Infrared light covers the range of wavelengths from 100 μm (very far infrared) to 0.7 μm (near infrared).

(5) Visible light occupies a very narrow region of the entire spectrum of electromagnetic radiation, from 500 nm to 700 nm. The light is visible because the rods and cones located in the human retina can detect it. These are not sensitive to wavelengths outside this range, which remain invisible to the human eye.

(6) Wavelengths shorter than visible light belong to the ultraviolet range: 100–500 nm. Beyond that region of the spectrum we find X-rays, whose wavelength is as low as 0.1 nm, and nuclear gamma rays of much shorter wavelengths.

The concept of color originates from the interaction of the human retina with the visible region of the electromagnetic spectrum. The sense of color is determined exclusively by the wavelength of the light. The color 'red' lies at one end of the visual spectrum (long wavelength), while 'blue' lies at the opposite end (short wavelength). The white daylight generated by the sun is a mixture of several basic colors and as such it is *polychromatic*. It can be dispersed into the basic rainbow colors by a prism (Figure 2). Other sources emit light of a precise individual wavelength. Such radiation sources are called *monochromatic*.

The atomic theory of light

Light is a form of energy generated, emitted or absorbed by atoms or molecules. To emit energy, the atom or molecule must be aroused to an excited energy level above its ground state (in which there is no excess energy to be discharged). Atoms, like human beings, cannot sustain excitement for long periods of time. Consequently, they have a natural tendency to rid themselves of the surplus energy, subsequently emitted in the form of particles or light wave packets called *photons*. The wavelength of the emitted photon is related to the energy surplus according to:

$$\lambda = \frac{hc}{E}$$

where h is a universal constant called Planck's constant, E is the energy surplus, c is the speed of light, and λ is the wavelength.

Each elementary atom or particular molecule possesses distinct and precisely determined excited energy levels. Consequently, different elements will emit photons of different energies, i.e. photons of different wavelengths. All these primary radiations are, therefore, monochromatic. The fact that sunlight is polychromatic indicates that the incandescent matter of which the sun is composed is a mixture of different elements (atoms).

Atoms can be excited by different mechanisms: they can be heated – a fact which on the atomic scale translates into intensification of their state of agitation, leading to an increase in mutual interatomic collisions; they can be excited by electrical discharge – which on the atomic scale means that they are bombarded by fast-moving charged particles; or they can be illuminated by electromagnetic radiation of a characteristic wavelength – which on the

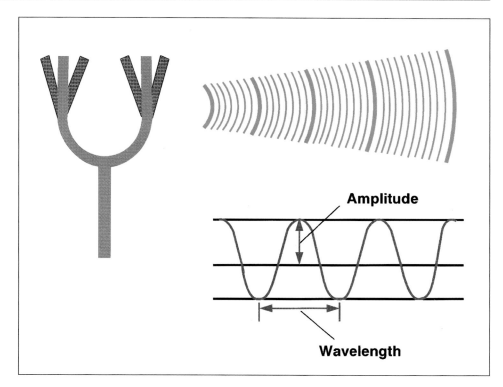

Figure 1   Sound wave generated by tuning fork

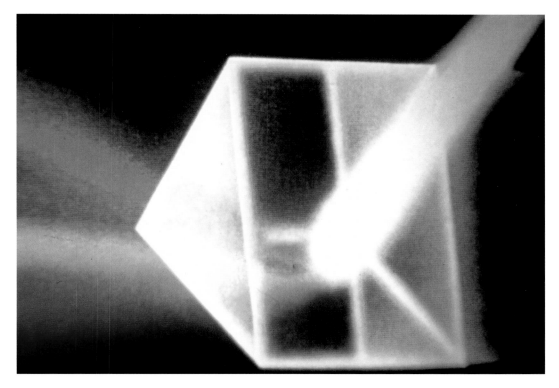

Figure 2   Dispersion of white light by a prism

atomic scale means that they absorb photons of selective wavelength.

Atoms decay from their excited to ground state levels in two different ways (Figure 3): spontaneous and stimulated emission. The normal mechanism is spontaneous emission. At the completion of a known and calculable period of time – the lifetime of the excited level – the atom returns to its ground state by emitting a characteristic photon of light.

In the early 1920s, Albert Einstein postulated and proved the existence of another mechanism – stimulated emission. An excited atom emits its characteristic photon instantaneously, even before the complete lifetime elapses, if it encounters on its journey a stimulating photon identical to and of the same wavelength as the one that it would have spontaneously emitted, should the lifetime have already elapsed.

Stimulated emission conforms to the following two laws:

(1) The stimulated photon travels in the same direction as its stimulator;

(2) The wave packet incorporated in the stimulated photon synchronizes itself to the wave packet of the stimulator. In other words, the two photons align their crests and troughs to act simultaneously, reinforcing rather than cancelling one another (which is the case when crests of one wave-packet align to the troughs of the other). Photons with aligned crests and troughs are called *coherent*.

The end result of stimulated emission is thus a pair of photons which are coherent and travel in tandem in the same direction. Stimulated emission constitutes the basis for the invention of the laser, effected some 30 years after Einstein's discovery.

Basic principle of laser operation

To illustrate the mechanism of laser light generation, imagine a perfectly straight tube or rod, housing a very large quantity of identical atoms or molecules. At each end of the tube reflecting mirrors are attached: the mirror at one end is totally reflective; at the other end (the output port of the laser tube), the mirror is only partially reflective (90% of the light is reflected back into the tube, while 10% is transmitted through the mirror and exits).

Imagine also that the atoms are excited to an elevated energy level by an external source (such as an illumination device or an electrical discharge). The exact instant of excitation varies from atom to atom and is governed by the rules of chance. This also applies to the spontaneous emission of photons at the end of the lifetime of each atom, which occurs at different points in time, randomly distributed. The emitted photons travel in various directions within the tube. Those hitting the tube walls are absorbed and vanish from the scene. On the other hand, a freshly emitted photon travelling in a direction parallel to the tube axis enjoys the probability of encountering another atom and thereby stimulating the emission of an additional photon, coherent with the stimulator and travelling in the same direction – namely, along the longitudinal axis of the tube. The two photons continue their journey, again enjoying the probability of giving rise, by a similar process, to two additional photons – all coherent with one another and all travelling along the same axis. The progression continues on and on, and eight, 16, 32, etc. photons are generated, all travelling in the same direction. This is clearly an *amplification* process that creates a very large flux of light photons.

To further enhance the amplification factor, photons that hit the totally reflective mirror, which is perpendicular to the tube axis, are reflected back into the tube, and they continue to travel along the same axis in the opposite direction. Every such photon will initiate a similar chain reaction, yielding a stream of coherent photons. Even when the partially reflective mirror is hit, 90% of the photons will be returned to the tube and will continue to contribute to the amplification sequence. The remaining 10% exit at the output port, constituting the source of laser radiation (Figure 4). They represent, in absolute terms, a very intense photon beam produced by the amplification chain.

The above description of the lasing process explains the acronym 'laser': Light Amplification by Stimulated Emission of Radiation. From the above description, we also learn what the unique properties of laser radiation are, that differentiate it from ordinary light:

(1) It is monochromatic because it is generated by a collection of identical atoms all emitting photons of the same wavelength;

(2) It is coherent by virtue of the stimulated emission which creates coherent photons; and

(3) The laser beam, being parallel to the longitudinal axis of the tube, features a very low angular divergence. (The divergence is never nil because, in practical terms, there is always some slight misalignment of the mirrors, as they cannot be positioned in precise perpendicularity to the axis).

The clinical implications of the first and last property are far-reaching. Monochromaticity and its consequences in surgery will be discussed in the next section. The low angular divergence of the laser beam enables the surgeon to take full advantage of the capabilities of classical optical systems, and to focus the laser beam precisely on the target area. The laws of physical optics imply that the size of the beam spot on the focal plane of an optical lens system is proportional to the angular divergence of the incoming beam. No matter how perfect the lens system, a largely divergent incoming

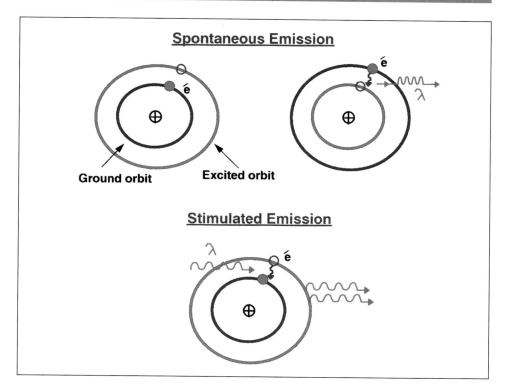

Figure 3 Photon emission modalities

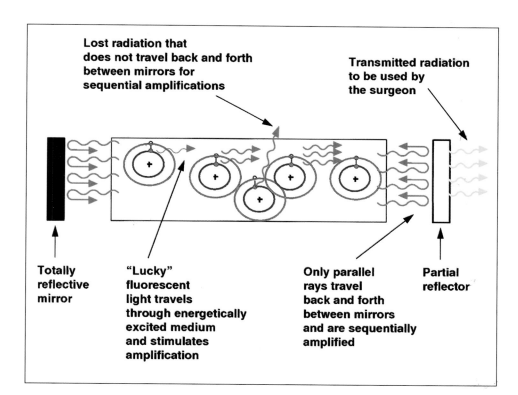

Figure 4 Operating principle of the laser

beam will result in a poorly focused output beam (large spot size). Conversely, a non-divergent or minimally divergent incoming beam, such as the laser, will converge at the focal plane of a high-quality optical system, into a very small spot size (Figure 5). The flux of the photons contained in the beam is the same in both instances. Consequently, in the case of the laser beam, the same flux of photons hits a target which is much smaller. Thus, the energy deposited per unit area is much higher than in the case of ordinary divergent light, and so is the effect on tissue. The laser beam, which in itself is an intense source of energy, is further down-focused to a minuscule spot size to strongly interact with the tissue. Two results are achieved: the target area is finely pin-pointed by a very precise beam, and the effect on tissue is very intense.

LASER–TISSUE INTERACTION

Physical effects of the laser on tissue

The laser effect on a tissue sample is one of transmission, reflection, scattering or absorption (Figure 6). The effect on tissue achieved by any laser commonly used in therapeutic medicine is a consequence of its absorption therein. In particular, the energy deposited by most of the commonly used lasers is transformed into heat, thereby obtaining a thermal effect on the tissue.

The types of lasers used in therapeutic medicine are confined to the visible, ultraviolet and infrared regions of the spectrum. Figure 7 presents a list of these lasers with their respective wavelengths.

Excimer lasers (a short form of excited dimers, which are short-lived unstable halogen molecules) emit light in the ultraviolet range (very short wavelength). Their absorption by the tissue leads to photochemical disintegration of large protein molecules, shaving away microstructures from the treated area. For this reason, excimers are used in cornea refractive surgery for the treatment of myopia (photokeratotomy).

Argon green lasers are used in ophthalmology for treating retinopathies related to vascular disorders of the retina bed. The monochromatic green light is selectively absorbed by the blood oxyhemoglobin, resulting in coagulation of the blood and sealing of the blood vessel.

Yellow dye and copper vapor lasers, also selectively absorbed by oxyhemoglobin, are used in dermatology and cosmetic surgery to treat vascular diseases of the skin such as port wine stains, telangiectasias and superficial hemangiomas.

The green dye laser is used in urological lithotripsy to pulverize ureteral stones (by a photoacoustical effect). The stones strongly absorb a green light of a very defined wavelength: 508 nm.

The green dye and copper vapor lasers are also strongly absorbed by the skin melanin. Consequently, they are used for treating pigmented lesions, such as café-au-lait or age spots.

Red light is selectively absorbed by the blue and black ink used to infiltrate the skin in the production of tattoos. Certain red-colored lasers, such as alexandrite or ruby, are employed for the removal of these otherwise indelible markings.

The infrared lasers constitute the primary subject of this book. They are widely recognized by the medical community as part of the armamentarium of modern surgery. We will, therefore, elaborate further on their interaction with biological tissue.

Figure 8 illustrates the relative absorption of light in water as a function of wavelength. Because water is a major component of the cellular structure, its interaction with the laser is predominant. The CO_2 laser features a wavelength of $10.6\,\mu m$ in the far infrared range. It is strongly absorbed by water, as indicated in Figure 9. CO_2 laser radiation is readily absorbed by the first few cellular layers of tissue, constituting the first $100\,\mu m$. Consequently, this is a laser used for superficial treatments.

The Nd:YAG laser (neodymium yttrium aluminum garnet) features a wavelength of $1.06\,\mu m$ (near infrared). Water is completely transparent to this type of radiation. Consequently, the Nd:YAG laser is ideal for the treatment of lesions located in liquid-filled cavities such as the bladder and the uterus (filled with a distension liquid). The Nd:YAG laser is, however, strongly scattered by the tissue. Penetrating beams are scattered and folded at multiple sites, increasing the effective path length of the beam through the tissue. Nd:YAG laser light, which is absorbed to some degree by the proteins within the tissue bed, deposits energy each time absorption takes place. The end result is the creation of a deep and laterally extended ball of affected tissue, 3–5 mm in diameter (Figures 1–8 and 10).

The Ho:YAG (holmium) and Er:YAG (erbium) lasers are lasers of the mid-infrared range, whose wavelength is approximately $2\,\mu m$. Both are pulsed, which means that the intense stream of photons is delivered during an extremely brief interval. These pulses are instantaneous and therefore very powerful, generating a shock-wave in the tissue. They are both absorbed by water, creating vapor microbubbles. The rapid expansion of the bubbles and their subsequent micro-explosion create the above-mentioned shock-wave effect. Er:YAG radiation is also strongly absorbed by hydroxyapatite, which has prompted its experimental use in bone surgery or in hard-tissue dental operations.

Thermal effects on tissue

Heat deposited in tissue elevates its temperature. Figure 9 summarizes how the tissue is affected, both visually and biologically, by the increase in its temperature. As long

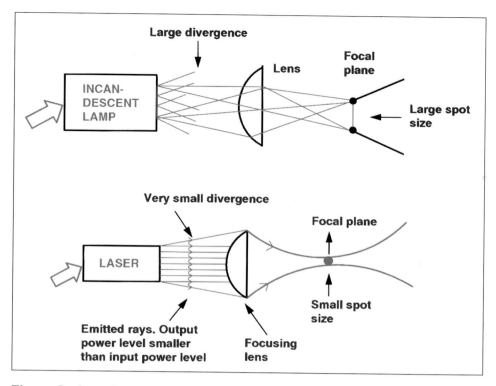

Figure 5 Spot size vs. angular divergence of the beam

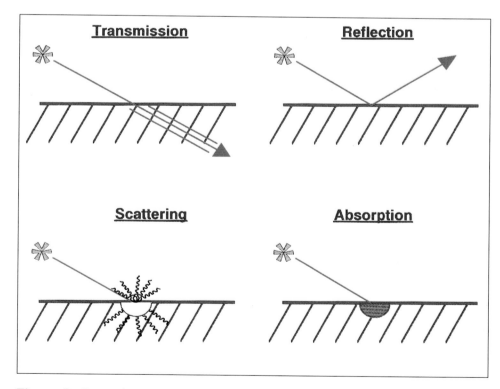

Figure 6 Laser–tissue interaction

	Name	Color	Wavelength
	Excimers	ultraviolet	200–400 nm
Visible	Argon	blue	488 nm
		green	515 nm
	532 YAG	green	532 nm
	Krypton	green	531 nm
		yellow	568 nm
	Dye laser	yellow/green	577 nm
		red	630 nm
	Helium neon	red	630 nm
	Gold vapor	red	630 nm
	Krypton	red	647 nm
	Ruby	deep red	694 nm
	Nd:YAG	infrared	1064 nm
		infrared	1318 nm
	CO_2	infrared	10600 nm

Figure 7 Lasers used in therapeutic medicine

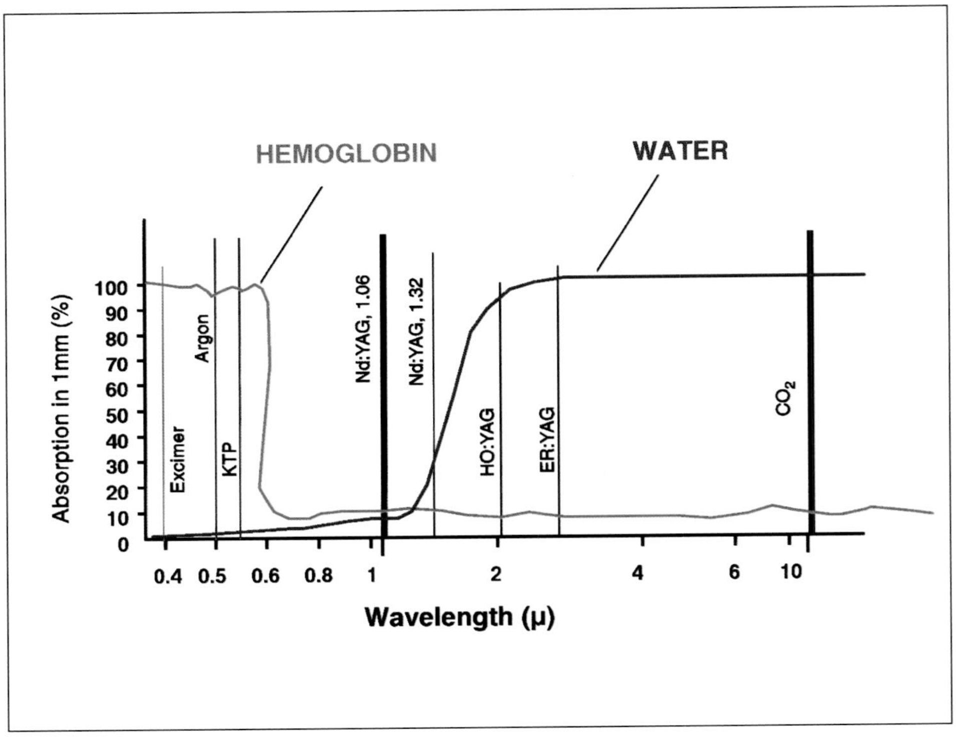

Figure 8 Absorption of laser radiation

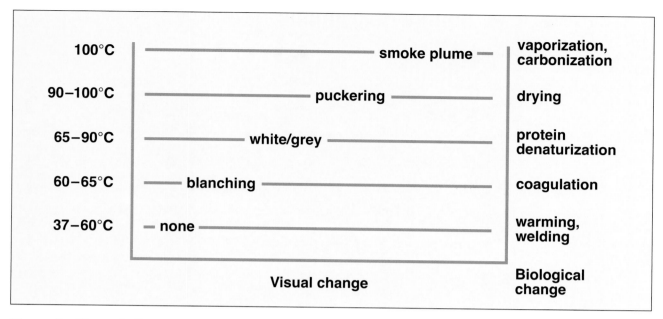

Figure 9 Thermal effects on tissue

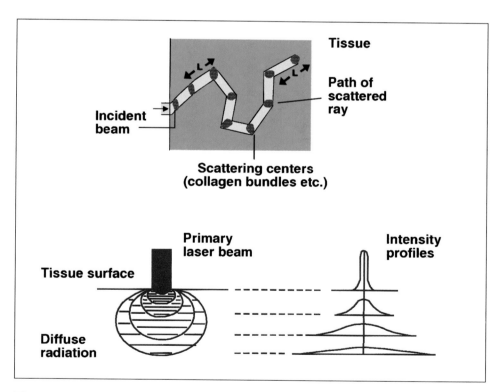

Figure 10 Scattering and penetration of Nd : YAG laser radiation

as the temperature does not reach 60°C, there is no visual change in the appearance of the tissue. Up to 45°C, the changes that occur are all reversible. Beyond that temperature, some of the cellular enzymes are destroyed and the functional operation of the cell is impaired. Between 60 and 65°C, capillary blood vessels shrink and the tissue undergoes extensive coagulation, showing distinct blanching.

It is noteworthy that the coagulation process induced by the CO_2 laser is rather different from that effected by the Nd:YAG laser. The shrinkage of the capillary vessel caused by the CO_2 laser is a result of vaporization of the water contained in the walls of the blood vessel. If, however, the CO_2 laser beam hits a vessel, it is readily absorbed by the blood liquid at its exit from the initially desiccated wall. Thus, it will never have the chance to hit the opposite wall, leaving the vessel open and thereby causing extensive bleeding. Hence, it is important to remember that the sharply focused beams of CO_2 lasers are inadequate for the treatment of highly vascular tissue. Conversely, Nd:YAG lasers are unhindered by the presence of the liquid medium; consequently, they can very effectively accomplish the complete coagulation of the bulk of the tissue. Nd:YAG lasers are excellent coagulators.

Temperatures between 65 and 90°C completely denature the proteins. The tissue turns a whitish color, indicative of dead cells, which subsequently slough off.

At 100°C, vaporization of the cellular water occurs. The high vapor pressure (generated by the rapid expansion of the cellular content that undergoes transformation from liquid to vapor) pushes against the cell membrane, which eventually ruptures, vigorously expelling the resulting fragments in an outgoing plume. The end effect of the entire process is the local removal of tissue matter (Figure 11).

If temperatures are raised much above boiling point, carbonization ultimately occurs.

Energy, power and power density

The rise in temperature of the tissue matter depends primarily on the amount of energy deposited on the target site, as well as on the capability of the tissue to rid itself of heat by dissipating it to surrounding areas. If a large quantity of energy is deposited in the tissue before it can dissipate the heat, a rise in temperature will occur.

Energy, power and power density are the physical parameters that determine the eventual rise in temperature. Energy is measured in joules. Power is the amount of energy delivered per second and is measured in watts (joules/s). The thermal effect of the laser is local. Thus, the physical quantity which governs the thermal response of the tissue is the amount of power delivered to a unit of area; this quantity is called *power density* and is measured in W/cm^2.

The higher the power density, the more rapid the temperature rise on and around the area where the laser beam impinges upon the tissue. In order to obtain the desired surgical effect, both power and power density can be adjusted easily. All commercial laser systems enable the user to vary the power on tissue in a continuous manner. At constant output powers, power density can be varied with the aid of optical devices, which either bring the laser beam into focus on the target site, or defocus it intentionally (Figure 12).

The shape of the cross-section of the beam of most commercial systems is approximately circular. The diameter of the beam can be decreased or increased by the respective focusing/defocusing method. Reducing the diameter of the beam spot by a factor of two represents a reduction of the spot area by a factor of four, and consequently, a fourfold increase in the power density (Figure 13).

The optical system through which the CO_2 laser beam is delivered incorporates specially designed lenses. This system is responsible for bringing the beam into focus on the tissue at the operative site. For a given optical system at a given power, the maximum power density is obtained when the beam is completely focused.

If the surgical circumstances require lower power densities (see below), the surgeon can achieve this by defocusing the beam – i.e. by increasing the diameter of the spot size and consequently increasing its area. Defocusing is normally effected by manually retracting the optical system from its focused position, or by employing a focusing/defocusing device.

High power densities are required when fine incisions must be performed. Traction is applied to the tissue on both sides of the desired incision and a focused beam is aimed at the required location. The depth of the incision is a function of the power delivered and of the dwell time of the laser on each and every point of the incision. The longer the dwell time, the larger the volume of tissue removed by the laser and, therefore, the deeper the cut. But the dwell time is inversely proportional to the speed of movement of the cutting tool. In short, the depth of the incision increases with the power of the beam and decreases with the speed of movement (Figure 14).

Vaporization is performed with a defocused beam. The surgeon moves the beam (scans) across the area to be vaporized in a cross-hatching pattern. The higher the power, the larger the volume of tissue vaporized during one complete scan of the lesion. If it is necessary to debulk a large and deeply penetrating lesion, the surgeon is well-advised to use the maximum available power. Conversely, if it is necessary to vaporize only a superficial layer and to control the depth of tissue removal, the surgeon must reduce the power accordingly.

Finally, in order to coagulate a bleeding point or an oozing area, the surgeon should defocus the laser beam, use low power and gently 'brush' the affected area.

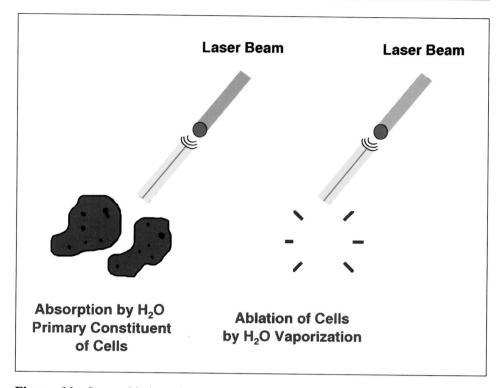

Figure 11 Laser ablation of cells by vaporization

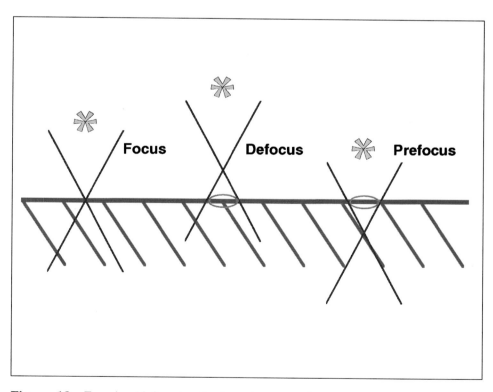

Figure 12 Focusing/defocusing the laser beam on tissue

LASER INSTRUMENTATION

CO$_2$ laser systems and accessories

The CO$_2$ laser beam is generated by a sealed gas-filled tube. The lasing gas is CO$_2$ and it is mixed with other types of gases which are required for different technological reasons. The excitation of the CO$_2$ molecules is effected by an electrical discharge.

One of the limitations of the CO$_2$ laser beam is that it cannot propagate very effectively through flexible fibers. Consequently, the delivery system ordinarily used in commercial products consists of a lightweight articulated arm, composed of straight hollow segmental tubes with reflective mirrors mounted at the joints. Hence, the CO$_2$ laser beam propagates in straight lines and bounces off each consecutive joint, eventually reaching the target tissue through an optical device attached to the end joint.

As the CO$_2$ laser is invisible to the human eye, each laser system is equipped with a red He–Ne (helium–neon) laser tube whose direction of propagation is coincident with the infrared beam. The red He–Ne beam enables the surgeon to aim at the target area and simulate visually on the tissue, the position and the extent of the therapeutic beam.

Manufacturers offer CO$_2$ laser units featuring different maximum powers from 15 to 100 W. CO$_2$ laser systems are composed of:

(1) A laser tube;

(2) A power supply which provides the necessary electrical energy to excite the lasing gas;

(3) A closed-circuit water-cooling system which removes excess heat from the tube and its surroundings;

(4) A control system based on a microcomputer;

(5) An articulated-arm delivery system; and

(6) A He–Ne laser tube.

Figures 15 and 16 show, respectively, a schematic diagram and a photograph of a state-of-the-art CO$_2$ laser system.

Accessories for CO$_2$ laser units are offered in different categories:

(1) Handpieces: attached to the end joint of the articulated arm and manipulated by the surgeon during the procedure (Figure 17). Usually, handpieces come in different focal lengths.

(2) Micromanipulators: devices coupled to the laser unit and mounted on the objective of an operative microscope/colposcope (Figure 18). The optical lens system enables both the red He–Ne beam and the infrared CO$_2$ beam to be focused at the desired distance. The surgeon observes the tissue through the objective of the microscope and steers the laser beam directly at the target tissue with the aid of a joystick that controls the gimballing of a reflective mirror.

(3) Rigid endoscopes: devices which incorporate operating channels through which the laser beam travels, as well as coupling devices which constitute the optical interface between the articulated arm of the CO$_2$ laser and the endoscope. A wide variety of endoscopes are available: laparoscopes (Figure 19), bronchoscopes, laryngoscopes, rectoscopes and anoscopes.

(4) CO$_2$ laser waveguides: rigid metallic or ceramic tubes through which the CO$_2$ laser beam propagates (Figure 20). They are either inserted through the operating channel of a laparoscope, or are supplied for freehand surgery to allow access to sites which are difficult to reach (such as nasal cavities when performing turbinectomies). The distal end of the rigid waveguide is brought into close proximity to the tissue and the laser beam is fired.

(5) Flexible CO$_2$ fibers (FlexiLase): recently introduced by Sharplan, they are a particular type of hollow flexible waveguide (Figure 21). Flexible fibers are used to enhance the maneuverability of the delivery device, to distance the body of the laser unit from the sterile field and to provide access to anatomical sites which are difficult to reach.

Recently, a revolutionary device – the SwiftLase – was introduced onto the market by Sharplan, enabling the surgeon to perform char-free vaporization of large areas. The absence of carbonization improves the visibility of the treated field, thereby enhancing the control the surgeon has over the operating procedure. Moreover, the SwiftLase enables the surgeon to control the depth of the thermal damage to surrounding tissue.

Nd : YAG laser systems and accessories

The Nd : YAG laser uses a solid-state rod (garnet) in which the neodymium atoms play the active lasing role. The exciting energy is supplied by a flashlight lamp which illuminates the rod. Both are housed in a container called the resonator. The shape of the resonator is ellipsoidal and its inner surface is coated with a highly reflective material. The lamp and the rod are placed at the two focal points of the ellipsoid. The light emitted by the lamp is reflected by the internal coating of the resonator and it is collected, almost in its entirety, by the rod positioned at the opposite focal point (Figure 22).

In contrast to the CO$_2$ laser, Nd : YAG laser beams propagate well through commercially available glass fibers, very much like visible light. The propagation is effected by a chain of internal reflections occurring at the boundaries of the glass fiber. Hence, the delivery

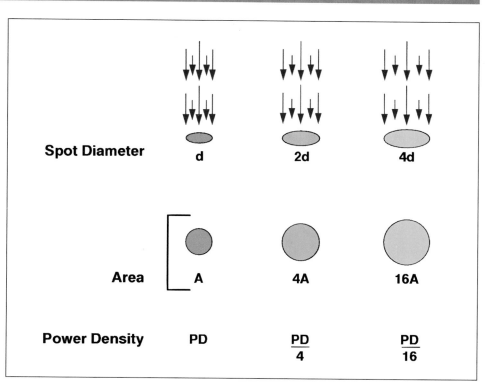

Figure 13 Diameter and area of the spot vs. power density

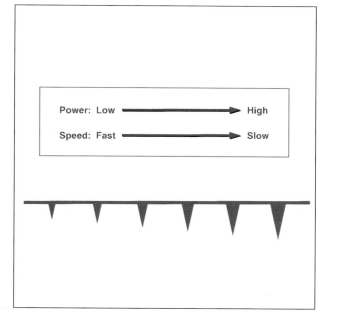

Figure 14 Depth of incision

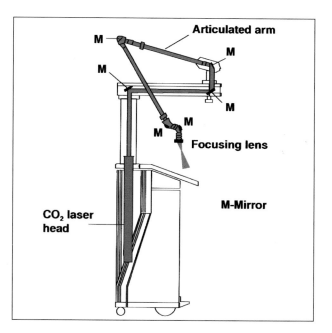

Figure 15 Schematic structure of a CO_2 laser

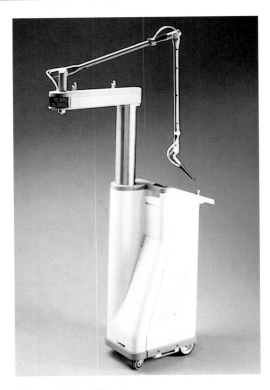

Figure 16 CO$_2$ laser system

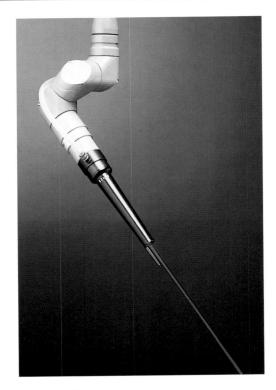

Figure 17 Focusing handpiece

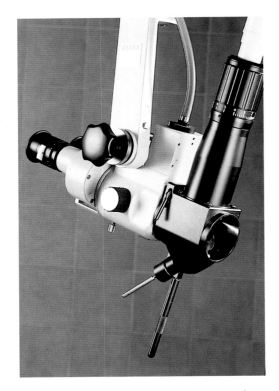

Figure 18 Micromanipulator mounted on an operative microscope

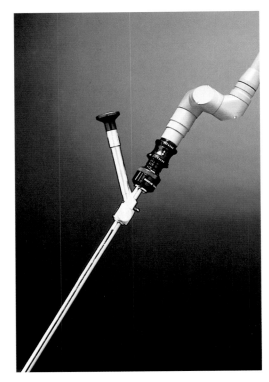

Figure 19 Laser laparoscope with laser coupler

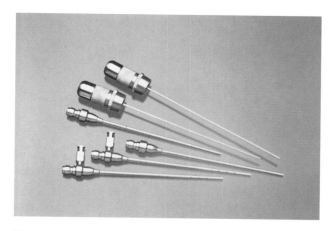

Figure 20 CO_2 laser waveguide set

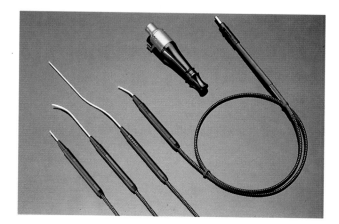

Figure 21 FlexiLase™ – CO_2 laser flexible fiber set

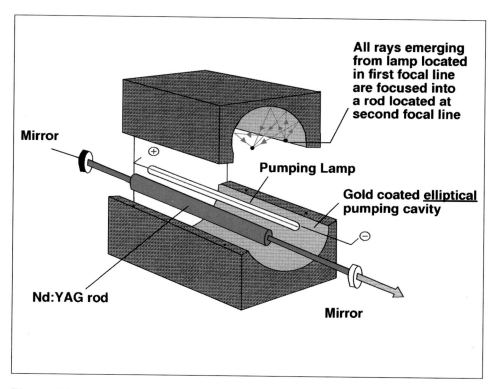

Figure 22 Internal structure of a Nd:YAG laser resonator

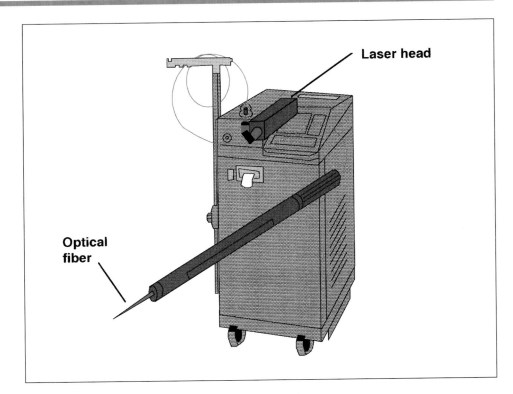

Figure 23 Schematic structure of a Nd:YAG laser

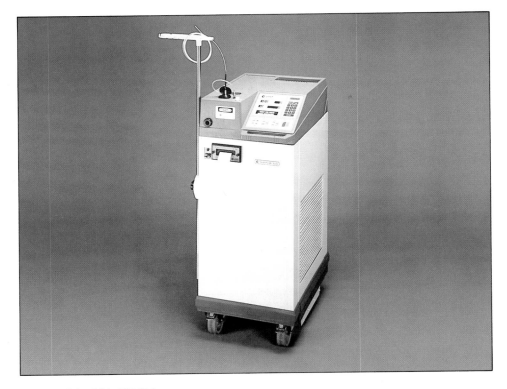

Figure 24 Nd:YAG laser system

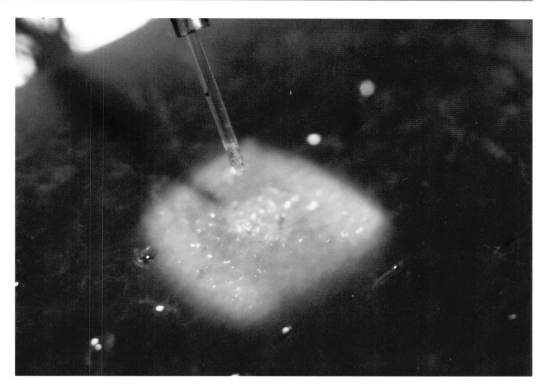

Figure 25   Coagulation effect of non-contact fiber

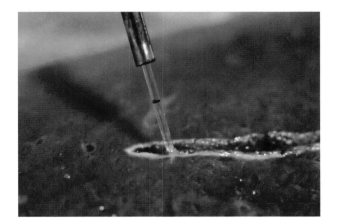

Figure 26   Cutting effect of a contact fiber

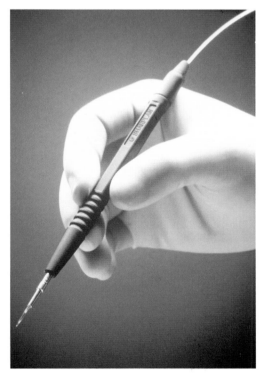

Figure 27   Freehand conical contact fiber

devices used in Nd : YAG lasers are a variety of fibers (see below) equipped with a connector that attaches to the output port of the laser system.

Manufacturers offer Nd : YAG laser units featuring different maximum powers, from 40 to 100 W. Nd : YAG laser systems are composed of:

(1) A laser head or resonator;

(2) A power supply, which furnishes the flashlight lamp with the necessary electrical energy;

(3) A closed-circuit water-cooling system, further chilled by a radiator which removes excess heat from the resonator;

(4) A control system, based on a microcomputer;

(5) A He–Ne laser tube; and

(6) An output-port optical assembly to which the external glass fiber is attached.

Figures 23 and 24 show, respectively, a schematic diagram and a photograph of a state-of-the-art Nd : YAG laser system. The accessories offered with Nd : YAG systems are almost exclusively fibers. They fall into two categories:

(1) Non-contact fibers, whose distal end is flat and highly polished. They operate at a short distance from the tissue, in order to create deep coagulation (Figure 25). A well-known example of their use is the treatment of superficial bladder tumors, where the fibers are inserted through a cystoscope. Non-contact fibers have no incision capability. These fibers are usually reusable. However, after a limited number of surgical procedures, they must be repolished with the aid of a special polishing kit.

(2) Contact fibers, featuring a sharpened sculpted conical tip. The laser radiation is concentrated at the very narrow tip and the fiber functions like a hot knife, capable of performing fine incisions when in contact with the tissue (Figure 26). Moreover, the tapered fiber prevents the rays from progressing forwards, while enabling their exit through the sides of the tip. The end result is that the forward penetration is reduced, much as in the case of the CO_2 laser. The side radiation, on the other hand, produces a hemostatic effect on the lateral surfaces of the wedge created by the incision. Contact fibers are used in a variety of configurations for freehand (Figure 27) and endoscopic applications. They feature different tip shapes (conical, hemispherical) and different diameters (400, 600, 800 and 1000 μm). They are offered as disposable, single-use, sterilized fibers.

Recently, new types of fibers have been introduced onto the market. These fibers possess a polished distal face which is inclined with respect to the fiber axis. This angle enables the fiber to emit the laser beam at right angles to its long axis. Employed transurethrally, these fibers are used to treat benign prostatic hypertrophy by coagulating the adenoma. Another type of fiber, emanating lateral diffusive radiation from an elongated segment located at its distal end, is used for the interstitial laserthermia of benign and malignant lesions.

Section I
Laser operative laparoscopy

Part 1
Endometriosis

Instrumentation and operational instructions

J. Donnez and M. Nisolle

Laser endoscopy has already been widely used in otolaryngology and gastroenterology and it is currently being investigated for clinical use in orthopedics, urology and gynecology. Prototype instruments for CO_2 laser laparoscopy appeared independently on three continents (developed by Bruhat and colleagues, Tadir and co-workers, Daniell and Brown, and Kelly and Roberts). The initial prototype proved to be inadequate because of loss of carbon dioxide, accumulation of intraperitoneal smoke, and an inability to keep the beam focused in the center of the channel. Fortunately, with the development of new laparoscopic instrumentation for CO_2 laser use, the majority of technical problems have been overcome. Instruments have been developed and tested in order to ensure safe, easy, accurate and effective procedures.

The operative laparoscope for laser laparoscopy is an instrument which is 12 mm in diameter with a 7.3-mm operative channel (Eder, USA; Wolff, Storz, Germany). To use the CO_2 laser through the laparoscope, the operator simply swings the articulated arm of the laser over the operative field and attaches the black coupler containing the alignment mirror and focusing lens to the operative channel of the laparoscope (Figure 1).

The laser coupler assembly (Figures 2 and 3) consists of the following:

(1) Coupler housing:

   (a) joystick control for manual adjustment of the laser beam within the lumen of the laparoscopic tube (Figure 2A);

   (b) tube attachment for quick and easy attachment/release of the laparoscopic tube (Figure 2B).

(2) Interchangeable lens housing (Figure 2C):

   (a) 200-mm working distance lens housing to match beam focal length to nominal length of standard second-puncture tube, giving spot size diameter of 0.64 mm;

   (b) 300-mm working distance lens housing to match beam length to nominal length of single-puncture tube (and optional 300-mm second-puncture tube), giving spot size diameter of 0.70 mm;

   (c) Each lens housing has a groove around it for convenient attachment of the sterile drape.

(3) Laser arm attachment (Figure 2D).

LASER COUPLER ADJUSTMENTS AND BEAM FOCUS/DEFOCUS

(1) Turn on the laser system. Aim the He–Ne beam at an appropriate thermal barrier such as a tongue depressor positioned approximately 1 cm distal to the tube.

(2) With the external illumination turned off, adjust the coupler joystick to obtain a full, round He–Ne spot without wall-reflection effects. The halo around the He–Ne spot could be symmetrical as well. Turn the external illumination back on.

(3) Viewing through the eyepiece, position the laparoscope away from the target site so that the He–Ne beam spot appears on the horizontal diameter of the viewing field, one-third of the way to the right of the viewing field center point, as shown in Figure 4. In this position the CO_2 beam is in focus 10 mm distal to the laparoscopic tube.

(4) To obtain a defocused CO_2 beam on the target site, move the laparoscopic tube away from the tissue. The He–Ne beam will move towards the center of the viewing field. At a distance of 80 mm from the tissue site, the He–Ne beam spot will appear at the center of the viewing field.

SWIFTLASE

The SwiftLase (Sharplan Model 757) is a miniature optomechanical scanner compatible with any CO_2 laser (Figure 5). The SwiftLase consists of two almost, but not exactly, parallel folding mirrors. Optical reflections of the CO_2 laser optical beam from the mirrors cause the beam to deviate from its original direction by an angle θ (Figure 6). The mirrors constantly rotate at slightly different angular velocity, thereby rapidly varying with time between zero and a maximal value, θ_{max}. By attaching the laparoscope focusing coupler of focal

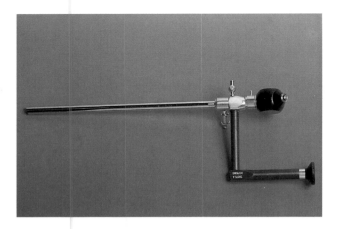

Figure 1 The single-puncture operative laparoscope for laser laparoscopy. The black coupler containing the alignment mirror and focusing lens is attached to the operative channel of the laparoscope

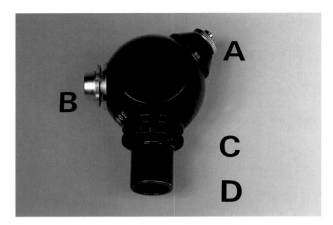

Figure 2 Laser coupler assembly: (A) Joystick; (B) tube attachment; (C) lens; (D) laser arm attachment

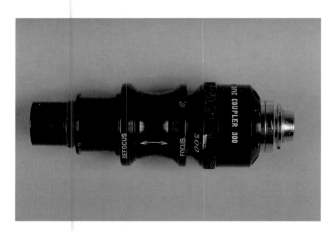

Figure 3 Laser 'direct' coupler

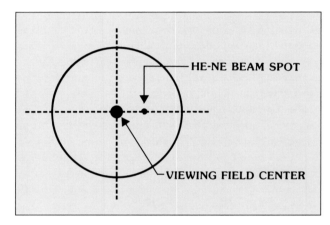

Figure 4 He-Ne beam spot ⅓ of the way to the right of viewing field center, indicating beam focus at 10 mm distal to laparoscopic tube

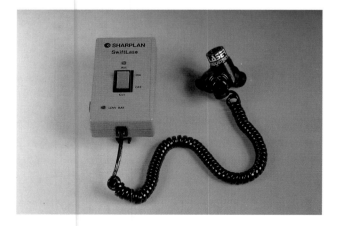

Figure 5(a) SwiftLase: optomechanical scanner consisting of two almost, but not exactly, parallel folding mirrors; (b) SwiftLase connected to the direct coupler

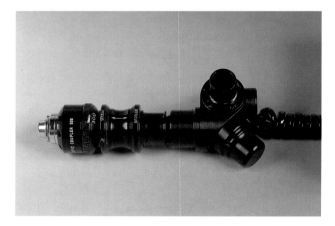

Figure 5(b) *See legend opposite*

length F to the Swiftlase, the CO_2 laser generates a focal spot which rapidly and homogeneously scans and covers a round area of diameter $2F\tan\theta_{max}$ at the distal end of the laparoscope. For a single-puncture laparoscope ($F = 300$ mm), θ_{max} was selected to provide a round treatment area of 2.5 mm in diameter. The rapid movement of the beam over the tissue ensures a short duration of exposure on individual sites within the area and very shallow ablation.

Since therapeutic CO_2 medical lasers typically generate a focused beam smaller than 0.9 mm in diameter at the laparoscope working distance, the use of the SwiftLase with a laser power level of 30 W will generate an optical power density of greater than 50 W/mm^2 on tissue. This is considerably higher than the threshold for vaporization of tissue without residual carbon charring (the threshold for char-free tissue ablation is about 30 W/mm^2). The time required for the SwiftLase homogeneously to cover a 2.5-mm round area is about 100 ms. During this time, the 30-W operating laser will deliver 3000 mJ to the tissue. Since the typical energy required to completely ablate tissue is about 3000 mJ/mm^3, keeping the laparoscope precisely on a single site for 0.1 s will generate a clean char-free crater of 0.2 mm in depth. However, the laparoscope can be moved smoothly and evenly across an extended lesion intended for treatment, consequently ablating a tissue layer as thin as 0.05–0.1 mm.

SMOKE EVACUATION

To allow a flow of fresh carbon dioxide down the beam channel, the CO_2 insufflation tubing is attached to this operative channel; the flow of carbon dioxide from the insufflator displaces smoke, which can reduce the power of the beam from the laser channel, and prevents fogging of the mirror and lens in the black coupler.

To evacuate smoke, a Veress needle can be inserted suprapubically under direct vision and transillumination, directing it towards the target site and connecting it to the smoke evacuation system. Auxilliary kits are available for synchronizing smoke evacuation with laser emission, providing automatic smoke evacuation from the target site. With the automatic smoke evacuation kit installed, smoke evacuation begins with actual laser emission and remains active for 3 seconds after the laser emission ceases.

If smoke disturbs the viewing field, the smoke evacuation flow can be increased, taking care not to cause a collapse of the pneumoperitoneum. The equilibrium state will be reached when the insufflation system is able to provide the amount of gas that the smoke evacuation port is releasing. If the smoke evacuation kit is installed, the expulsion of gas (smoke) can be regulated using a sterile infusion drip kit.

SECOND-PUNCTURE PROBES

The present second-puncture probe which permits the use of the CO_2 laser with the laparoscope is a doubling-ring probe that is 8 mm in external diameter with a 5.6-mm operating channel. The second-puncture laparoscope is based on two tubes. The inner tube contains the operating channel and the insufflation port as well as the locking device for securing it to the outer tube. Two distinct outer tubes are provided: open-end and hook-tipped (Figure 7). The outer tube includes a smoke evacuation port with stopcock. This assembly provides the user with a double-lumen second-puncture laparoscope that is easily disassembled for cleaning purposes. The hook-tipped outer tube is recommended for use in clinical situations that require a back-stop to protect healthy tissue beyond the treatment site. The probe attaches to the same laser coupler assembly that is used with the operative laparoscope. A 200-mm working-distance lens is then used.

WAVE GUIDES

Rigid stainless-steel CO_2 laser probes (Figure 8) with an outer diameter of 4.9 mm were also developed recently (Baggish and co-workers and Tadir and associates). The probe is attached to the articulated arm of a CO_2 laser system. Optical transmission throught these probes is not affected by manipulating the articulated arm. A conventionally used He–Ne aiming beam is transmitted coaxially through the probe. The short focal length (focal place: > 0.4 mm < 2 cm from the probe top) yields a beam that defocuses within a short distance beyond the focal plane. This is expressed by a sharp drop in power density and may serve as an optical backstop.

ACCESSORIES

Third-puncture probes are shown in Figure 9. The following operating instruments were developed in our department in collaboration with the Storz Company:

(1) Atraumatic probe;

(2) Hook for fimbrioplasty;

(3) Probe with backstop for use in vaporizing adhesions near the blood vessels;

(4) Smoke suction and rinsing tube; and

(5) Double-channel probe for rinsing the pelvis and for suction.

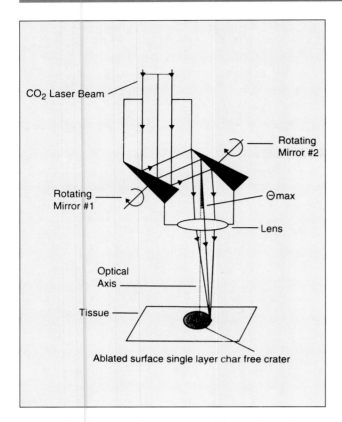

Figure 6 Optical reflections of the beam from the two mirrors cause it to be deflected from its original direction by θ°

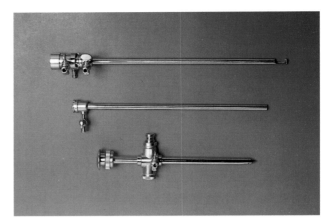

Figure 7 Second-puncture probes: (upper) hook-tipped; (middle) open end; (lower) trocar

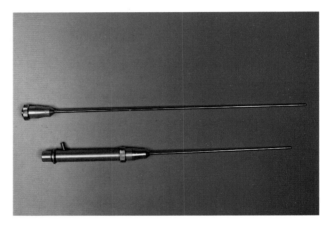

Figure 8 Rigid stainless steel CO_2 laser probes

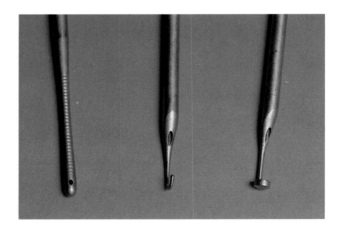

Figure 9 Third-puncture probes: Left, atraumatic probe; center, hook for fimbrioplasty; right, probe with backstop. An inner channel is used for rinsing the operating field

Peritoneal endometriosis: evaluation of typical and subtle lesions

M. Nisolle, F. Casanas-Roux and J. Donnez

Endometriosis most commonly affects the pelvic peritoneum close to the ovaries, including the uterosacral ligaments, the peritoneum of the ovarian fossa and the peritoneum of the cul-de-sac. The increased diagnosis of endometriosis at laparoscopy can be explained by the increased experience and ability of the surgeon to detect such lesions. The greatest change has been in the case of 'subtle' lesions, the diagnosis of which increased from 15% in 1986 to 65% in 1988[1-6]. The diagnosis of peritoneal endometriosis at the time of laparoscopy is often made by the observation of typically puckered black or bluish lesions. There are, in addition, numerous subtle appearances of peritoneal endometriosis; these lesions, frequently non-pigmented, were diagnosed as endometriosis following biopsy confirmation by Jansen and Russell in 1986[2].

TYPICAL LESIONS

The typical black peritoneal endometriotic lesion (Figure 1) results from tissue bleeding and retention of blood pigment, producing brown discoloration of tissue. Puckered black lesions are a combination of glands, stroma and intraluminal debris (Figure 1c).

Evolution

The macroscopic appearance of ectopic endometrium is probably dependent upon the longevity of the process. Viable cells may implant and the initial appearance may be an irregularity or discoloration of the peritoneal surface – the earliest sign being hemosiderin staining of the peritoneal surfaces. Initially, these lesions may appear hemorrhagic, but menstrual shedding from a viable endometrial implant initiates an inflammatory reaction which provokes a scarification process; this, in turn, encloses the implants. The presence of entrapped menstrual debris is responsible for the typical black or bluish appearance. If the inflammatory process obliterates or devascularizes the endometrial cells, eventually this discoloration disappears. A white plaque of old collagen is all that remains of the ectopic implant. Scarring of the peritoneum around endometrial implants is a typical finding. In addition to encapsulating an isolated implant, the scar may deform the surrounding peritoneum or result in the development of adhesions.

SUBTLE APPEARANCES

Sometimes the subtle endometriotic lesions can be the only lesions seen at laparoscopy. The subtle forms are more common and may be more active than the puckered black lesions (Table 1).

Table 1 Different appearances of peritoneal endometriosis

Color	Description
Black	typical puckered black lesions
Red	red flame-like lesions[2]
	glandular excrescences[2]
	petechial peritoneum[7]
	areas of hypervascularization[7]
White	white opacification[2]
	subovarian adhesions[2]
	yellow-brown peritoneal patches[2]
	circular peritoneal defects[1]

The non-pigmented endometriotic peritoneal lesions include the following:

(1) White opacification of the peritoneum (Figure 2a), which appears as peritoneal scarring or as circumscribed patches, often thickened and sometimes raised. Histologically, white opacified peritoneum is due to the presence of an occasional retroperitoneal glandular structure and scanty stroma surrounded by fibrotic tissue or connective tissue (Figure 2b and c).

(2) Red flame-like lesions of the peritoneum (Figure 3a) or red vesicular excrescences, more commonly affecting the broad ligament and the uterosacral ligaments. Histologically, red flame-like lesions and vesicular excrescences are due to the presence of active endometriosis surrounded by stroma (Figure 3b–d).

(3) Glandular excrescences on the peritoneal surface (Figure 4a), which in color, translucency and consistency closely resemble the mucosal surface of the endometrium seen at hysteroscopy. Biopsy reveals the presence of numerous endometrial glands (Figure 4b).

(4) Subovarian adhesions (Figure 5a) or adherence between the ovary and the peritoneum of the ovarian fossa, which are distinctive from adhesions characteristic of previous salpingitis or peritonitis. Histologically,

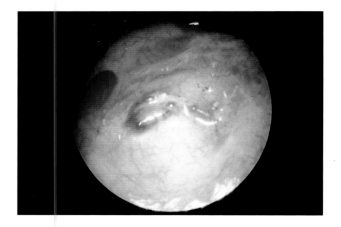

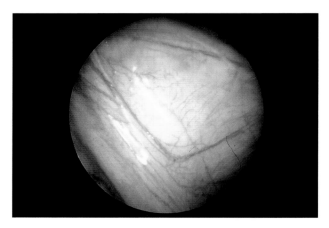

Figure 1 Puckered black lesion, laparoscopic aspect: (a) black lesion without and (b) with fibrosis; (c) histology: presence of endometrial glands and typical stroma. Note the presence of intraluminal debris (Gomori's trichrome × 110)

Figure 2 White opacification of the peritoneum: (a) laparoscopic aspect; (b) and (c) histology: rare retroperitoneal glandular structure and scanty stroma surrounded by fibrotic tissue (Gomori's trichrome × 56, × 110)

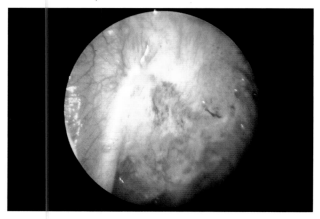

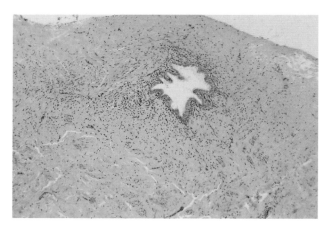

Figure 1(b)   *See legend above*

Figure 2(b)   *See legend above*

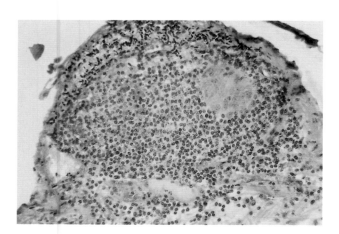

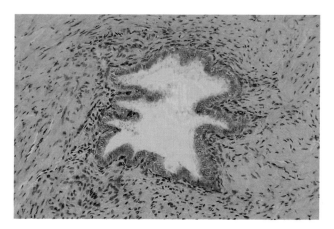

Figure 1(c)   *See legend above*

Figure 2(c)   *See legend above*

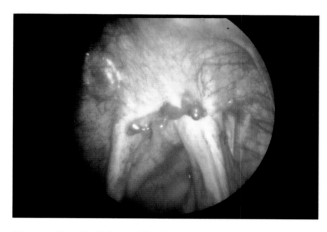

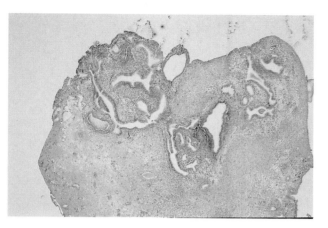

Figure 3 Red flame-like lesion of the peritoneum: (a) laparoscopic aspect; (b)–(d) histology: active endometriotic glands surrounded by stroma (Gomori's trichrome × 25, × 56, × 110)

Figure 3(b) *See legend opposite*

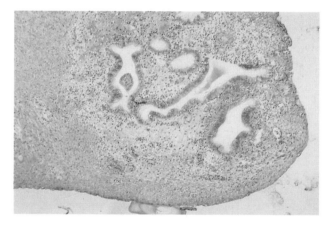

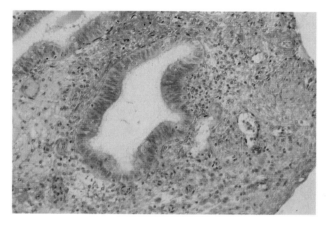

Figure 3(c) *See legend above*

Figure 3(d) *See legend above*

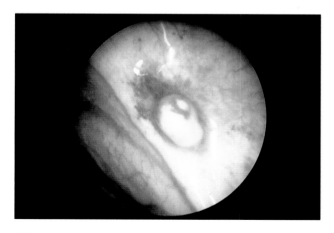

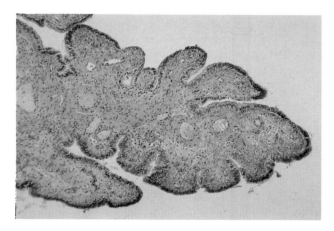

Figure 4 Glandular excrescences on the peritoneal surface: (a) laparoscopic aspect; (b) histology: presence of numerous endometrial glands (Gomori's trichrome × 56)

Figure 4(b) *See legend opposite*

connective tissue with sparse endometrial glands is found (Figure 5b).

(5) Yellow-brown peritoneal patches (Figure 6a) resembling 'café au lait' patches. The histological characteristics are similar to those observed in white opacification, but in the yellow-brown patches, the presence of the blood pigment hemosiderin among the stroma cells produces the 'café au lait' color (Figure 6b).

(6) Circular peritoneal defects (Figure 7a) as described by Chatman[1]. Serial section demonstrates the presence of endometrial glands in more than 50% of cases (Figure 7b).

(7) Areas of petechial peritoneum (Figure 8a) or areas with hypervascularization (Figure 9a), which were diagnosed as endometriosis in our recent study[6,7]. These lesions resemble the petechial lesions resulting from manipulation of the peritoneum or from hypervascularization of the peritoneum. They most generally affect the bladder and the broad ligament; histologically, red blood cells are numerous and endometrial glands are very rare (Figures 8b and c, 9b).

HISTOLOGICAL STUDY OF PERITONEAL ENDOMETRIOSIS

Typical lesions

The morphological characteristics of peritoneal endometriosis were studied in 109 biopsies with histologically proved endometriosis[6] (Table 2). An endometriotic lesion was considered 'active' when typical glandular epithelium appeared as either proliferative or completely unresponsive to hormones, with typical stroma. Such a lesion was found in 76% of cases. Areas of oviduct-like epithelium with ciliated cells were demonstrated in 55% of peritoneal endometriotic foci. The epithelial height and the mitotic index were calculated in typical glandular epithelium. Epithelial height was measured with a micrometer and the mitotic index was calculated by counting mitotic figures per 2000 epithelial cells, as previously described[8]. Their values were $14.8 \pm 3.2\,\mu m$ and 0.6‰, respectively.

Table 2 Morphological characteristics of peritoneal endometriosis

Biopsies ($n = 109$)	Number
Typical glandular epithelium and stroma	109 (100%)
Active endometriosis	83 (76%)
Oviduct-like epithelium	46 (55%)
Epithelial height (μm)	14.8 ± 3.2
Mitotic index (‰)	0.6

Subtle lesions

Confirmation of endometriosis in subtle lesions was made by Jansen and Russell[2]. Endometriosis was confirmed in 81% of white opacified lesions, 81% of red flame-like lesions, 67% of glandular lesions, 50% of subovarian adhesions, 47% of yellow-brown patches and 45% of circular peritoneal defects. Later, Stripling and colleagues[4] confirmed endometriosis in 91% of white lesions, 75% of red lesions, 33% of hemosiderin lesions, and 85% of other lesions. In our study, we confirmed the presence of endometriosis in non-pigmented lesions of the peritoneum in more than 50% of cases.

Unsuspected peritoneal endometriosis

In a recent study[6], biopsies were taken from visually normal peritoneum of 32 women undergoing laparoscopy for infertility, in whom neither typical nor subtle appearances of endometriosis were found (group II). In another group of 52 women with apparent endometriosis, biopsies were also taken from visually normal peritoneum (group I).

The peritoneum was considered normal if no lesion, as previously described, was seen. A biopsy was taken from the normal peritoneum of the uterosacral ligaments. Histological study revealed the presence of endometriotic tissue in two cases (6%) in the group of 32 infertile women without endometriosis. This rate was less than one-half the rate (13%) observed in normal peritoneum taken from women with visible endometriosis (Table 3).

Identification of endometriosis in biopsy specimens from areas of normal peritoneum in patients with known endometriosis was reported by Murphy and colleagues[9]. By scanning electron microscopy, 25% of their specimens, which appeared normal by gross inspection, were found to contain evidence of endometriosis. In our study, by light microscopy, we reported a rate of 13%[6]. Moreover, histological study of biopsies from visually normal peritoneum in infertile women without any typical or 'subtle' endometriotic lesions revealed the presence of endometriosis in 6% of cases[6]. Unsuspected peritoneal endometriosis can thus be found in the visually normal peritoneum of infertile women, with or without known associated endometriosis. Although the rate (13%) in women with visible endometriosis was twice the rate observed in women without endometriosis, the difference was not significant. The size of the endometriotic lesions in visually normal peritoneum ($313 \pm 185\,\mu m$) probably explains why the peritoneum had a normal aspect and why the lesion was not visible, even though a meticulous inspection was made to identify small and non-hemorrhagic lesions[6].

As recently demonstrated in infertile women, the diagnosis of endometriosis at laparoscopy has increased.

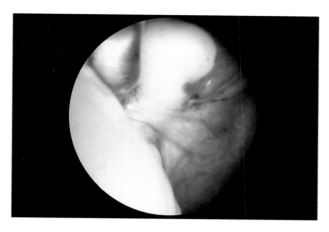

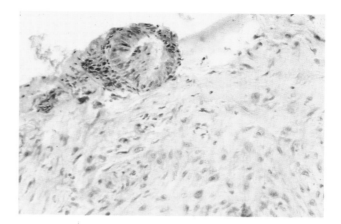

Figure 5 Subovarian adhesions: laparoscopic aspect: adherence between ovary and peritoneum of the ovarian fossa; (b) histology: connective tissue with sparse endometrial glands (Gomori's trichrome × 110)

Figure 5(b)   *See legend opposite*

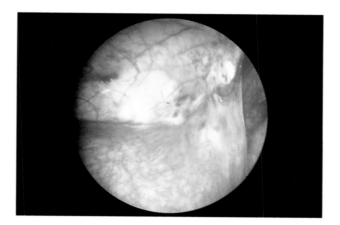

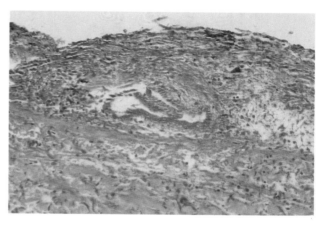

Figure 6 Yellow-brown peritoneal patches of the peritoneum: (a) laparoscopic aspect; (b) histology: the presence of blood pigment (hemosiderin) among the stroma cells produces the 'cafe au lait' color (Gomori's trichrome × 110)

Figure 6(b)   *See legend opposite*

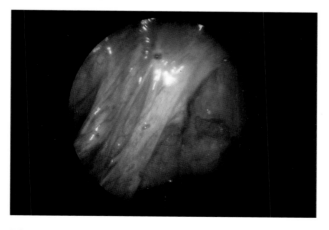

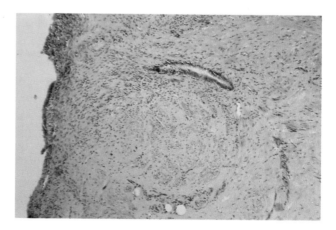

Figure 7 Circular peritoneal defects: (a) laparoscopic aspect; (b) histology: the typical endometrial glands are found in more than 50% of cases (Gomori's trichrome × 25)

Figure 7(b)   *See legend opposite*

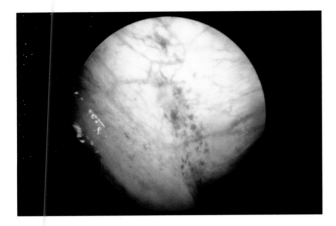

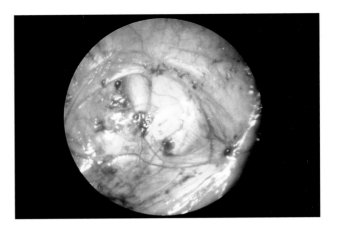

Figure 8 Areas of petechial peritoneum: (a) laparoscopic aspect; (b) histology: note the typical endometrial glands and stroma (Gomori's trichrome × 56, × 110)

Figure 9 Areas of hypervascularization: (a) laparoscopic aspect; (b) histology: red blood cells are numerous and endometrial glands are very rare (Gomori's trichrome × 110)

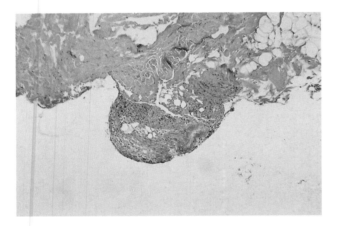

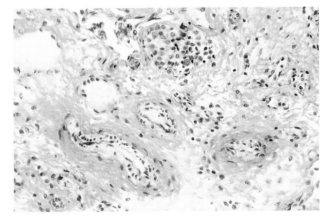

Figure 8(b) *See legend above*

Figure 9(b) *See legend above*

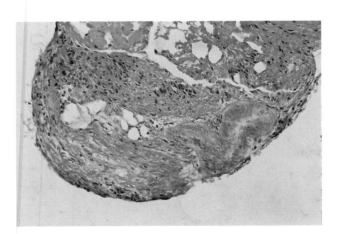

Figure 8(c) *See legend above*

Table 3 Peritoneal endometriosis and infertility; biopsies were taken from the peritoneum of women with (group I) and without (group II) apparent endometriosis; all the women were undergoing laparoscopy for infertility

	Group I (n = 52)	Group II (n = 32)
Number of biopsies		
from visible endometriotic lesions*	86	—
from normal-appearing peritoneum*	52	32
Histological proof of endometriosis		
in visible lesions*	80/86 (93%)	—
in normal-appearing peritoneum*	7/52 (13%)	2/32 (6%)

*, Refers to the macroscopic appearance

However, our data confirm that the operating surgeon did not make the diagnosis in at least 6% of cases, despite the significant increase in the diagnosis and documentation of endometriosis.

Hormonal independence

Using qualitative histochemistry, the microscopic changes[10] present in endometrium have been observed in ectopic implants, but endometrial implants do not demonstrate the characteristic ultrastructural changes of normal endometrium[11]. The fact that endometrial implants can undergo cyclical histological changes, similar to those found in normal endometrium, demonstrates that ectopic endometrium responds to gonadal hormones. But the majority of implants do not demonstrate histological changes synchronous with the comparable uterine endometrium[12]. Some of the reasons[13] may be:

(1) The deficiency in steroid receptors;

(2) The influence of the surrounding scarification process;

(3) The pressure atrophy; and

(4) The hormonal independence of ectopic endometrial glands.

The evaluation of steroid receptors in ectopic endometrial implants could be difficult because of the small number of glandular and stromal cells within the implant, and the heterogeneity of the tissue. While most implants can be demonstrated to possess progesterone receptors[14], only 30% have estrogen receptors. In the ovary, implants have far fewer estrogen and progesterone receptors than does normal epithelium[15,16]. Castration, menopause, pregnancy or therapeutic suppression of gonadal function can dramatically alter the pattern of the disease. We have recently shown[17] that hormonal treatment is unable to eradicate endometriosis. Indeed, both in peritoneal endometriosis and in ovarian endometriosis, microscopic examination of specimens (taken after 6 months of therapy) revealed a high incidence of active endometriosis, without signs of degeneration. Mitotic activity was found, and this suggested the presence of hormonally independent glands in endometriotic foci.

MORPHOMETRIC STUDY OF THE VASCULARIZATION

Vascularization

Vascularization of endometriotic implants is probably one of the most important factors in the growth and invasion of endometrial glands into other tissue. A stereometric analysis was applied in order to study, precisely, the vascularization in peritoneal endometriotic foci[18,19].

Vascularization of typical and subtle lesions

We histologically evaluated the vascularization of typical peritoneal endometriosis and its modifications, according to the macroscopic appearance of peritoneal endometriosis.

Methods

In a series of 135 women who were undergoing laparoscopy for infertility, 220 peritoneal biopsies of 3–5 mm in size were taken from areas of the pelvic peritoneum bearing foci of endometriosis, with a biopsy punch forceps (26-175 DH, Storz, Tuttlingen, Germany). In all cases, a biopsy was taken from the typical (puckered black) endometriotic implants (n = 135, group Ia). Laparoscopy and biopsy were systematically carried out during the early luteal phase.

In the same series, a peritoneal biopsy was taken from an area with subtle appearances. The different subtle appearances of endometriosis were classified as red lesions: vesicular lesions, red flame-like lesions and glandular excrescences (group Ib, $n = 35$); and white lesions: white opacification, yellow-brown patches and circular peritoneal defects (group Ic, $n = 150$).

All biopsy specimens were fixed in formaldehyde and embedded in paraffin; $4\,\mu m$ serial sections were stained with Gomori's trichrome and examined on a blind basis with a Leitz Orthoplan microscope (Leitz, Wetzlar, Germany). A two-dimensional image analysis program set on a Vidas computer (Kontron Bildanalyse GmBH, Eching, Germany) was completed by the interactive counting of 262 144 points.

All endometriotic lesions ($n = 220$) were analyzed, field by field, using the objective 40 x of an Axioskop light microscope (Zeiss, Oberkochen, Germany) and a television camera (Dage-MTI, Michigan City, IN, USA). The histological features were displayed on a television monitor and stored in the memory for processing by the measuring program. The mean of fields analyzed in each case was 13.3 ± 6.7. Histological structures of interest such as the stroma, the glandular epithelium and lumen, the capillaries and the lymphocytes were drawn moving a cursor (Figure 10a). Each different structure was discriminated and gray level images were transferred to binary images (Figure 10b). The interactive measurements of the selected parameters (number of structures, area and perimeter of the structures per field) were appended and stored at the end of an existing database.

Data management and evaluation were checked according to specific search criteria on the Videoplan (Kontron Bildanalyse GmBH, Eching, Germany), and displayed on the television monitor and printed. In all cases, the mitotic index was calculated as previously described[8], by counting mitotic figures (prometaphase, metaphase, anaphase and telophase) for 2000 epithelial cells per biopsy. This is the only method available for women because administration of colchicine or tritiated thymidine is not ethical. The contingency table method, the χ^2 (chi-square) test, the t-test and the median test were used for statistical analysis.

Results

Biopsies taken from typical puckered black or bluish peritoneal lesions showed the presence of endometrial elements (glands and stroma) in all cases (100%).

The results concerning the capillaries are shown in Table 4. The number of capillaries per mm^2 of stroma, their mean surface area and the surface area ratio (capillaries/stroma) were calculated. In group Ia, the number of capillaries per mm^2 of stroma was 243. Their mean surface area was $118 \pm 84\,\mu m^2$, and the ratio of capillaries/stroma surface area was 2.4%.

When compared to group Ia, a significant difference in the number of capillaries per mm^2 of stroma was observed in groups Ib and Ic ($p < 0.001$ and $p < 0.05$, respectively). Both the mean surface area and the ratio of capillaries/stroma surface area found in group Ic were significantly reduced when compared to groups Ia and Ib ($p < 0.001$). The capillary mean surface area was significantly higher ($p < 0.001$) in group Ib, compared to group Ia.

The contingency table method was used in order to compare the surface area occupied by the capillaries in each field. In group Ia, the surface area per field occupied by the capillaries reached $3000\,\mu m^2$. However, in group Ic, the surface area did not exceed $500\,\mu m^2$. The difference in values is statistically significant ($p < 0.05$). Not only the capillary mean surface area, but also the surface area per field occupied by the capillaries was significantly reduced in group Ic, when compared to group Ia.

The mitotic index was calculated in glandular epithelium and its value was 0.1‰ and 0.61‰ in groups Ia and Ib, respectively. In group Ic (white lesions), no mitosis was observed.

Table 4 Morphometric study of the stromal vascularization

	Typical lesions (black) group Ia ($n = 135$)	*Red lesions group Ib* ($n = 35$)	*White lesions group Ic* ($n = 50$)	*Treated typical lesions group Id* ($n = 45$)
Number of capillaries/mm^2 stroma	243	147*[†]	206[†]	225
Capillary mean surface area (μm^2)	118 ± 84	234 ± 192*[†]	78 ± 43[†]	71 ± 40[†]
Capillaries/stroma relative surface (%)	2.4	3.2*[†]	1.5[†]	1.4[†]

*, Significantly different from group Ic and Id ($p < 0.05$); [†], significantly different from group Ia ($p < 0.001$)

Influence of GnRH agonist on the vascularization

The vascularization of typical peritoneal endometriosis was evaluated in 45 patients after gonadotropin releasing hormone (GnRH) agonist therapy. The results concerning the capillaries are shown in Table 4. The number of capillaries per mm^2 of stroma, their mean surface area and the surface area ratio (capillaries/stroma) were calculated. There was no significant difference in the number of capillaries per mm^2 of stroma between the treated and untreated patients. However, in the treated group, their mean surface area (71 ± 40 µm^2) was significantly different ($p < 0.001$) from the value observed in the untreated group (118 ± 84 µm^2). The capillaries/stroma ratio was significantly lower ($p < 0.002$) in the treated group (1.4%) than in the untreated group (2.4%).

Comments on vascularization

The method of descriptive and computerized interactive morphometry for different tissue was applied to the study of endometriotic foci, in order to evaluate the stromal vascularization[19]. Our study demonstrated significant differences between the typical (black or bluish) lesion and the 'subtle' lesion. Subtle lesions were classified as red lesions (vesicular, red flame-like and glandular excrescences) and white lesions (white opacification, yellow-brown patches and circular peritoneal defects). When compared to typical lesion data, the vascularization was found to be significantly higher in red lesions and significantly lower in white lesions. This change was due to an increase (red) or a decrease (white) in the volume occupied by the vessels, as proved by both the mean capillary surface area and the ratio of capillaries/stroma surface area. This change was more evident in the group of red lesions, where the number of capillaries/mm^2 was significantly lower than in the other subgroups.

Thus, in the red lesions, the increased level of vascularization is due to a greater number of larger vessels than in the other groups. In white lesions, there was a greater number of smaller vessels; the number of capillaries was higher than in red lesions.

The mitotic index was also significantly different in the three groups. Mitotic processes permit the maintenance and growth of peritoneal endometriosis. The absence of mitosis in white lesions proves their low 'activity'[6,18,19].

According to our data, we can suggest that there are probably different types of peritoneal endometriotic lesions, in different stages of development. Red flame-like lesions and glandular excrescences are probably the first stage of early implantation of endometrial glands and stroma.

The growth and aggressiveness of endometrial glands in the stroma has recently been demonstrated by a three-dimensional evaluation[18]. Indeed, in this group, a higher incidence of glands with ramifications was observed when compared to typical and white lesions. The significantly higher stromal vascularization and epithelial mitotic index could be responsible for the invasion of ectopic sites by glands and stroma.

Thereafter, menstrual shedding from viable endometrial implants could initiate an inflammatory reaction, provoking a scarification process which encloses the implant. The presence of intraluminal debris is responsible for the typical black coloration of the same lesion. This scarification process is probably responsible for the reduction in vascularization, as proved by the significant decrease in the capillaries/stroma relative surface area. Thereafter, the inflammatory process devascularizes the endometriotic foci, and white plaques of old collagen are all that remain of the ectopic implant.

Concerning the white lesions, our study demonstrated the absence of mitosis, and poor vascularization, although a similar number of capillaries were found when compared to typical lesions. Our hypothesis is that white opacification and yellow-brown lesions are latent stages of endometriosis. They are probably non-active lesions which could be quiescent for a long time[18,19].

Some morphological changes in endometriotic foci after hormonal therapy have been described previously[17]. The mitotic index has been found to be significantly reduced. One of our hypotheses concerning the mechanism of action was the reduction in the vascularization of glandular epithelium after GnRH agonist therapy. Macroscopically, preoperative hormonal therapy results in the reduction of pelvic vascularity and inflammation diagnosed at the time of the second-look laparoscopy.

Our results demonstrated that there was a significant decrease in the vascularization of the endometriotic foci after GnRH agonist therapy[19]. This change was due, not to a reduction in the number of capillaries in the lesion, but to a decrease in the area of the vessels. Indeed, in the treated patients (group II), a predominance of smaller vessels was observed when compared with the untreated patients (group I). This vascularization decrease, observed histologically, was in accordance with the observations made by laparoscopy after hormonal therapy. Vascular effects of the GnRH agonist on the uterine arteries have also been demonstrated by Doppler[20]. The hypoestradiol state induced by GnRH agonist therapy could also have an effect on the vascularization of the endometriotic stroma.

The reduction in the vascularization after hormonal therapy could account for the decrease in the inflammatory reaction observed around the endometriotic foci.

In conclusion, the evaluation of the stromal vascularization permitted the differentiation and classification of the different appearances of peritoneal endometriosis, according to their vascularization level. Our study proves that the 'activity' of peritoneal endometriosis is related to the vascularity. This concept must be taken

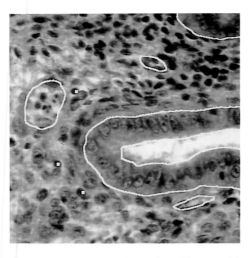

Figure 10 A two-dimensional image: (a) histological structures are traced by a digitizer: glandular epithelium, lumen, stroma and capillaries

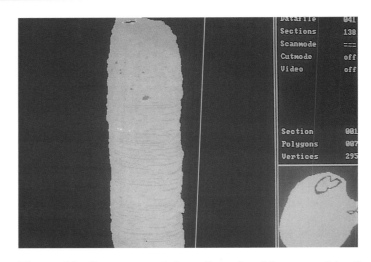

Figure 11 Reconstructed three-dimensional image models of the elements of a peritoneal endometriotic lesion indicated as a solid structure: (a) stroma (pink); (b) epithelium (green); (c) lumen (blue)

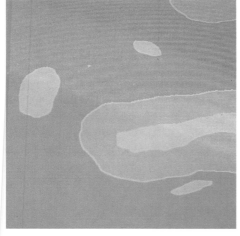

Figure 10(b) Grey level image of the same field

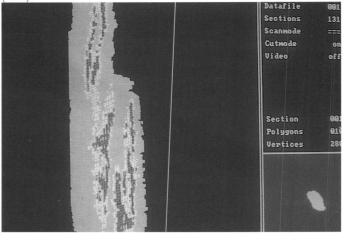

Figure 11(b) *See legend above*

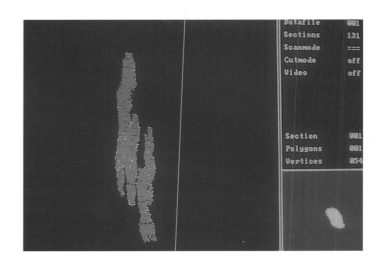

Figure 11(c) *See legend above*

into account in the further discussions of the American Fertility Society Endometriosis Classification. Typical, red, and white lesions are three different stages of the peritoneal disease and their relative relation to infertility probably also differs.

THREE-DIMENSIONAL ARCHITECTURE OF ENDOMETRIOSIS

In order to further elucidate the biological characteristics of peritoneal endometriotic lesions – for example, how they stereologically develop *in vivo*, and how glandular epithelium and stroma are related to the surrounding tissue – a recently advanced stereographic computer technology[18] was applied for the investigation of the three-dimensional (3-D) architecture of peritoneal endometriosis.

Methods

All biopsy specimens were fixed in formaldehyde and embedded in paraffin; 6-μm serial sections were stained with Gomori's trichrome and examined on a blind basis, with a Leitz Orthoplan microscope (Leitz, Wetzlar, Germany). The histological features of the sections were displayed using an Axioskop microscope (Zeiss, Oberkochen, Germany) through a CCD 72 E camera (Dage-MTI, Michigan City, IN, USA) on a monitor, on which two-dimensional figures drawn with a digitizer were superimposed using a computer (Vidas, Kontron Bildanalyse GmBH, Eching, Germany). Computer-assisted reconstruction of three-dimensional models was developed with two main aims in mind: to generate a complete multicolored model of a complex structure which can be rotated and viewed from any angle or orientation; and to calculate the volumes and surfaces within the 3-D model automatically.

The major features of the program[18] include:

(1) Input of serial section data by manual tracing, or automatic contour finding;

(2) Alignment of sections;

(3) Editing and reassignment of contours of individual sections;

(4) Storing contour data in a file;

(5) Selecting a range of sections and/or a range of elements to be used for reconstruction;

(6) Reconstructing models in a wire frame and/or a solid modelling mode by using parallel projection;

(7) Rotating the reconstruction in the x, y and z plane at variable magnifications;

(8) Viewing inside a model by cutting away part of the reconstruction using an 'electronic knife';

(9) Calculating surfaces and volumes; and

(10) Plotting the reconstruction on a matrix or laser printer.

With this program, outlines of glandular structure and endometrial stroma in the serial histological sections were traced by the digitizer, sections were aligned and contour data stored in a file; once all the serial outlines had been digitized and stored, reconstructed (3-D) image models of these *in vivo* structures were displayed on the television monitor. The 3-D reconstruction could generate a complete multicolored model of the complex structure, which could be rotated and viewed from any angle or orientation.

Volumes of the reconstructed glandular and stromal structures were obtained by a calculation function in the same program. Lumen volume was also calculated. Ratios of lumen volume/epithelial volume/stromal volume were determined for each specimen. The χ^2 test was used for statistical analysis.

Results

In 42 women who were undergoing laparoscopy for infertility, peritoneal biopsies of 3–5 mm in size were taken from areas of the pelvic peritoneum bearing foci of endometriosis, with a biopsy punch forceps (26-175 dh, Storz, Tuttligen, Germany). Biopsies were taken from the typical (puckered black) endometriotic implants in all cases.

Group I consisted of 26 women with peritoneal endometriosis who had not previously received any hormonal therapy. All of them underwent laparoscopy during the early luteal phase.

Group II consisted of 17 women who had received GnRH agonist therapy (Zoladex, ICI, Cambridge, UK) for 12 weeks before biopsy. After an initial stimulation of estradiol (E$_2$) secretion, GnRH agonist administration resulted in a range of levels of postmenopausal E$_2$ secretion (15 ± 6 pg/ml).

Histologically, all the biopsy specimens showed typical epithelium and stroma of the endometrial type. The reconstructed 3-D image models of the structures in the peritoneal endometriotic lesions were displayed, and a pink color was applied for the stroma (Figure 11a), a green color for the epithelium (Figure 11b) and a blue color for the lumen (Figure 11c).

The 3-D image models were usually shown as a solid structure (Figure 11); however, models could be displayed as a transparent structure, when they were simultaneously shown with their stromal and epithelial structures (Figure 12).

Stereographically, two types could be easily recognized and classified. The first type (Figure 13) was composed of cylinder-like glands without ramifications. The lesion showed a regular distribution of the glandular epithelium in the stromal structure, which was also regular.

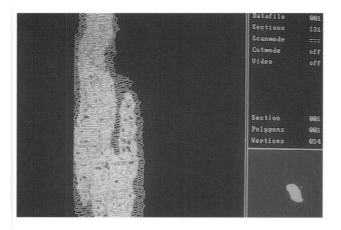

Figure 12 The three-dimensional image models displayed as a transparent structure; the stromal, epithelial and luminal structures are shown simultaneously

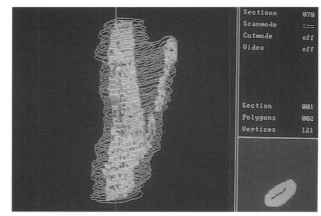

Figure 15 (a) and (b) Luminal structures are interconnected

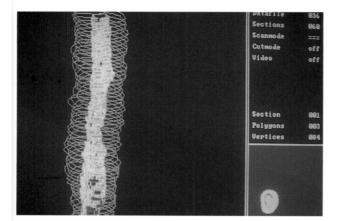

Figure 13 Cylinder-like gland; regular distribution of the glandular epithelium in the stroma

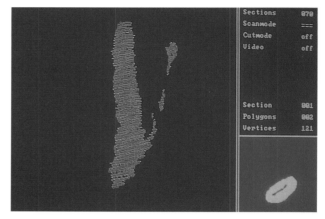

Figure 15 (b) *See legend above*

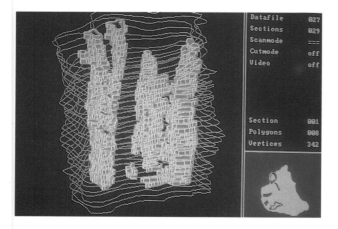

Figure 14 Glands with ramifications; luminal structures are interconnected (three-dimensional)

Table 5 Stereometry of volumes of three-dimensional structures: percentage of the lesion attributed to the epithelium, stroma or lumen

Ratio	Group I (n = 26)	Group II (n = 16)
Epithelium/lesion	19.9%	14.9%
Stroma/lesion	62.2%	51.8%
Lumen/lesion	13.2%	25.2%

The second type (Figure 14) was composed of glands with ramifications.

Luminal structures were interconnected (Figure 15). Epithelial structures appeared like fingers and seemed to invade the stroma. The distribution of glandular structures in the stroma was not regular. Many glandular structures formed inside luminal structures, whose diameter varied from 22 to 185 μm.

In all groups, the 'external' stromal surface was regular. Like normal uterine epithelial structures, the glandular epithelium had a markedly regular luminal surface. In some cases, the lumen was dilated; in others, especially when the ramifications were numerous, the lumen was narrow. The incidence of the first type was 44% in group I and 46% in group II. The incidence of the second type was 56% and 54%, respectively. The volumes of epithelial, stromal and luminal structures were measured separately by computer stereometry, and the results are shown in Table 5. The stroma/lesion ratio was 62.2% and 51.8% in groups I and II, respectively. Although there was a decrease in stroma/lesion ratio in group II as compared to group I, the difference was not significant. The epithelium/lesion ratio was 19.9% and 14.9%, respectively. The lumen/lesion ratio was 13.2% in group I and 25.2% in group II. These values were significantly different ($p < 0.01$).

Comments

Recently, computer stereographic studies of skin tissues[21-23] have been reported describing the advantages of the computer-generated 3-D models of tissue structures. As far as we know, there has been no publication on the subject of endometriosis, using computer graphic mechanical methods of reconstruction.

When compared with the 3-D models demonstrated in other studies, the present 3-D models seemed to be much better and to show more realistic appearances of structures, since the structures of the reconstructed models were colored. Furthermore, the transparent display of our 3-D models was excellent for the observation of their interior structures. The present

study demonstrates that two different types of peritoneal endometriotic lesions can be differentiated: a first type without ramification of the glands, and a second type in which glands are ramified and connected (Figures 13 and 14). Further studies are needed in order to evaluate whether the two different types could be correlated either to the different degree of 'aggressiveness' or to the different appearances of peritoneal endometriosis.

From the present stereographic findings, one may consider that the apparently multifocal occurrence (in two-dimensional views) of glandular epithelium in one lesion is not confirmed by the 3-D study. Indeed, in each peritoneal lesion, epithelial glands are interconnected by luminal structures. It is probable that in each peritoneal lesion, epithelial structures occur in a single focus of the stroma, and then may gradually develop, elongate and swell, forming luminal structures, occasionally with endometrial debris inside. During the expansion, all glands are connected and no peripheral epithelial structures become independent by loss of interconnection.

Since each of the peritoneal lesions, stereographically reconstructed in the present study, was only a part of the peritoneal endometriosis of one patient, it is far too soon to reach any conclusion; however, in the future, the 3-D analysis of stereographically reconstructed lesions could contribute to the understanding of the *in vivo* development of endometriosis.

This stereometric study of volumes of 3-D structures revealed the volume distribution in peritoneal endometriosis. The ratios of epithelium, stroma and lumen/lesion observed in groups I and II indicate a more powerful effect of the GnRH agonist therapy on the stroma than on the epithelium. This effect could be due to the reduction in stromal vascularization, induced by the GnRH agonist. The stromal capillary network can also be reconstructed in 3-D. In active lesions, the 3-D evaluation of the capillary network reveals the presence of a great number of larger vessels (Figure 16). After GnRH agonist therapy (as well as in white lesions), the network is composed of smaller vessels (Figure 17).

The present stereographic and stereometric study has shown some new characteristics of peritoneal endometriosis. Further studies are under way to investigate the variations in the 3-D architecture of peritoneal endometriotic lesions among different patients, patients of differing ages, and patients with different types of peritoneal endometriosis, before and after hormonal therapy.

HYPOTHESIS

Figure 18 illustrates a hypothesis of the evolution of a peritoneal endometriotic lesion. Red flame-like lesions and glandular excrescences are probably the first stage of early implantation of endometrial glands and stroma.

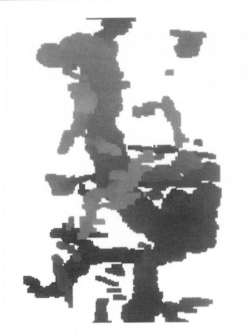

Figure 16 The three-dimensional evaluation of the capillary network; a great number of larger vessels can be seen

Figure 17 The three-dimensional evaluation of the capillary network; smaller vessels are seen after gonadotropin releasing hormone agonist therapy or in white lesion

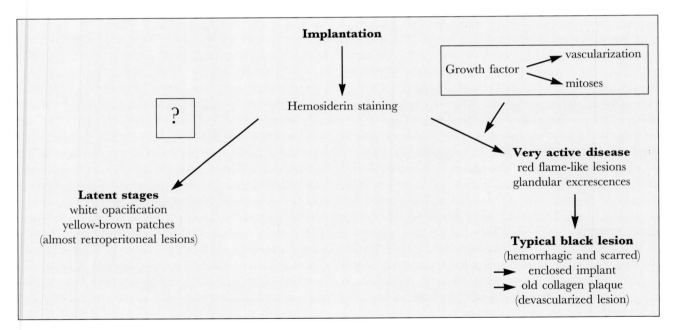

Figure 18 Hypothesis of peritoneal endometriotic lesion evolution

Their significantly higher vascularization is responsible for the invasion. Indeed, mitotic activity has been proved to be related to the vascularization[17]. This could explain the growth and aggressiveness of recently implanted endometrial cells. Thereafter, menstrual shedding from viable endometrial implants could initiate an inflammatory reaction, provoking a scarification process which encloses the implant. The presence of intraluminal debris is responsible for the typical black coloration of the same lesion. This scarification process causes a reduction in vascularization, as proved by the significant decrease in the capillaries/stroma relative surface area.

Thereafter, the inflammatory process devascularizes the endometrial cells, and white plaques of old collagen are all that remain of the ectopic implant. The vascularization of this scarred endometriotic tissue was found to be significantly reduced in our study (relative surface 1.5%). White opacification and yellow-brown lesions could be latent stages of endometriosis as suggested by the poor vascularization observed. They are probably non-active lesions which could be quiescent for a long time.

REFERENCES

1. Chatman, D.L. (1981). Pelvic peritoneal defects and endometriosis; Allen-Masters syndrome revisited. *Fertil. Steril.*, **36**, 751

2. Jansen, R.P.S. and Russell, P. (1986). Non-pigmented endometriosis: clinical laparoscopic and pathologic definition. *Am. J. Obstet. Gynecol.*, **155**, 1154

3. Redwine, D.B. (1987). The distribution of endometriosis in the pelvis by age groups and fertility. *Fertil. Steril.*, **47**, 173–5

4. Stripling, M.C., Martin, D.C., Chatman, D.L., Vander Zwaag, R. and Poston, W.M. (1988). Subtle appearances of pelvic endometriosis. *Fertil. Steril.*, **49**, 427,

5. Martin, D.C., Hubert, G.D., Vander Zwaag, R. and El-Zeky, F. (1989). Laparoscopic appearances of peritoneal endometriosis. *Fertil. Steril.*, **51**, 63

6 Nisolle, M., Paindaveine, B., Bourdon, A., Berlière, M., Casanas-Roux, F. and Donnez, J. (1990). Histologic study of peritoneal endometriosis in infertile women. *Fertil. Steril.*, **53**, 984–8

7. Donnez, J. and Nisolle, M. (1988). Appearances of peritoneal endometriosis. In *Proceedings of the IIIrd International Laser Surgery Symposium*, Brussels

8. Donnez, J., Casanas-Roux, F., Caprasse, E.J., Ferin, J. and Thomas, K. (1985). Cyclic changes in ciliation, cell height, and mitotic activity in human tubal epithelium during reproductive life. *Fertil. Steril.*, **43**, 554–9

9. Murphy, A.A., Green, W.R., Bobbie, D., de la Cruz, Z.C. and Rock, J.A. (1986). Unsuspected endometriosis documented by scanning electron microscopy in visually normal peritoneum. *Fertil. Steril.*, **46**, 552

10. Brosens, I., Vasquez, G. and Gordts, S. (1984). Scanning electron microscopic study of the pelvic peritoneum in unexplained infertility and endometriosis. *Fertil. Steril.*, **41**, 215

11. Lox, C.D., Word, L. and Heine, M.W. (1984). Ultrastructural evaluation of endometriosis. *Fertil. Steril.*, **41**, 755

12. Roddick, J.W., Conkey, G. and Jacobs, E.J. (1960). The hormonal response of endometriotic implants and its relationship to symptomatology. *Am. J. Obstet. Gynecol.*, **79**, 1173–7

13. Donnez, J., Nisolle, M., Casanas-Roux, F. and Clerckx, F. (1993). Endometriosis: rationale for surgery. In Brosens, I. and Donnez, J. (eds.) *The Current Status of Endometriosis Research and Management*, pp.385–96. (Carnforth, UK: Parthenon Publishing)

14. Jänne, O., Kauppila, A. and Kokko, E. (1981). Estrogen and progestin receptors in endometriosis lesions: comparison with endometrial tissue. *Am. J. Obstet. Gynecol.*, **141**, 562–6

15. Bergqvist, A., Rannevik, G. and Thorell, J. (1981). Estrogen and progesterone cytosol receptor concentration in endometriotic tissue and intrauterine endometrium. *Acta Obstet. Gynecol. Scand.*, **101**, 53–8

16. Tamaya, T., Motoyaha, T. and Ohono, Y. (1979). Steroid receptor levels and histology of endometriosis and adenomyosis. *Fertil. Steril.*, **31**, 394–400

17. Nisolle, M., Casanas-Roux, F. and Donnez, J. (1988). Histologic study of ovarian endometriosis after hormonal therapy. *Fertil. Steril.*, **49**, 423

18. Donnez, J., Nisolle, M. and Casanas-Roux, F. (1992). Three dimensional architectures of peritoneal endometriosis. *Fertil. Steril.*, **57**, 980

19. Nisolle, M, Casanas-Roux, F., Anaf, V., Mine, J.M. and Donnez, J. (1993). Morphometric study of the stromal vascularization in peritoneal endometriosis. *Fertil. Steril.*, **59**, 681

20. Matta, W.H.M., Stabille, I., Shaw, R.S. and Campbell, S. (1988). Doppler assessment of uterine blood flow changes in patients with fibroids receiving the GnRH agonist Buserelin. *Fertil. Steril.*, **49**, 1083

21. Braverman, M.S. and Braverman, I.M. (1986). Three-dimensional reconstructions of objects from serial sections using a microcomputer graphic system. *J. Invest. Dermatol.*, **86**, 290–4

22. Marchevsky, A.M., Gil, J. and Jeanty, H. (1987). Computerized interactive morphometry in pathology: current instrumentation and methods. *Hum. Pathol.*, **18**, 320–31

23. Ito, M., Yokoyama, H., Ikeda, K. and Sat, Y. (1990). Stereographic analysis of syringomas. *Arch. Dermatol. Res.*, **282**, 17–21

The association of endometriosis with pelvic pain

4

D.C. Martin

INTRODUCTION

Sampson was unable to find a relationship between the extent of disease and the severity of pain and compared this with the lack of correlation for adhesions in general[1]. Many subsequent studies have shown no correlation between symptoms such as pain, dysmenorrhea and dyspareunia and the stage of endometriosis[2–5]. Others have suggested a similar lack of correlation between symptoms and absence or presence of various pathological findings[4,6–8].

The lack of relation may be due to patient response to endometriosis, a lack of study focus, or study bias. This lack can be manifest in clinical care by adaptation of therapeutic models related to the type of referral population[9]. Of the problems in study design, the easiest to quantitate is the tertiary center bias between psychiatric orientation and surgical orientation. In a report from a psychiatric center, only 48% of women with pelvic pain had organic pathology while 64% reported childhood sexual abuse[10]. On the other hand, in patients referred to a surgical practice, 98% had pelvic pathology while no patients (0%) were questioned regarding childhood sexual abuse[11]. These differences are significant with p values of < 0.001 (Tables 1 and 2) and appear to represent a difference both in the type of patients referred and in the center's approach.

Although early studies of the surface appearance of peritoneal lesions did not add to our understanding of pain[12], recent studies have pointed out a correlation between the relative peritoneal location and fluid concentrations of CA-125 and placental protein (PP)14[13]. Moreover, increasing size or depth of fibrotic scars was associated with pain and tenderness[12,14–20] while typical lesions were commonly associated with dyspareunia[21]. Although histological documentation can be difficult, this has been accomplished in up to 98% of patients[22,23].

Also, a recent study limited to patients with infertility documented that dyspareunia, pelvic pain and moderate or severe dysmenorrhea were associated with revised American Fertility Society (rAFS) staging[24,25]. A separate study documented that severe dysmenorrhea was highly predictive of endometriosis[26].

DISCUSSION

Numerous theories have been proposed to explain the mechanism of pain mediation by endometriotic tissue,

Table 1 There is a statistically significant difference between the findings at surgery in patients seen in a psychiatric practice[10] and those seen in a surgical practice[11].

	Walker[10]	Martin[11]	Total
Pathology noted	12	111	123
No pathology noted	13	2	15
Total	25	113	138

$\chi^2 = 48.2$, $p < 0.001$

Table 2 There is a statistically significant difference between the histories of childhood sexual abuse in patients seen in a psychiatric practice[10] and those seen in a surgical practice[10,11]

	Walker[10]	Martin[11]	Total
History of childhood sexual abuse noted	16	0	16
No history of childhood sexual abuse noted	9	113	122
Total	25	113	138

$\chi^2 = 48.2$, $p < 0.001$

including production and release of prostaglandins; inflammatory mediators (kinins, histamine, interleukins, etc.); fibrosis; cyclical hemorrhage; and compression, distension and distortion of tissues innervated by the visceral and somatic pathways[27,29]. None are consistent in explaining the various clinical findings seen with endometriosis. Several investigators have demonstrated the variable gross appearance[11,23,30–32] and biochemical activity[33,34] of endometriotic lesions.

An early theory of pain production proposed by Sturgis[15] suggested that both fibrotic reaction and functional glands were required for pain mediation. Previous trichrome stain study of these white lesions demonstrated fibrous and muscular components[23]. Further analysis using trichrome stain may show microscopic fibrosis associated with lesion types other than those with gross fibrosis. An additional stain which may be helpful is one to demonstrate neural tissue[27].

Redwine[35] has documented a progression of lesions in different age-groups from clear at a median age of

21.5 years, to red at 26.3 years, to scarred white at 29.5 years, to black at 31.9 years. Lesions in younger age-ranges include those which have previously been identified as producing increased prostaglandin[34]. These bioactive lesions may be responsible for generalized pain and dysmenorrhea, while fibrotic lesions may create more focal tenderness. Presently, the influence of lesions of differing gross appearances is of unknown clinical significance.

Accurate assessment of symptoms is difficult because of the effect that emotional and psychological factors have on the patient's perception and reporting of pain. In fact, even when psychological evaluation and symptom mapping are performed preoperatively, the extent of disease at laparoscopy does not show a significant correlation with the pain ratings[6].

There may be no way to determine the ability of a pathological stimulus to produce pain, since it is a subjective experience of multideterminate cause. This is part of the conclusion in one study of women with chronic pelvic pain in whom pathological findings had little or no relevance, as the pain was due primarily to the past and present psychological problems of the patient[10]. However, only 52% of the patients had pathological findings while 57% of the controls had infertility.

Studies often conclude that the extent or stage of endometriosis does not correspond with the severity of symptoms[2,3,5,8,27]. However, quantitation of dysmenorrhea into mild, moderate and severe categories documented prevalence rates for endometriosis of 32, 41 and 95%, respectively. Thus, severe dysmenorrhea was highly predictive of endometriosis[26]. Furthermore, focal tenderness was found in 61% of patients with endometriosis and also appears to be of limited predictive value for the location or extent of disease[18].

Tenderness on examination has been shown to be predictive of pelvic adhesions[36] and fibrotic pelvic pathology[13,18]. Focal pelvic tenderness may allow more objective and reproducible prediction of the location and possibly the extent of endometriosis[19,20]. In addition, tenderness may be associated with biological activity and depth of infiltration[16,18,19] as well as with a scarred black appearance[21].

Of statistical significance is the difference in depth and volume of tender vs. non-tender endometriosis[18]. This confirms a corollary to previous studies suggesting that the volume of disease is directly related to patient symptoms[16,17]. Many of the previously proposed mechanisms of pain mediation could be applied here to explain the relationship of depth and volume to tenderness. The presence of preoperative tenderness should allow the surgeon to anticipate extensive excision or ablation if endometriosis is confirmed. However, whether surgical treatment of these tender lesions will relieve the tenderness or symptoms remains to be evaluated.

PROPOSED INSTRUMENT

Reviews of the current knowledge of endometriosis suggest the need for ongoing study[37]. The American Fertility Society subcommittee on the classification of endometriosis in the presence of pelvic pain has published an instrument confirmed by the 1993 Annual Meeting of The American Fertility Society. This instrument uses a combination of preoperative assessment and operative descriptions[38].

The instrument uses patients' descriptions of pain and is quantitated as mild, discomforting, distressing, horrible or excruciating. Other descriptions and limitations are noted. There is a description for the quality of tenderness caused on palpation, the extent of nodularity, the diffuse or focal distribution, and/or any fixation of the uterus or adnexa. An anatomical drawing is used to demonstrate the affected areas (Figure 1)[38].

At the time of surgery, adhesions and lesions are described separately. Adhesions are described as avascular/thin, thick/dense, bands/string-like, or sheet-like. These are drawn on a schematic diagram of the pelvis (Figure 2)[25,38].

The operative findings are noted with a measurement of mean diameter and depth in millimeters. The visual appearance is described as clear, vesicular/bleb-like, pink, flame-like/red, black/blue, yellow/brown, white or fibrotic. These findings are noted on a similar schematic diagram of the pelvis. Furthermore, each lesion is noted on a table demonstrating the size in millimeters, depth, appearance, final histology and quadrant of location.

CONCLUSIONS

Of the many questions that can be asked, two appear at the opposite ends of the spectrum. The first is: Does endometriosis cause pain and tenderness in a significant number of women? Data show that the answer to this question is yes[12,14–21]. The second question is a more specific question regarding a select patient population: Do patients with 'chronic pelvic pain' have a significant amount of that pain caused by endometriosis? This is more difficult to answer because the concept and definition of 'chronic pelvic pain' vary significantly from one researcher to another. However, if we look at patients who are referred to centers specializing in a psychosomatic approach to chronic pelvic pain, it appears that endometriosis is not commonly a main component of the pain. This does not address the problem of 'chronic pelvic pain' in the general obstetrical/gynecological population; nor does it discuss dysmenorrhea, cyclic pelvic pain, pelvic tenderness or dyspareunia.

Although some studies have shown no relationship between symptoms and the stage of endometriosis, other studies of specific groups have shown a correlation.

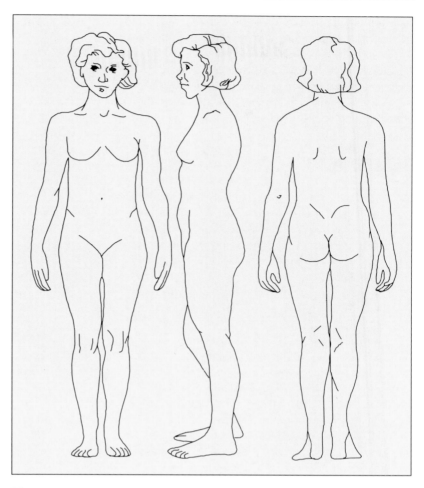

Figure 1 Patients and physicians chart signs and symptoms on a body map (from reference 39, with permission)

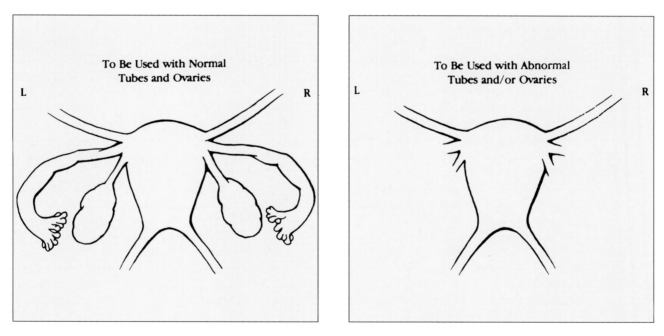

Figure 2 The physician draws the pelvic finding at surgery (adapted from the Revised American Fertility Society classification, reference 25)

In a population limited only to infertility, dyspareunia, pelvic pain, moderate dysmenorrhea and severe dysmenorrhea have been associated with rAFS staging. It is hoped that the AFS instrument[38] will be useful in further delineating the association of endometriosis with the various signs and symptoms attributed to this condition and to other pelvic pathology.

REFERENCES

1. Sampson, J.A. (1921). Perforating hemorrhagic (chocolate) cysts of the ovary. Their importance and especially their relation to pelvic adenomas of the endometrial type ('adenomyoma' of the uterus, rectovaginal septum, sigmoid, etc.). *Arch. Surg.*, **3**, 245–323

2. Gray, L.A. (1958). The conservative operation for endometriosis: a report of its use in 200 cases. *J. Ky. Med. Assoc.*, **56**,1219

3. Buttram, V.C. (1979). Conservative surgery for endometriosis in the infertile female: a study of 206 patients with implications for both medical and surgical therapy. *Fertil. Steril.*, **31**, 117–23

4. Cunanan, R.G., Courey, N.G.M. and Lippes, J. (1983). Laparoscopic findings in patients with pelvic pain. *Am. J. Obstet. Gynecol.*, **146**, 589–91

5. Fedele, L., Parazzini, F., Bianchi, S., Arcaini, L. and Candiani, G.B. (1990). Stage and localization of pelvic endometriosis and pain. *Fertil. Steril.*, **53**, 155–8

6. Stout, A.L., Steege, J.F., Dodson, W.C., and Hughes, C.L. (1991). Relationship of laparoscopic findings to self-report of pelvic pain. *Am. J. Obstet. Gynecol.*, **164**, 73–9

7. Franssen, A.M.H.W., Kauer, F.M., Chadha, D.R., Zijlstra, J.A. and Rolland, R. (1989). Endometriosis: treatment with gonadotropin-releasing hormone agonist buserelin. *Fertil. Steril.*, **51**, 401–8

8. Kresch, A. (1984). Laparoscopy in 100 women with chronic pelvic pain. *Obstet. Gynecol.*, **64**, 672

9. Steege, J.F., Stout, A.L. and Somkuti, S.G. (1993). Chronic pelvic pain in women: toward an integrative model. *Obstet. Gynecol. Surv. Rev.*, **48**, 95–110

10. Walker, E., Katon, W., Harrop-Griffiths, J., Holm, L., Russo, J. and Hickok, L.R. (1988). Relationship of chronic pelvic pain to psychiatric diagnoses and childhood sexual abuse. *Am. J. Psychiatry*, **145**, 75–80

11. Martin, D.C., Hubert, G.D., Vander Zwaag, R. and El-Zeky, F.A. (1989). Laparoscopic appearances of peritoneal endometriosis. *Fertil. Steril.*, **51**, 63–7

12. Ripps, B.A. and Martin, D.C. (1991). Focal pelvic tenderness, pelvic pain and dysmenorrhea in endometriosis. *J. Reprod. Med.*, **36**, 470–2

13. Koninckx, R.P., Riittinen, L., Seppala, M. and Cornillie, F.J. (1992). CA-125 and placental protein 14 concentrations in plasma and peritoneal fluid of women with deeply infiltrating pelvic endometriosis. *Fertil. Steril.*, **57**, 523–30

14. Hasson, H.M. (1981). Classification for endometriosis. *Fertil. Steril.* (letter), **35**, 368

15. Sturgis, S.H. and Call, B.J. (1954). Endometriosis peritonei – relationship of pain to functional activity. *Am. J. Obstet. Gynecol.*, **68**, 1421

16. Cornillie, F.J., Oosterlynck, D., Lauweryns, J.M. and Koninckx, P.R. (1990). Deeply infiltrating pelvic endometriosis: histology and clinical significance. *Fertil. Steril.*, **53**, 978–83

17. Koninckx, P.R., Meuleman, C., Demeyere, S., Lesaffre, E. and Cornillie, F. J. (1991). Suggestive evidence that pelvic endometriosis is a progressive disease, whereas deeply infiltrating endometriosis is associated with pelvic pain. *Fertil. Steril.*, **55**, 759–65

18. Ripps, B.A. and Martin, D.C. (1992). Correlation of focal pelvic tenderness with implant dimension and stage of endometriosis. *J. Reprod. Med.*, **37**, 620–4

19. Koninckx, P.R. and Martin, D.C. (1992). Deep endometriosis: a consequence of infiltration or retraction or possibly adenomyosis externa? *Fertil. Steril.*, **58**, 924–8

20. Koninckx, P.R. and Cornillie, F.J. (1993). Infiltrating endometriosis: infiltration, retraction or adenomyosis externa? In Martin, D.C. (ed.) *Atlas of Endometriosis*, pp.9.1–9.8. (London: Gower Med. Publ.)

21. Vercellini, P., Bocciolone, L., Vendola, N., Colombo, A., Rognoni, M.T. and Fedele, L. (1991). Peritoneal endometriosis. Morphologic appearance in women with chronic pelvic pain. *J. Reprod. Med.*, **36**, 533–6

22. Martin, D.C. and Berry, J.D. (1990). Histology of chocolate cysts. *J. Gynecol. Surg.*, **6**, 43–6

23. Stripling, M.C., Martin, D.C., Chatman, D.L., Vander Zwaag, R. and Poston, W.M. (1988). Subtle appearance of pelvic endometriosis. *Fertil. Steril.*, **49**, 427–31

24. Fedele, L., Bianchi, S., Bocciolone, L., Di Nola, G. and Parazzini, F. (1992). Pain symptoms associated with endometriosis. *Obstet. Gynecol.*, **79**, 767–9

25. American Fertility Society: Revised American Fertility Society classification of endometriosis: 1985. *Fertil. Steril.*, **43,** 351–3

26. Naish, C.E., Kennedy, S.H. and Barlow, D.H. (1992). Correlation between pain symptoms and laparoscopic findings. Presented at *3rd World Congress on Endometriosis*, p.065 (abstract). (Brussels: Ipsen)

27. Hurst, B.S. and Rock, J.A. (1989). Endometriosis: pathophysiology, diagnosis and treatment. *Obstet. Gynecol. Surv.*, **44**, 297–304

28. Schenken, R.S. (1989). *Endometriosis: Contemporary Concepts in Clinical Management.* (Philadelphia: JB Lippincott)

29. Sturgis, S.H. and Call, B.J. (1954). Endometriosis peritonei – relationship of pain to functional activity. *Am. J. Obstet. Gynecol.*, **68**, 1421

30. Chatman, D.L. (1981). Pelvic peritoneal defects and endometriosis: Allen-Masters syndrome revisited. *Fertil. Steril.*, **36**, 751–6

31. Jansen, R.P.S. and Russell, P. (1986). Nonpigmented endometriosis: clinical, laparoscopic, and pathologic definition. *Am. J. Obstet. Gynecol.*, **155**, 1154–9

32. Vasquez, G., Cornillie, F. and Brosens, I.A. (1983). Peritoneal endometriosis: scanning electron microscopy and histology of minimal pelvic endometriotic lesions. *Fertil. Steril.*, **42**, 696–703

33. Moon, Y.S., Leung, P.C.S., Yuen, B.H., *et al.* (1981). Prostaglandin F in human endometriotic tissue. *Am. J. Obstet. Gynecol.*, **141**, 344

34. Vernon, M.W., Beard, J.S., Graves, K. and Wilson, E.A. (1986). Classification of endometriotic implants by morphologic appearance and capacity to synthesize prostaglandin F. *Fertil. Steril.*, **46**, 801–6

35. Redwine, D.B. (1987). The distribution of endometriosis in the pelvis by age groups and fertility. *Fertil. Steril.*, **47**, 173–5

36. Stovall, T.G., Elder, R.F. and Ling, F.W. (1989). Predictors of pelvic adhesions. *J. Reprod. Med.*, **34**, 345–8

37. Rock, J.A. (1990). Endometriosis: overview and future directions. *J. Reprod. Med.* (Suppl.), **35**, 76–81

38. The American Fertility Society (Groff, T.R., Shaw, R.M., Buttram, V.C. Jr, Brosens, I., Martin, D.C., Rock, J.A., Donnez, J.G. and Canis, M.) (1993). Management of endometriosis in the presence of pelvic pain. *Fertil. Steril.*, **60**(6), 952–5

39. Martin, D.C. (1990). *Laparoscopic Appearance of Endometriosis*, 2nd Edn. (Memphis: Resurge Press)

Laser uterine nerve ablation

C.J.G. Sutton

5

The treatment of dysmenorrhea has undergone some curious changes during the past 30 years reflecting new developments in medicine and surgery. For many years the operation of presacral neurectomy was employed for patients with intractable dysmenorrhea but yielded disappointing results with failure rates of about 11–15% in primary dysmenorrhea and 25–40% in secondary dysmenorrhea [1,2]. In 1952 White [3] pointed out that the nerve supply to the cervix is not usually interrupted by the presacral neurectomy procedure and for this reason, and with the development of new drugs to suppress ovulation, the procedure was abandoned by most gynecologists.

The actual incidence of dysmenorrhea is difficult to assess and depends on many complex and variable factors including prevailing social and sexual attitudes in different societies. Prevalence rates vary in different studies from 3 to 90% but probably the best population study comes from Sweden, where all 19-year-old girls from the town of Gothenburg were questioned with a 90% response rate [4]. A total of 73% of the girls suffered from primary dysmenorrhea and 15% had severe dysmenorrhea which affected their working ability and could not be controlled adequately by analgesics or ovulation suppression. It is for this group of patients that surgery is recommended, either by the paracervical uterine denervation technique of Doyle [5] or, more simply, by laser uterine nerve ablation (LUNA) at the time of laparoscopy. Before describing this technique, it behoves us to consider the relevant anatomy and to look in some detail at Doyle's procedure [5] which we are trying to imitate with the laser rather than the scalpel.

ANATOMY OF THE UTERINE NERVE SUPPLY

The sensory parasympathetic fibers to the cervix and the sensory sympathetic fibers to the corpus traverse the cervical division of the Lee-Frankenhauser plexus [6] which lies in, under and around the attachments of the uterine ligament to the cervix. Sympathetic fibers which have reached the cervix by accompanying the uterine arteries can also be found in this area.

The parasympathetic components originate from the first to the third and fourth sacral nerves, reaching the plexus by the pelvic nerves (nervi erigentes). In a study of 33 cadavers, Campbell [7] confirmed the findings of earlier workers [8,9] by identifying parasympathetic fibers in the anterior two-thirds of the uterosacral ligaments and

demonstrated the presence of small ganglia around the area where the ligaments attach to the cervix. Theoretically, therefore, division of the uterosacral ligaments at the point of their attachment to the cervix should lead to interruption of most of the cervical sensory fibers and some of the corporal sensory fibers and lead to a diminution in uterine pain at the time of menstruation.

DOYLE'S PROCEDURE

In 1963 Joseph Doyle described the procedure of paracervical uterine denervation which bears his name [10]. The procedure could be performed vaginally or abdominally and the authors suggested that gynecologists may be more comfortable with the former approach while general surgeons would prefer the latter. Employing the vaginal approach, a suture was placed through the posterior lip of the cervix at the apex of the vagina and traction of this suture increased the distance of the cervix from the ureter, which is clearly demonstrated in his article by a very convincing radiograph of a cervico-uretogram. The attachments of the uterosacral ligaments to the cervix were then divided between two Heaney clamps and to prevent regrowth of the bisected nerve trunks, the posterior leaf of the peritoneal incision was interposed between them. The abdominal approach was recommended if endometriosis was suspected or any gross pathology, such as fibroids, was felt. The pathological tissue was then excised (which may, of course, have had a significant effect on the results) and then traction was applied to the uterosacral ligaments by means of a suture placed in the cervix just above the point of their insertion. Doyle carefully scrutinized the course of the ureters and found them rarely to lie close to the ligaments, usually running 1–2 cm laterally. As before, the ligaments were divided between two clamps and in further refinement of the technique, he sutured the ligaments together with stainless steel sutures to the isthmus of the cervix in the midline, about 1 cm higher than their original attachment.

Doyle's results were extremely impressive, with complete pain relief in 63 out of 73 cases (86%); 35 had primary dysmenorrhea (85.7% success) and 33 had secondary dysmenorrhea (86.8% success). Relief was partial in six cases and there were four failures [5,11]. With such a satisfactory outcome it is difficult to see why the operation sank into obscurity. Possibly the advent of powerful prostaglandin synthetase inhibitors reduced the demand for relatively drastic forms of intervention. Interest in Doyle's work has recently revived with the development of surgical lasers which can be used endoscopically to perform much the same tissue effect without the need for major surgery.

LASER LAPAROSCOPIC UTERINE NERVE ABLATION

Uterine neurectomy can be performed on patients with either primary or secondary dysmenorrhea at the same time as a diagnostic laparoscopy is performed. The procedure was initially performed by electrocautery but there was always concern about the spread of the electric current in this area due to the close proximity of the ureter and the uterine artery.

The pelvis is inspected carefully for associated pathology, particularly endometriosis, and if this is found it should be carefully vaporized with carbon dioxide laser energy transmitted directly through the operating channel of the laparoscope or via a second laser probe inserted suprapubically or in the right or left iliac fossa. A further puncture is required for a suction/irrigation instrument to wash off residual carbon deposits using heparinized Rinter's lactate solution, and to evacuate the smoke which is produced in large amounts during a laser neurectomy. This probe is also useful to exert pressure on the posterior aspect of the cervix between the insertions of the uterosacral ligaments, thus serving to accentuate them in much the same way as traction on the posterior cervical suture as described by Doyle in his original technique[5].

The posterior leaves of the broad ligaments are carefully inspected to try to identify the course of the ureters which can rarely lie close to the uterosacral ligaments but usually run 1–2 cm laterally. They can usually be 'palpated' via a probe and often the characteristic peristaltic movements can be recognized beneath the peritoneal surface. The operator should also take note of some thin-walled veins which often lie just lateral to the uterosacral ligaments, because if they are accidentally punctured they can cause troublesome bleeding which can be very difficult to stop with the carbon dioxide laser. Hemostatic clips, bipolar diathermy or an endocoagulator should be immediately available if required.

Once the operator has noted these potential hazards, the uterosacral ligaments are encouraged to 'stand out' by the assistant manipulating the uterus with an 8-mm Hegar dilator to one or the other side, and at the same time using the probe to put pressure on the posterior aspect of the cervix as described above. The laser is set at a relatively high power density setting of 10 000–15 000 W/cm^2 and the uterosacral ligaments are vaporized near the point of their attachment to the posterior aspect of the cervix. The idea of the procedure is to destroy the sensory nerve fibers and their secondary ganglia as they leave the uterus; because of the divergence of these fibers in the uterosacral ligament, they should be vaporized as close to the cervix as possible. A crater about 2 cm in diameter and 1 cm deep is formed, and great care must be taken to vaporize medially rather than laterally to avoid damage to the vessels already identified coursing alongside the uterosacral ligaments (Figure 7). A further refinement is to superficially laser the posterior aspects of the cervix between the insertion of the ligaments to interrupt fibers crossing to the contralateral side[12]. It is relatively easy to vaporize to the correct depth when the uterosacral ligaments are well formed but sometimes their limits are poorly defined and the procedure is less than satisfactory, simply because it is difficult to be sure that the area vaporized is in the same place as the uterine nerve fibers.

RESULTS

We have been using the carbon dioxide laser laparoscopically for the past 7 years at St Luke's Hospital in Guildford, UK, and have treated over 600 patients[13]. Most of the patients treated have suffered from endometriosis and about one-fifth of the patients have had laser laparoscopic uterine nerve ablation performed for secondary dysmenorrhea associated with endometriosis, or for primary dysmenorrhea unresponsive to oral contraceptives or non-steroidal anti-inflammatory drugs (NSAIDs), usually Ponstan forte (Parke Davis) or Synflex (Syntex Pharmaceuticals). Patients with primary dysmenorrhea were asked to record the intensity of their pain on a linear analog scale, marked from 0 to 10, before the operation and again before the follow-up visit 4 months later. All patients were warned that the first period might be slightly more uncomfortable, possibly due to edema around the nerve fibers during the healing process after laser surgery. The follow-up interview was conducted by one of the vocational trainees from general practice in order to minimize subjective bias that might have been introduced had the surgeon himself seen the patient at the follow-up visit. Patients with secondary (congestive) dysmenorrhea were informed that if endometriosis was discovered at diagnostic laparoscopy, all visible implants would be vaporized and the uterosacral ligaments also vaporized if this was technically feasible. Sometimes only one of the ligaments was anatomically obvious and in that case the procedure was recorded as a partial LUNA only.

During the past 5 years we have treated 126 patients with laser uterine nerve ablation laparoscopically. The results are summarized in Table 1: 26 had primary dysmenorrhea, and 100 had congestive dysmenorrhea in association with endometriosis. We deliberately did not

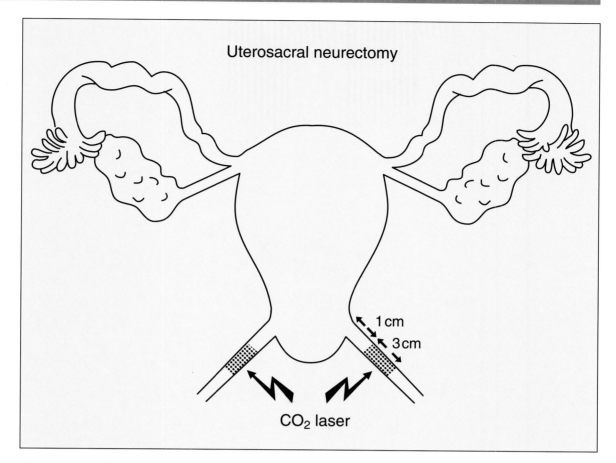

Figure 1(a)   The technique of laser laparoscopic uterine nerve ablation; (b) and (c) a crater about 2 cm in diameter and 1 cm deep is formed

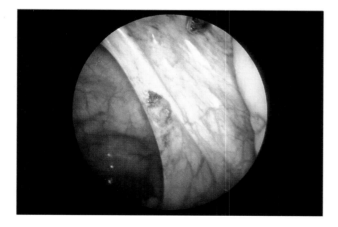

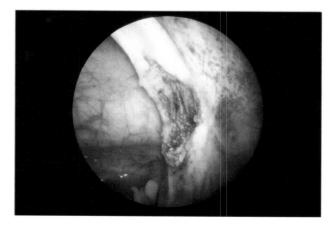

Figure 1(b)   *See legend above*

Figure 1(c)   *See legend above*

Table 1 Laser uterine nerve ablation (LUNA) results with carbon dioxide laser. LFU, lost to follow-up

	LFU	Improved	Same	Worse
Endometriosis (n = 100)	6	81 (86%)	13	—
Primary dysmenorrhea (n = 26)	4	16 (73%)	6	—
Total (n = 126)	10	97 (84%)	19	—

include patients with secondary dysmenorrhea due to other causes such as fibroids or pelvic congestion.

In patients with primary dysmenorrhea we used the linear analog scale to judge the response to treatment. The initial score was on average 9.2, and in 16 patients (73%) the symptoms were improved with an average score among the successful patients of 3.4. Of these, 15 had a complete neurectomy and one had a partial neurectomy due to poor formation of the uterosacral ligament on one side.

No patients were made worse by the procedure but six patients failed to show any improvement; in three of these, a partial neurectomy was performed, suggesting an element of technical failure. Of the three patients who failed to show any improvement, one subsequently had a hysterectomy and the pathologist noted marked adenomyosis in the myometrium (endometriosis interna), explaining her lack of response to nerve severance. Four patients were lost to follow-up.

Of the 100 patients with secondary dysmenorrhea associated with endometriosis, six were lost to follow-up; 81 (86%) reported an improvement in symptoms, even though 26 (32%) of them had a partial (unilateral) neurectomy. In three patients the symptoms returned 6 months to 1 year following the procedure. No patients were made worse but 13 reported no improvement and, interestingly, nine of these had incomplete or partial neurectomies.

There were no serious complications in this group of patients and all were treated on a day case or overnight stay basis. Troublesome bleeding was encountered in two patients requiring endocoagulation or hemostatic clips and the insertion of a redivac drain in the pelvis for 12 h.

DISCUSSION

Although many women are able to cope with the symptoms of dysmenorrhea, there remains a sizeable proportion of the female population who have to take to their beds for a few days each month; in the USA it has been estimated that 600 million work hours are lost annually to this affliction[14]. Before 1960, many patients were treated surgically with the interruption of the inferior hypogastric nerve plexus (presacral neurectomy)[15,16] or simple division of the uterosacral ligament, performed either abdominally or vaginally[11]. With the advent of oral contraceptives and NSAIDs in the 1960s, these procedures virtually fell into disuse in spite of the fact that at least 20% of dysmenorrheic patients fail to respond to NSAID therapy[17–19].

With the increasing popularity of operative laparoscopy in recent years, there has been a revival of interest in Doyle's procedure[5,10,11] because it is possible to perform the transection or destruction of the uterosacral ligaments either with diathermy coagulation and laparoscopic scissors[20], the carbon dioxide laser[21–23], or the KTP/532 laser[12].

The study of Lichten and Bombard[20] is particularly interesting because it is one of the few, or indeed the only randomized prospective double-blind study performed in this rapidly developing branch of operative gynecology. A relatively homogeneous group of women were selected who had severe or incapacitating dysmenorrhea, who had no demonstrable pelvic pathology at laparoscopy and who were unresponsive to NSAIDs and oral contraceptives prescribed concurrently. Co-existing psychiatric illness was evaluated with the Minnesota Multiphasic Personality Inventory and those with abnormal psychological profile were excluded from the study. The remaining 21 patients were randomized to the uterine nerve ablation or control group at the time of diagnostic laparoscopy. Neither the patient nor the clinical psychologist who conducted the interview and the follow-up was aware of the group to which the patient had been randomized. No patient in the control group reported relief from dysmenorrhea, whereas nine of the 11 patients (81%) who had LUNA reported almost complete relief at 3 months and five of them had continued relief from dysmenorrhea 1 year after surgery. Interestingly, those who reported surgical success also reported relief from associated symptoms of nausea, vomiting, diarrhea and headaches.

Although there were no reported complications in the above study, the numbers involved were small; the use of thermocautery in this area is potentially hazardous because of the proximity to the ureter. We have chosen preferentially the carbon dioxide laser because of its ability to vaporize tissue precisely, causing a zone of thermal necrosis only 500 μm beyond the impact site[24]. The main disadvantage of this laser lies in its absorption by blood, rendering it ineffective in stopping anything more than small vessel hemorrhage. Great care must therefore be taken to control the laser beam and to avoid puncturing the thin-walled vessels lying lateral to the uterosacral ligaments. If bleeding does occur, attempts should be made to stop it by the usual techniques of pressing on the bleeding point with a blunt probe, lowering the power density and defocusing the beam in order to char the vessels. If this is unsuccessful, equipment should be available to use other endoscopic techniques of hemostasis such as endocoagulation[25], bipolar desiccation[26,27] or hemostatic clips[28]. If there is any doubt about hemostasis a redivac drain should be introduced and left in the pelvis for several hours after the operation to prevent pelvic hematoma formation and to monitor the amount of blood lost. Not only should hemostatic equipment be available, but any gynecologist attempting the procedure of laser uterine nerve ablation should be able to employ endoscopic operative skills to deal with these problems or otherwise be prepared to perform a laparotomy to stop the bleeding; also, the patient should be forewarned of this possible complication. Without wishing to belabor this point unduly, there have been at least two deaths reported from North America directly attributable to bleeding from the transection of the uterosacral ligaments with the carbon dioxide laser, and for this reason Daniell[12] prefers to use the KTP/532 laser. This laser is in fact a frequency-doubled Nd:YAG laser and emits an emerald-green light (532 nm) which photocoagulates tissue and therefore has better hemostatic properties than the carbon dioxide laser. Daniell's results are shown in Table 2. He carefully counsels his patients and tells them that the first period might still be painful and that some of them may be made worse by the procedure; with 4% of the endometriosis patients and 10% of primary dysmenorrhea patients this does appear to be the case. The relatively high number in this latter group without pelvic pathology suggests that considerable psychological overlay must be operating here. We do not tell patients that the procedure may make their periods worse and so far no patients have complained of a deterioration of dysmenorrhea.

Although this technique is frequently used by laser laparoscopists, there are only a few reported series in the literature. Feste[22] reported his results with 12 patients in a review of 202 patients treated by laser laparoscopy. In a review article Daniell and Feste[21] reported on their combined results with carbon dioxide laser laparoscopy in a series of 50 patients; 64% with endometriosis and 50% with primary dysmenorrhea were cured, and 19 and 21%, respectively, were unchanged. With this laser 6% with endometriosis but none with primary dysmenorrhea were made worse. The numbers are too small to draw any worthwhile conclusions but the more precise vaporization obtainable with the carbon dioxide laser may be an important factor.

Donnez has reported a series of 100 patients who have been followed for more than 1 year[23]. There was complete relief from symptoms in 50% of the patients while 41% reported mild to moderate relief. There was no change in the symptoms in 9% of cases but no patients said their dysmenorrhea was worse following the procedure.

In this study they found too that many patients complaining of dyspareunia also experienced relief from this symptom; we also have noticed this in the absence

Table 2 Laser uterine nerve ablation (LUNA) results with KTP laser (from reference 12)

	Improved (%)	Same (%)	Worse (%)
Endometriosis (n = 80)	60 (75)	17 (21)	3 (4)
Primary dysmenorrhea (n = 20)	12 (60)	6 (30)	2 (10)
Total (n = 100)	72 (72)	23 (23)	5 (5)

of endometriosis, especially in patients with very taut and well-demarcated uterosacral ligaments. Donnez and colleagues[23] may, however, have another explanation for this finding, since they found histological evidence of endometriosis in biopsies of the uterosacral ligaments in 52% of patients with pelvic pain. In about 10% of them, there was no laparoscopic evidence of the disease. There is considerable controversy in the literature about the significance of random peritoneal biopsies, but if it is eventually shown that endometriosis exists without its usual outward appearances[29], it calls into question the whole philosophy of vaporizing the deposits with lasers or electrocautery and certainly explains some of our treatment failures.

SUMMARY

The use of the carbon dioxide or fiberoptic laser at laparoscopy offers a simple and relatively safe approach to the treatment of dysmenorrhea, both primary and secondary. The procedure takes about 5 minutes to perform and generates a large amount of smoke, but as long as care is taken in recognizing the pelvic anatomy before the laser is fired, there should be little possibility of damage to the ureters or the thin-walled veins coursing just medial to the uterosacral ligaments.

Prospective double-blind randomized controlled studies have shown that laparoscopic transection of the uterosacral ligaments close to their insertion on the posterior aspect of the cervix is an effective treatment for dysmenorrhea that has been unresponsive to drug therapy. Further trials are needed on larger numbers of patients to establish the long-term results but available evidence suggest that this relatively simple procedure is a useful technique in laparoscopic surgery.

REFERENCES

1. Tucker, A.W. (1947). Evaluation of pre-sacral neurectomy in the treatment of dysmenorrhoea. *Am. J. Obstet. Gynecol.*, **53**, 336
2. Ingersoll, F. and Meigs, J.V., (1948). Presacral neurectomy for dysmenorrhoea. *N. Engl. J. Med.*, **238**, 357

3. White, J.C. (1952). Conduction of visceral pain. *N. Engl. J. Med.*, **246**, 686–90

4. Andersch, B. and Milsom, I. (1982). An epidemiologic study of young women with dysmenorrhoea. *Am. J. Obstet. Gynecol.*, **144**, 655

5. Doyle, J.B. (1954) Paracervical uterine denervation for dysmenorrhoea. *Trans. N. Engl. Obstet. Gynecol. Soc.*, **8**, 143

6. Frankenhauser, G. (1864). Die Bewegungenerven der Gebarmutter. *Z. Med. Nat. Wiss.*, **1**, 35

7. Campbell, R.M. (1950). Anatomy and physiology of sacro-uterine ligaments. *Am. J. Obstet. Gynecol.*, **59**, 1

8. Laterjet, A. and Roget, P. (1922). Le plexus hypogatrique chez la femme. *Gynecol. Obstet.*, **6**, 225

9. Davis, A. (1936). Intrinsic dysmenorrhoea. *Proc. R. Soc. Med.*, **29**, 931

10. Doyle, J.B. and Des Rosiers, J.J. (1963). Paracervical uterine denervation for relief of pelvic pain. *Clin. Obstet. Gynecol.*, **6**, 742–53

11. Doyle, J.B. (1955). Paracervical uterine denervation by transection of the cervical plexus for the relief of dysmenorrhoea. *Am. J. Obstet. Gynecol.*, **70**, 1

12. Daniell, J.F., (1989). Fibreoptic laser laparoscopy. In Sutton, C. (ed.) *Laparoscopic Surgery. Baillières Clinical Obstetrics and Gynaecology.* (London: Baillière Tindall)

13. Sutton, C.J.G. (1989). Laser uterine nerve ablation. In Donnez, J. (ed.) *Laser Operative Laparoscopy and Hysteroscopy*, pp.43–52. (Leuven: Nauwelaerts)

14. Ylikorkala, O. and Dawood, Y.M. (1978). New concepts in dysmenorrhoea. *Am. J. Obstet. Gynecol.*, **130**, 833

15. Black, W.T. Jr (1964). Use of pre-sacral sympathectomy in the treatment of dysmenorrhoea: a second look after 25 years. *Am. J. Obstet. Gynecol.*, **89**, 17

16. Counseller, V. (1934). The treatment of dysmenorrhoea by resection of the pre-sacral nerves: evaluation of end results. *Am. J. Obstet. Gynecol.*, **28**, 161

17. Henzl, M.R. (1985). Dysmenorrhoea: achievements and challenges. *Sex. Med. Today*, **9**, 8

18. Dawood, Y.M., (1985). Dysmenorrhoea. *Pain Analg.*, **1**, 20

19. Dawood, M.Y., (1985). Overall approach to the management of dysmenorrhoea. In Dawood, M.Y., McGuire, J.L. and Demers, L.M. (eds.) *Premenstrual Syndrome and Dysmenorrhoea*, pp. 177–204. (Baltimore: Urban and Schwarzenberg)

20. Lichten, E.M. and Bombard, J. (1987). Surgical treatment of dysmenorrhoea with laparoscopic uterine nerve ablation. *J. Reprod. Med.*, **32**, 37–42

21. Daniell, J.F. and Feste, J. (1985). Laser laparoscopy. In Keye, W.R. (ed.) *Laser Surgery in Gynaecology and Obstetrics*, Ch.11, pp.147–65. (Boston, Mass: G.K. Hall)

22. Feste, J.R. (1985). Laser laparoscopy. *J. Reprod. Med.*, **30**, 414

23. Donnez, J. and Nisolle, M. (1989). Carbon-dioxide laser laparoscopy in pelvic pain and infertility. In Sutton, C. (ed.) *Laparoscopic Surgery. Baillière's Clinical Obstetrics and Gynaecology*, pp.525–44. (London: Baillière Tindall)

24. Bellina, J.H., Hemmings, R., Voros, I.J. and Ross, L.F. (1984). Carbon dioxide laser and electro-surgical wound study with an animal model. A comparison of tissue damage and healing patterns in peritoneal tissue. *Am. J. Obstet. Gynecol.*, **148**, 327

25. Semm, K. and Mettler, L. (1980). Technical progress in pelvic surgery via operative laparoscopy. *Am. J. Obstet. Gynecol.*, **138**, 121

26. Reich, H. (1987). Laparoscopic oophorectomy and salpingo-oophorectomy in the treatment of benign tubo-ovarian disease. *Int. J. Fertil.*, **32**, 233

27. Reich, H. (1989). Advanced operative laparoscopy. In Sutton, C. (ed.) *Laparoscopic Surgery. Baillière's Clinical Obstetrics and Gynaecology*, pp.655–82. (London: Baillière Tindall)

28. Semm, K. and Freys, I. (1989). Conventional operative laparoscopy. In Sutton, C. (ed.) *Laparoscopic Surgery. Baillière's Clinical Obstetrics and Gynaecology*, Ch.2. (London: Baillière Tindall)

29. Nisolle, M., Paindavine, B., Boudon, A. and Donnez, J. (1990). Histological study of peritoneal endometriosis in infertile women. *Fertil. Steril.*, **53**, 984–8

Endometriosis: rationale for surgery

J. Donnez, M. Nisolle and F. Casanas-Roux

In this chapter, we will try to classify the different indications for surgery and/or combined (medico-surgical) therapy in:

(1) Peritoneal endometriosis;

(2) Ovarian endometriosis;

(3) Deep-infiltrating endometriosis of the rectovaginal septum;

(4) Ureteral endometriosis; and

(5) Digestive endometriosis.

MEDICAL THERAPY AND ENDOMETRIOSIS

Many studies have reported that medical therapy is unable to eradicate endometriosis.

Laparoscopic evaluation

In the last decade, three new agents – danazol, gestrinone and gonadotropin releasing hormone (GnRH) agonists – have created further options in the hormonal treatment of endometriosis. In one of our studies, the use of different hormonal agents was evaluated in order to compare the evolution of the disease after a 6-month course of therapy.

Laparoscopy was used to evaluate the effect of medical therapy and a variable degree of resolution was described after long-term therapy. Ovarian endometriosis regressed in only 30% of cases after danazol therapy. Buttram and colleagues[1] also found that ovarian disease > 1 cm (typically invasive endometrioma) responded less well to danazol than did peritoneal and superficial ovarian endometriosis.

The results obtained with lynestrenol were slightly better, but the results obtained with gestrinone were similar to those obtained with danazol. When all of these agents were compared, GnRH agonist emerged superior to danazol, lynestrenol or gestrinone treatment[2,3]. Indeed, ovarian endometriotic lesions regressed more often after GnRH agonist therapy, in moderate as well as in severe endometriosis. When administered subcutaneously, the GnRH agonist was found to be the most efficacious[4].

In moderate and severe endometriosis, when the scores before and after hormonal therapy were compared, the most significant difference in scores was found among women treated with a GnRH agonist[2,3]. The data were in agreement with a previous study in which a lower mitotic index was found in ectopic glandular epithelium after buserelin therapy than that observed after either lynestrenol or gestrinone therapy[5].

As suggested in a previous study[2,3], the advantage of an effective hormonal treatment is a reduction in the pelvic vascularity and inflammation which are often present around endometriotic foci. The improved pelvic environment facilitates the technical aspect of surgery and reduces the risk of postoperative adhesion formation.

Despite its relatively superior efficacy when compared to other drugs, the GnRH agonist was unable to completely suppress endometriotic cells because the ectopic foci are not governed by the normal control mechanisms governing the uterine endometrial glands and stroma. This suggests the need for surgical removal of invasive ovarian endometriosis.

Thus, there was a reduction in the American Fertility Society (AFS) or Revised AFS (r-AFS) score following medical therapy, but the score never reached zero[2-4]. Moreover, very often the observations made at the time of the second-look laparoscopy at the end of the medical therapy were too optimistic. Indeed, in 1987, Evers[6] demonstrated by laparoscopy carried out 2 months after cessation of therapy, that there was no significant difference in the size and number of implants when compared to the initial score (at first-look laparoscopy). This study proved a swift recurrence after cessation of medical therapy.

Histology

We reported a histological examination of residual ovarian endometriotic lesions after hormonal treatment (either danazol, lynestrenol, gestrinone, buserelin nasal spray (n.s.) or buserelin subcutaneous (s.c.) implant)[2,3]. In most cases, glandular epithelium was found. These data were not in agreement with many reports published previously, which described a recurrence rate of only about 30–40% after hormonal treatment.

A high incidence of active endometriosis without any signs of degeneration was found in all groups except after a GnRH agonist implant[5].

Mitotic figures were found, although others described the absence of mitosis in such implants. Histological study showed that a lower mitotic index of ovarian

Table 1 Rationale for surgery in endometriosis; the leading Board members of the *Third World Congress on Endometriosis* were asked to evaluate the rationale for surgery and to find five major indications for surgery (see Conclusion in text)

Rationale	Buttram[1]	Canis*	Donnez[7]	Evers[6]	Querleu*	Rolland*	Schweppe*
Adhesions	+	+	+	+**	+	+	
Rectovaginal septum endometriosis (deep-infiltrating endometriosis)	+	+	+	+	+	+	+
Endometriotic cyst	+	+	+	+	+	+†	+
Intestinal endometriosis	+					+	+
Peritoneal endometriosis	+	+	+	+**			+‡
Uterosacral ligaments (invasive endometriosis)	+	+	+	+	+		

*, Personal communication; **, in cases of infertility; †, if > 5 cm in diameter; ‡, if persistent or recurrent after medical therapy

endometrial epithelium was observed in the GnRH agonist group.

Mitotic processes account for the persistence of ovarian endometriosis despite the administration of hormonal therapy. The ectopic foci are more or less autonomous, not governed by the normal control mechanisms governing the uterine endometrial glands and stroma.

The precise reason why a number of implants or cells do not respond to hormonal therapy is unknown but three hypotheses[2-4] have been proposed:

(1) The drug does not gain access to the ovarian endometriotic foci because fibrosis surrounding the foci prevents access locally.

(2) Endometriotic cells may have their own genetic programming, while an endocrine influence appears to be only secondary and dependent on the degree of differentiation of the individual cell.

(3) The low number of endometriotic steroid receptors and their different regulatory mechanisms in ectopic and eutopic endometrium may result in deficient endocrine dependency. The nuclear estrogen binding sites seen in foci of endometriosis do not appear to change during the menstrual cycle, whereas these sites in the uterine endometrium down-regulate during the secretory phase.

RATIONALE FOR SURGERY

The leading Board members of the *Third World Congress on Endometriosis* were asked to evaluate the rationale for surgery in cases of endometriosis and to find five major indications for surgery. The results of the consensus can be seen in Table 1.

Peritoneal endometriosis

The relationship between endometriosis and infertility is not clear although many mechanisms have been suggested.

In cases of infertility, we suggest vaporizing the endometriotic implants found at the time of diagnostic laparoscopy. Vaporizing an endometriotic implant provokes the bubbling of old blood, followed by the appearance of a curdy white material representing vaporization of the stromal layer. After the endometriotic lesion has been vaporized, retroperitoneal fat is encountered, and the appearance of bubbling confirms the complete vaporization of the lesion. Recently, the use of the SwiftLase has allowed the surgeon to ablate the endometriotic lesion layer by layer (Donnez and colleagues, unpublished report).

If a lesion is overlying a vital structure such as the ureter, urinary bladder, colon or larger blood vessels, a retroperitoneal injection of fluid (aquadissection and aquaprotection)[8,9] provides safer vaporization of the lesions.

A recent randomized study[10] has demonstrated that surgical excision (coagulation or laser vaporization) results in a higher pregnancy rate than that observed after expectant management.

In cases of peritoneal endometriosis associated with pelvic pain, laser uterine nerve ablation (LUNA) and endometriotic implant vaporization have been found to be efficacious[11].

In peritoneal endometriosis, the preoperative use of a GnRH agonist must be considered only in cases of very severe inflammatory disease and in cases of red lesions, mostly exclusive and numerous. In this case, the preoperative use of a GnRH agonist will facilitate surgical excision or vaporization by reducing the vascularization and inflammation[3,12,13]. However, in most cases there is no need to use a GnRH agonist preoperatively for mild or minimal endometriosis.

Results of the consensus

Of the seven members of the Board, three concluded that peritoneal endometriosis should be treated by surgery and two more agreed with this in cases of infertility (see Table 1).

Ovarian endometriosis

Three different types of ovarian endometriosis can be identified:

(1) Superficial hemorrhagic lesions;

(2) Hemorrhagic cysts (endometriomas); and

(3) Deeply infiltrating ovarian endometriosis (infrequent).

Superficial lesions

Superficial ovarian lesions are small vesicular lesions covering the ovarian cortex, or small implants, usually found on the lateral surface of the ovary. Adhesions between the ovary and the broad ligament are often observed.

From a histopathological point of view, the endometrial cyst may be lined with free endometrial tissue, similar histologically and functionally to eutopic endometrium[14]. Active ectopic endometrial tissue can cover the inner surface of a small cavity in the ovary. In some instances, atypical epithelium and ciliated cells are found[5].

Endometriomas

The term 'chocolate cyst' was applied by Sampson[15] to describe the endometrial cyst of the ovary.

In large endometriomas, the cyst is often lined with a flattened endometrial epithelium (Figure 1). The cyclical changes of these enclosed lesions are less significant than those in the free-growing lesions, and late secretory changes and menstrual bleeding are absent. The mobilization of the cysts from their fixed position provokes the rupture and subsequent spillage of contents[8,12,13].

As pointed out by Hughesdon[18], the internal surface of a chocolate cyst is really the external surface of the ovary; the ovarian cortex is identifiable by the presence of primordial follicles.

Ovarioscopy has recently been described by Brosens[14]; ovarian endometriomas appear as dark fibrotic areas with hemosiderin pigmentation that alternate with highly vascularized areas with focal bleeding. The vessels in these areas are often congested and tend to be larger at the hilus of the ovary.

According to Brosens's hypothesis, the hemorrhagic content of many 'chocolate cysts' may originate from chronic focal bleeding from congested blood vessels rather than from endometrial shedding.

Three months after drainage of the endometrioma and GnRH agonist therapy (which provokes amenorrhea), chocolate-colored fluid is still present[4-13]. This fact proves that endometrial shedding is not responsible for chocolate-colored fluid formation. In our opinion, its origin could be:

(1) Cyst wall exudation (Donnez);

(2) Congested cyst wall blood vessels (Brosens)[14];

(3) Inflammation around persistent intracystic endometrial foci which are resistant to medical therapy[3,5].

Deep-infiltrating ovarian endometriosis

Deep-infiltrating ovarian endometriosis is characterized by the presence of very active endometrial glands which invade the ovarian cortex (Figure 2). In this type of ovarian endometriosis, areas of oviduct-like epithelium with ciliated cells were demonstrated in 62% of cases[5]. Endometriotic lesions were considered to be active when typical glandular epithelium appeared to be either proliferative, or completely unresponsive to hormones with typical stroma. Such a lesion was found in 84% of cases. The mitotic index was calculated in typical glandular epithelium and its value was 3.9‰. This type of endometriotic implant was found to be completely hormonally independent in our series.

Rationale for surgery

The relationship between infertility and ovarian endometriomas is clearer than for endometriosis in general. Indeed, an ovarian endometriotic cyst can disturb the follicular maturation and rupture and provoke adhesions.

Small (<1 cm in diameter) endometriotic implants of the ovary were vaporized until follicles containing fluid were encountered or no further pigmented tissue was seen.

Large (<3 cm in diameter) endometriomas were destroyed as follows. After washing, the interior wall of the cyst was carefully examined to confirm the absence of any intracystic lesion suspected to be malignant (ovarian cystoscopy). The interior wall of the cyst was then vaporized to destroy the mucosal lining of the cyst. The vaporization continued until no further pigment could be seen. After copious irrigation, the ovaries were left open.

During diagnostic laparoscopy, a large endometrial cyst (>3 cm in diameter) was washed out with irrigation

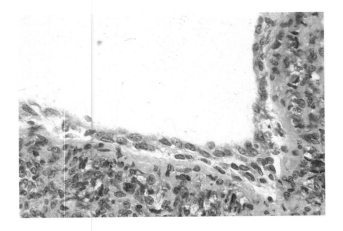

Figure 1 Ovarian endometriotic cyst (chocolate cyst): the cyst is lined with a flattened endometrial epithelium (Gomori's trichrome, × 110)

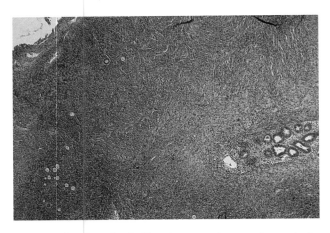

Figure 2 Deeply infiltrating ovarian endometriosis: very active endometrial glands are found, invading the ovarian cortex deeply (Gomori's trichrome); (a) ovarian follicles are seen less than a few millimeters from deeply infiltrating endometriosis (× 25)

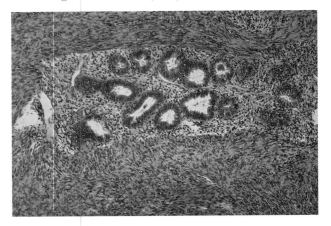

Figure 2(b) Very active glands found invading the ovarian cortex deeply (× 56)

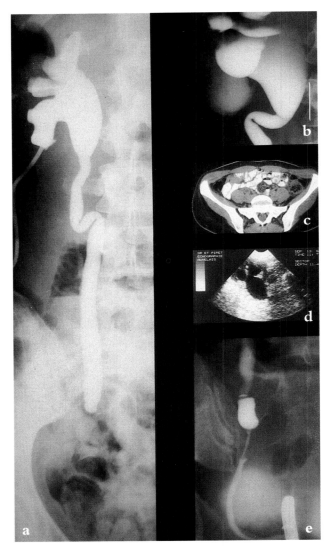

Figure 3(a) Ureteral occlusion was proved by pyelography; ureteral dilatation was diagnosed by (b) intravenous pyelography, (c) CT scan and (d) renal echography; (e) retrograde catheterization of the ureter indicated the level of occlusion

fluid (saline solution), and a biopsy was taken. Then, GnRH agonist (Zoladex®, Decapeptyl®) therapy was given for 12 weeks to decrease the cyst size. Thereafter, a second-look laparoscopy was carried out. If the diameter of the residual endometrial cyst was < 3 cm after GnRH agonist therapy, the interior wall of the cyst was vaporized as previously described[13].

To close the ovary, Tissucol (fibrin sealant) (Immuno AG, Vienna, Austria) was injected transabdominally into the intraovarian vaporized area, and the edges of the ovarian cyst were approximated with atraumatic forceps for 2–3 minutes[13].

Ovarian endometriosis must be classified according to its laparoscopic aspect: superficial implants can be destroyed easily, as can small endometriomas (less than 3 cm in diameter). However, in the case of large endometriomas of more than 3 cm in diameter, we have proved that the opening, washing and rinsing of the ovarian cyst is ineffective. Indeed, 3 months after this type of drainage, the cyst has returned to its original size. The most effective approach in size reduction is drainage followed by GnRH agonist therapy. We have shown that this approach provokes a 50% reduction of the original diameter[7,13,17].

In ovarian endometriosis, the preoperative use of a GnRH agonist must be considered in cases of ovarian cysts measuring more than 3 cm in diameter and in cases of multiple and inflammatory superficial lesions with inflammatory adhesions. GnRH agonist therapy should not be considered, however, in cases of endometriotic cysts less than 3 cm in diameter and in superficial ovarian implants.

This three-step therapy offers several advantages, such as a decrease in cyst diameter, reduced inflammation, a decrease in cyst wall thickness and the absence of follicles and corpus luteum, all of which facilitate the surgical procedure.

Consensus

All seven Board members considered that surgery *must* be performed in cases of endometriotic cysts and in cases of periovarian endometriotic adhesions related to infertility (Table 1).

Deep-infiltrating endometriosis of the rectovaginal septum

In cases of deep-infiltrating endometriosis of the rectovaginal septum, which is probably another type of the disease (adenomyosis), surgical excision is required (see Chapter 8).

All seven Board members considered this pathology as an absolute indication for surgery. The use of a GnRH agonist preoperatively is more debatable. In our

opinion, its preoperative use should not be systematic but can be suggested to facilitate the complete removal of the lesion.

Ureteral endometriosis

There are two types of ureteral occlusion provoked by endometriosis:

(1) The 'true' ureteral endometriosis: endoluminal (Figure 3); from a histological point of view, not only endometrial glands are found in the ureteral wall, but also endoluminal endometrial polyps are seen protruding into the lumen (Figure 4).

(2) The ureteral pseudo-occlusion provoked by a peritoneal endometriotic lesion covering the ureter (Figure 5).

Preoperative use of a GnRH agonist could be useful as a diagnostic tool or to facilitate the surgical procedure in cases of pseudo-occlusion. By decreasing the size of the lesion and the inflammation surrounding the lesion, GnRH agonist therapy allows the surgeon to remove the peritoneal lesion covering the ureter *without* segmental ureteral resection.

Digestive endometriosis

Deep-infiltrating endometriosis or adenomyosis (Chapter 8) can provoke signs of rectal perivisceritis with partial involvement of the rectal muscularis. But sometimes, severe endometriosis invades the rectum deeply and provokes an occlusion, requiring a partial bowel resection (Figures 8 and 9). Histology reveals the presence of very active endometrial glands invading the entire rectal wall (Figure 10).

Very rarely, cecal endometriosis is found. In the case shown in Figures 11 and 12, a pelvic examination and CT scan led to the suspicion of an ovarian endometriotic cyst. Laparoscopy revealed two normal ovaries but an inflammatory mass surrounding the cecum.

Radiography of the colon permits the diagnosis of endometriosis of the cecum and of the terminal portion of the small bowel. For this type of pathology, surgical bowel resection is indicated.

CONCLUSION

This chapter reviews the major indications for surgery in cases of endometriosis:

(1) Ovarian cysts, adhesions and rectovaginal endometriosis are absolute indications for surgery.

(2) Peritoneal endometriosis (mild or minimal) is considered by approximately half of the experts to

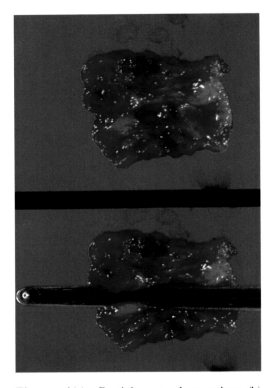

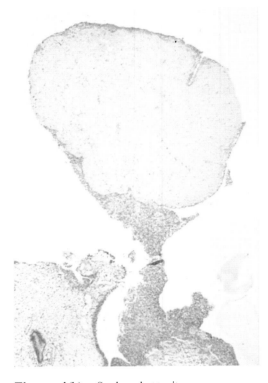

Figure 4(a) Partial ureteral resection; (b) polypoid endometrial glands were found in the ureteral lumen; (c) and (d) typical endometrial epithelium and stroma were found invading the ureteral wall

Figure 4(b) *See legend opposite*

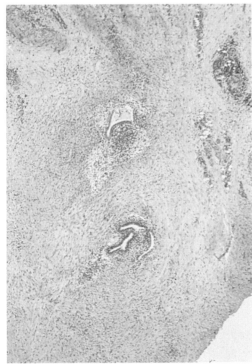

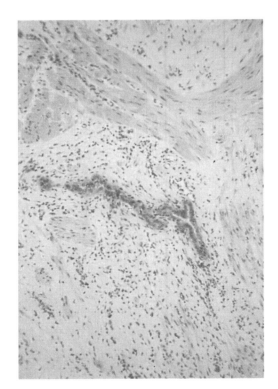

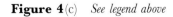

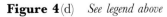

Figure 4(c) *See legend above*

Figure 4(d) *See legend above*

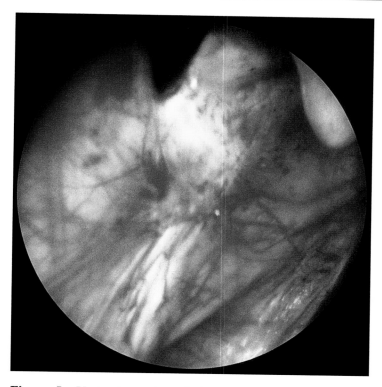

Figure 5 Ureteral pseudo-occlusion provoked by endometriotic peritoneal lesion covering the ureter

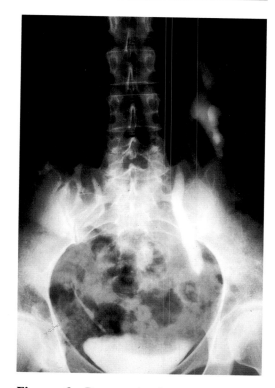

Figure 6 Preoperative intravenous pyelography (IVP) showing the dilatation of the left ureter

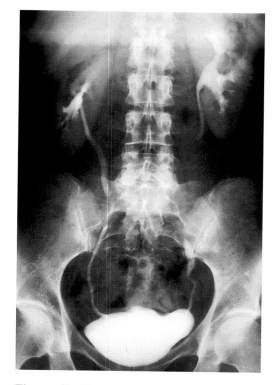

Figure 7 Postoperative IVP showing the recovery of the left ureter, 3 months after laparoscopic removal with the CO_2 laser of the peritoneal lesion covering the ureter (Figure 5)

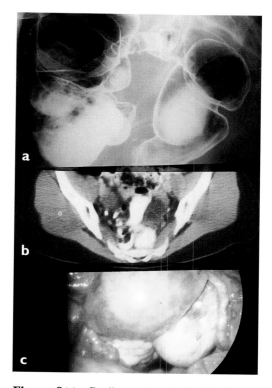

Figure 8(a) Radiography of colon leading to diagnosis of rectal endometriosis as suspected by (b) CT scan; (c) laparoscopy confirms the diagnosis of an endometriotic cyst with rectal infiltration

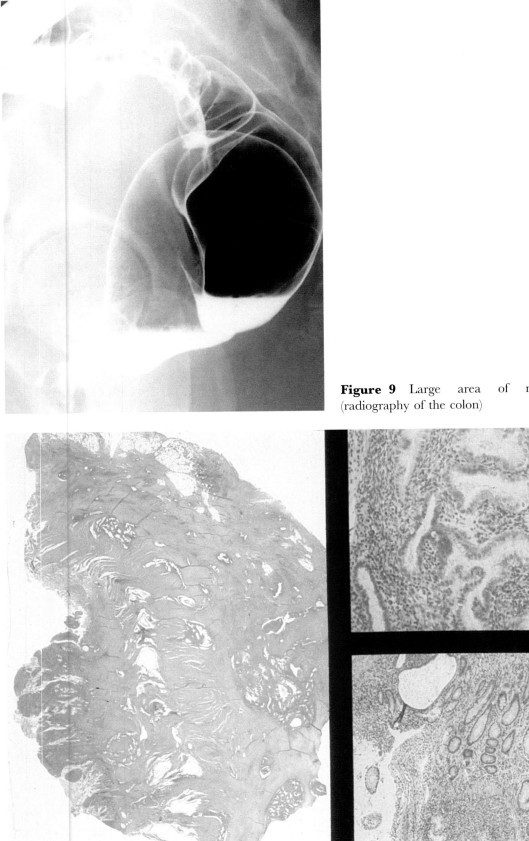

Figure 9 Large area of rectal endometriosis (radiography of the colon)

Figure 10 Partial bowel resection; histology reveals the presence of endometrial epithelium and stroma in the entire wall of the rectum

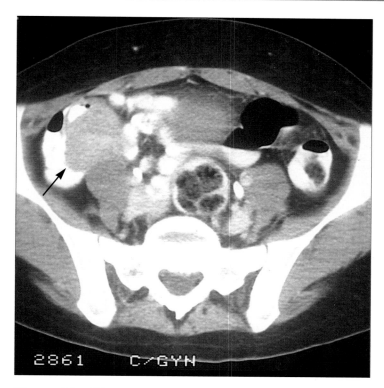

Figure 11 CT scan: presence of endometriotic lesion close to the cecum

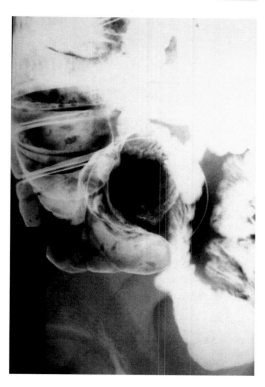

Figure 12 Radiography of the colon reveals the presence of endometriosis in the cecum and in the terminal portion of the small bowel

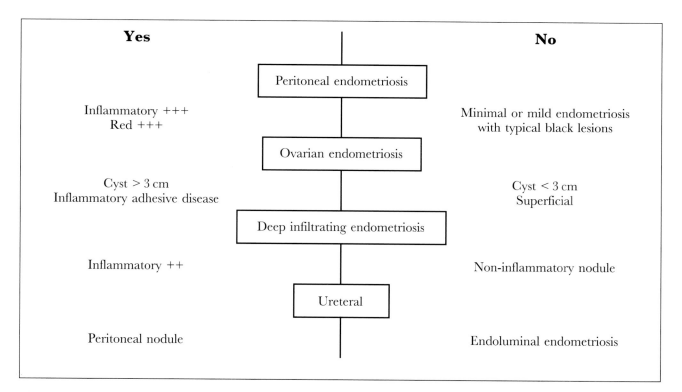

Figure 13 Indications for preoperative use of GnRH agonist

be an indication for surgery. Randomized studies must be carried out in order to decide this question.

(3) Ureteral and/or digestive endometriosis are indications for surgery if a ureteral or intestinal occlusion with deep wall involvement is diagnosed.

In some instances, a gonadotropin releasing hormone (GnRH) agonist must be given before surgery and considered as a chemotherapy before debulking surgery (Figure 13).

REFERENCES

1. Buttram, V., Reiter, R. and Ward, S. (1985). Treatment of endometriosis with danazol: report of a 6-year prospective study. *Fertil. Steril.*, **43**, 353

2. Donnez, J., Nisolle, M., Clerckx, F. and Casanas-Roux, F. (1989). Combined therapy in endometriosis: preoperative use of danazol, gestrinone, lynestrenol, buserelin spray and buserelin implant. In Boutaleb, Y. and Gzouli, A. (eds.) *Treatment of Endometriosis – Recent Developments in Fertility and Sterility* series, p.312. (Carnforth, UK: Parthenon Publishing)

3. Donnez, J., Nisolle, M. and Casanas-Roux, F. (1990). Endometriosis-associated infertility: evaluation of preoperative use of danazol, gestrinone and buserelin. *Int. J. Fertil.*, **42**, 128

4. Donnez, J., Nisolle, M. and Casanas-Roux, F. (1989). Administration of nasal buserelin as compared with subcutaneous buserelin implant for endometriosis. *Fertil. Steril.*, **52**, 27–30

5. Nisolle, M., Casanas-Roux, F. and Donnez, J. (1988). Histologic study of ovarian endometriosis after hormonal therapy. *Fertil. Steril.*, **49**, 423–6

6. Evers, J.L.H. (1987). The second-look laparascopy for evaluation of the result of medical treatment of endometriosis should not be performed during ovarian suppression. *Fertil. Steril.*, **47**, 502–4

7. Donnez, J., Nisolle, M., Casanas-Roux, F. and Clerckx, F. (1993). Endometriosis: rationale for surgery. In Brosens, I. and Donnez, J. (eds.) *The Current Status of Endometriosis Research and Management*, p.385. (Carnforth, UK: Parthenon Publishing)

8. Donnez, J. (1987). CO_2 laser laparoscopy in infertile women with adhesions or endometriosis. *Fertil. Steril.*, **48**, 390–4

9. Nezhat, C., Crowgey, S.R. and Garrison, C.P. (1986). Surgical treatment of endometriosis via laser laparoscopy. *Fertil. Steril.*, **45**, 778–83

10. Tulandi, T. and Mouchawar, M. (1991). Treatment-dependent and treatment-independent pregnancy in women with minimal and mild endometriosis. *Fertil. Steril.*, **56**, 790–1

11. Sutton, C. (1989). Laser uterine nerve ablation. In Donnez, J. (ed.) *Laser Operative Laparoscopy and Hysterscopy*, pp.43–52. (Leuven: Nauwelaerts Printing)

12. Donnez, J., Nisolle, M. and Casanas-Roux, F. (1989). CO_2 laser laparoscopy in infertile women with adnexal adhesions and women with tubal occlusion. *J. Gynecol. Surg.*, **5**, 47–53

13. Donnez, J. and Nisolle, M. (1991). Laparoscopic management of large ovarian endometrial cysts: use of fibrin sealant. *J. Gyncol. Surg.*, **7**, 163–7

14. Brosens, I. and Gordon, A. (1989). Endometriosis: ovarian endometriosis. In Brosens, I. and Gordon, A. (eds.) *Tubal Infertility*, pp.313–17. (London: Gower Medical Publishing)

15. Sampson, J.A. (1927). Peritoneal endometriosis due to the menstrual dissemination of endometrial tissue into the peritoneal cavity. *Am. J. Obstet. Gynecol.*, **14**, 422–69

16. Hughesdon, P.E. (1957). The structure of endometrial cysts of the ovary. *J. Obstet. Gynecol. Br. Empire*, **64**, 481–7

17. Donnez, J., Nisolle, M. and Casanas-Roux, F. (1992). Three-dimensional architectures of peritoneal endometriosis. *Fertil. Steril.*, **57**, 980–3

Endoscopic management of peritoneal and ovarian endometriosis

7

J. Donnez, M. Nisolle, V. Anaf, M. Smets, S. Bassil and F. Casanas-Roux

Advanced operative laparoscopy techniques for laser adhesiolysis and vaporization of endometriotic implants have been developed, and laser surgeons are now able to remove endometriosis from the reproductive structure with precision. There are at least three advantages of laser laparoscopy over conventional operative laparoscopy: precise destruction of diseased tissue, minimal bleeding and minimal damage to the adjacent normal tissue. Tissue reaction and postoperative adhesion formation have been shown to be no greater than with conventional methods[1].

LASER SURGERY

The endoscopic use of the laser is not new in medicine, and several types of operative procedures have been carried out with the CO_2 laser laparoscope for the treatment of reproductive pathology. The most frequent indication is endometriosis, which can be vaporized by means of CO_2 laser laparoscopy with highly satisfactory postoperative pregnancy rates[2-6]. Laser surgeons have removed endometriosis with great precision from the reproductive structure. But vaporization of the endometriotic peritoneal lesion or of the endometriotic cyst wall provokes residual carbon charring. Expensive high-power operating lasers are required for the vaporization of tissue without residual carbon charring. The SwiftLase, which allows a char-free ablation, even when using a 30-W operating laser, will be described in this chapter.

Endoscopic techniques

From 1982 to 1991, 6250 laser laparoscopies were carried out in our department. In the series, 2912 patients underwent laparoscopy for endometriosis.

Peritoneal endometriotic implants

In general, a power setting of 40–50 W is used. The debulking of endometriotic implants is best performed using a continuous firing mode. If a lesion is overlying a vital structure such as the ureter, urinary bladder, colon, or larger blood vessels, a retroperitoneal injection of fluid (aquadissection and aquaprotection) provides safer vaporization of the lesions. This duration allows a 100–200-μm depth of vaporization, thus substantially

limiting the depth of penetration. Vaporizing an endometriotic implant (Figure 1(a) and(b)) provokes the bubbling of old blood, followed by a curdy white material representing vaporization of the stromal layer. After the endometriotic lesion has been vaporized, retroperitoneal fat is encountered, and the appearance of bubbling confirms the complete vaporization of the lesion. Absorption of the CO_2 laser by water (contained in fatty tissue) for a few seconds after the complete destruction of the implant prevents deeper penetration of the laser beam.

Ovarian endometriosis < 3 cm

Ovarian endometriosis is treated during first-look laparoscopy if a penetration of no more than 3 cm into the ovary is observed and if the cyst diameter is no larger than 3 cm (Figures 2–4).

Small (< 1 cm in diameter) endometriotic implants of the ovary were vaporized until follicles containing fluid were encountered or no further pigmented tissue was seen. Large (< 3 cm in diameter) endometriomas were destroyed as follows. A 3–4-mm portion of the top of the cyst was excised, the chocolate-colored material was aspirated, and the cyst was washed out with irrigation fluid (Figure 3(a) and (b)). After washing, the interior wall of the cyst was examined carefully to confirm the absence of any intracystic lesion suspected to be malignant (ovarian cystoscopy). With a power setting of 40 W and continuous mode application, the interior wall of the cyst was then vaporized to destroy the mucosal lining of the cyst (Figure 4(a) and (b)). The vaporization continued until no further pigment could be seen. After copious irrigation, the ovaries were left open.

Ovarian endometriosis > 3 cm

In our series of 2912 patients with endometriosis, ovarian endometriomas larger than 3 cm in diameter (Figures 5–9) were found in 481 patients. During diagnostic laparoscopy, the endometrial cyst was washed out with irrigation fluid (saline solution), and a biopsy was taken. Then, gonadotropin releasing hormone (GnRH) agonist (Zoladex, ICI, UK) therapy was given for 12 weeks to decrease the cyst size. A decrease of 50% in cyst diameter was observed after drainage followed by a 12-week course of a GnRH agonist (Figure 5).

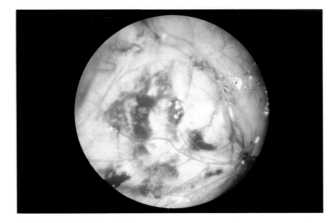

Figure 1(a)   Peritoneal endometriotic lesion, typical red lesion; (b) after vaporization with the SwiftLase (CO_2 laser). Note the absence of carbonized areas (char-free ablation)

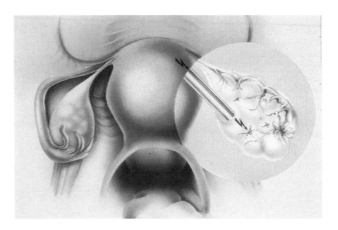

Figure 2(a)–(c)   Small and superficial ovarian implants are vaporized

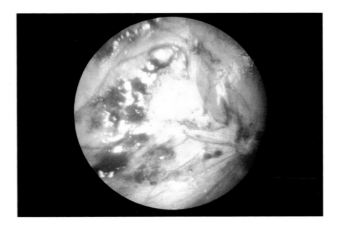

Figure 1(b)   *See legend above*

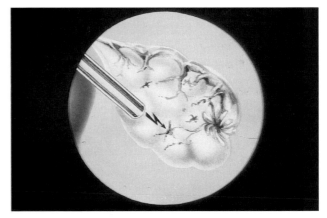

Figure 2(b)   *See legend above*

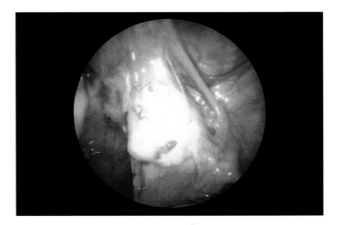

Figure 2(c)   *See legend above*

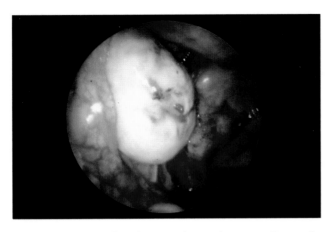

Figure 3(a)   Ovarian endometrioma < 3 cm in diameter; (b)–(e) the ovarian cyst is washed out with saline solution

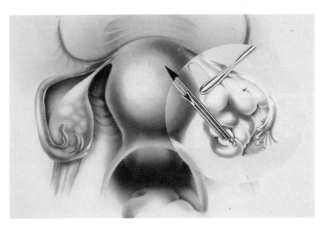

Figure 3(b)   *See legend opposite*

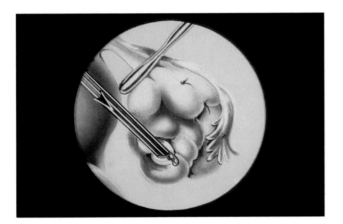

Figure 3(c)   *See legend above*

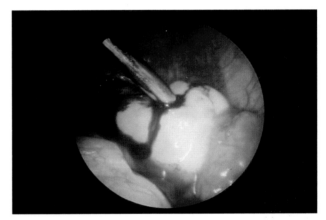

Figure 3(d)   *See legend above*

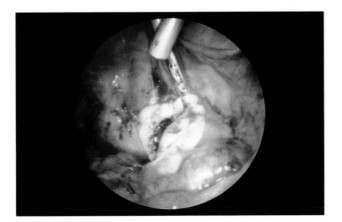

Figure 3(e)   *See legend above*

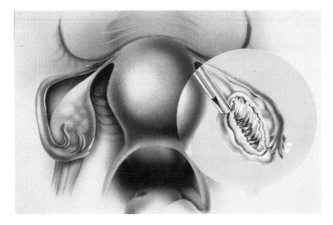

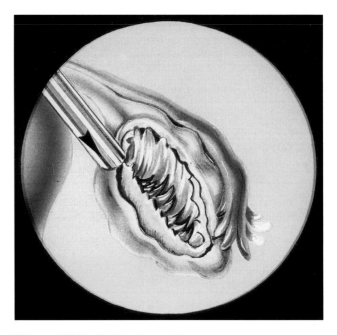

Figure 4(a)–(c)   The mucosal lining of the endometrial cyst is vaporized

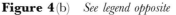

Figure 4(b)   *See legend opposite*

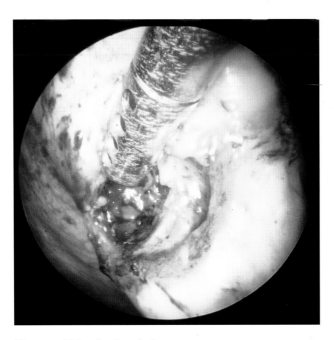

Figure 4(c)   *See legend above*

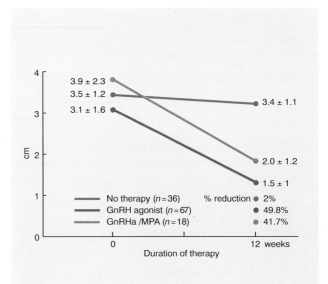

Figure 5   Comparative evaluation of cyst diameter after drainage alone, and after drainage followed by GnRH agonist therapy. Drainage of ovarian endometriotic cyst is ineffective if not associated with GnRH agonist. After drainage and GnRH agonist a decrease of 50% in cyst diameter is observed

Drainage alone (if not associated with GnRH agonist) was ineffective; indeed, 12 weeks after drainage, the ovarian cyst diameter was found to be unchanged when compared to the diameter observed before drainage.

Thereafter, a second-look laparoscopy was carried out. If the diameter of the residual endometrial cyst was < 3 cm after GnRH agonist therapy ($n = 233$), the interior wall of the cyst was vaporized as previously described. If the diameter of the residual cyst was > 3 cm after GnRH agonist therapy (Figure 6) another technique was proposed. In this series, the range of the ovarian cyst sizes was 3–8 cm. A portion of the ovarian cyst was first removed by making a circular cut over the protruded ovarian cyst portion, using the CO_2 laser. Partial cystectomy was then carried out (Figure 7). Ovarian cystoscopy (Figure 8) was performed for evaluation of the interior cyst wall, and a biopsy was taken. The residual endometrial cyst wall was then vaporized with the CO_2 laser, equipped with the SwiftLase (Figures 9 and 10). The ovary was left open in a first series of 20 patients. In a consecutive series of 62 patients, the ovary was not left open. To close the ovary[5], Tissucol (fibrin sealant) (Immuno AG, Vienna, Austria) was injected transabdominally into the intraovarian vaporized area, and the edges of the ovarian cyst were approximated with atraumatic forceps for 2–3 minutes (Figure 11). (After clotting occurs, further mechanical stress should be avoided for 3–5 minutes). At the end of the procedure, copious irrigation of the pelvic cavity was carried out to prevent deposits of carbon and glue. Thereafter, 100–200 ml of 32% Dextran 70 was instilled into the peritoneal cavity in all patients of both groups. Recently, the closure of the ovarian edges has been performed using special new titanium clips (Figure 12) (Endohernia®, Autosuture). The clips permit an excellent approximation of ovarian edges. Very often, two or three clips are sufficient to close the ovary.

USE OF SWIFTLASE

The SwiftLase (Sharplan Model 757) is a miniature optomechanical scanner compatible with any CO_2 laser (Figure 13). The SwiftLase consists of two almost, but not exactly, parallel folding mirrors. Optical reflections of the CO_2 laser optical beam from the mirrors cause the beam to deviate from its original direction by an angle θ (see Figure 6, Chapter 2, p.24). The mirrors constantly rotate at slightly different angular velocities, thereby varying rapidly with time, between zero and a maximal value θ_{max}. By attaching the laparoscope focusing coupler of focal length F to the SwiftLase, the CO_2 laser generates a focal spot which rapidly and homogeneously scans and covers a round area of diameter $2F \tan \theta_{max}$ at the distal end of the laparoscope (Figure 14). For a single-puncture laparoscope ($F = 300$ mm), θ_{max} was

selected to provide a round treatment area of 2.5 mm in diameter. The rapid movement of the beam over the tissue ensures a short duration of exposure on individual sites within the area and very shallow ablation.

Since therapeutic CO_2 medical lasers typically generate a focused beam smaller than 0.9 mm in diameter at the laparoscope working distance, using the SwiftLase with a laser power level of 30 W will generate an optical power density of above 50 W/mm^2 on tissue. This is considerably higher than the threshold for vaporization of tissue without residual carbon char (the threshold for char-free tissue ablation is about 30 W/mm^2). The time required for the SwiftLase to homogeneously cover a 2.5-mm round area is about 100 ms. During this time, the 30-W operating laser will deliver 3000 mJ to the tissue. Since the typical energy required to completely ablate tissue is about 3000 mJ/mm^3, keeping the laparoscope precisely on a single site for 0.1 s will generate a clean char-free crater of 0.2-mm depth. However, the laparoscope can be moved smoothly and evenly across an extended lesion intended for treatment, consequently ablating a tissue layer as thin as 0.05–0.1 mm.

Results

The operating time varied from 45 to 80 min. Vaporization of the mucosal lining was facilitated by the preoperative therapy (GnRH agonist administered subcutaneously)[7]. Indeed, the interior wall of the endometrial cyst seen during ovarian cystoscopy was found to be less hemorrhagic and more atrophic than before therapy. These data were confirmed by ovarian biopsy. An endometriotic lesion was considered 'active' when typical glandular epithelium was either proliferative, or completely unresponsive to hormonal therapy with typical stroma. Such a lesion was found significantly more often (84% of cases, $p < 0.001$) before GnRH agonist therapy than after such therapy (44% of cases)[3,5,7–9].

In a first series of 20 patients with residual ovarian cysts > 3 cm in diameter, the technique was used successfully to vaporize the endometriotic ovarian lesions, and the ovary was left open; 3 months after the procedure, a third-look laparoscopy was performed in nine patients. Dense and fibrous adhesions between the vaporized area of the ovary and the broad ligament, the bowel, and the Fallopian tube were found in eight out of nine patients. Laparoscopic salpingo-ovariolysis was carried out.

In a second series of 62 patients with residual ovarian cysts > 3 cm in diameter, vaporization of the mucosal lining was performed, and Tissucol was used to close the ovary[5]. Of the 62 women, 15 underwent a laparoscopy in the 3 months after the procedure. In all cases, periovarian adhesions were absent, and the healing of

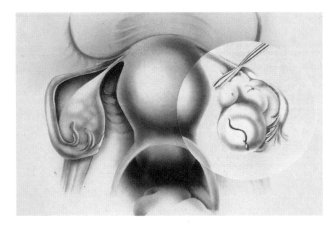

Figure 6(a)–(c) Ovarian endometrioma > 3 cm in diameter

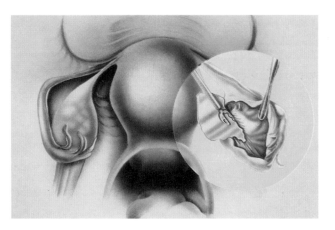

Figure 7(a)–(c) A circular cut over the protruded ovarian cyst portion and partial cystectomy are carried out

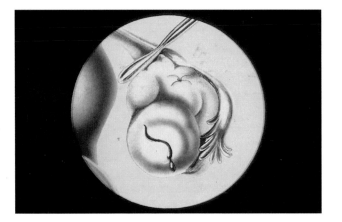

Figure 6(b) *See legend above*

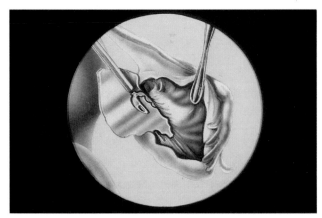

Figure 7(b) *See legend above*

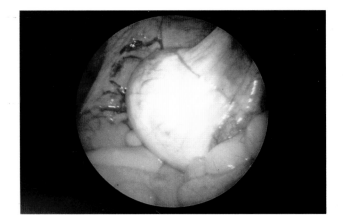

Figure 6(c) *See legend above*

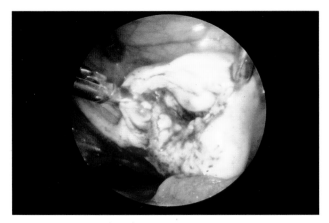

Figure 7(c) *See legend above*

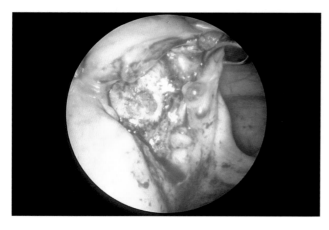

Figure 8 Ovarian cystoscopy: the interior wall is carefully examined. The epithelial lining of the cyst wall appears atrophic and less inflammatory after GnRH agonist therapy

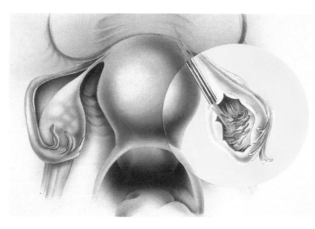

Figure 9(a)–(c) Residual endometrial cyst wall is vaporized with the SwiftLase which permits a char-free ablation, layer by layer. It reduces the carbonization and the thermal damage to the normal ovarian cortex

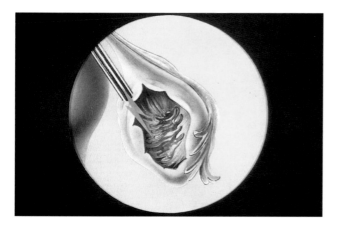

Figure 9(b) *See legend above*

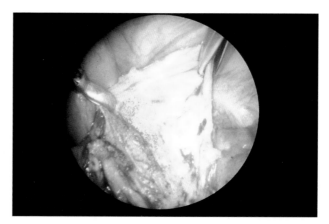

Figure 9(c) *See legend above*

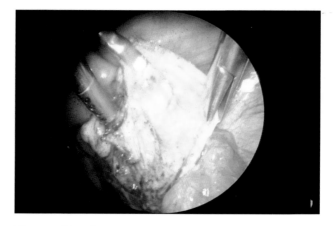

Figure 10 Complete vaporization is achieved

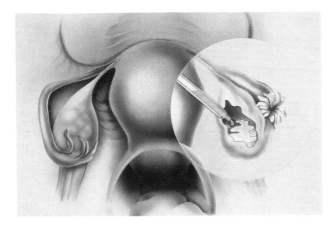

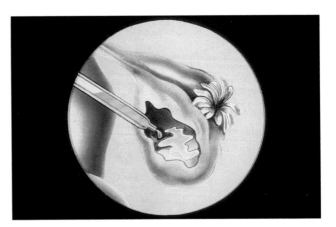

Figure 11(a)–(c)   Ovarian closure with Tissucol® (fibrin glue); (d)–(f) the edges are approximated with atraumatic forceps; (g) final aspect

Figure 11(b)   *See legend opposite*

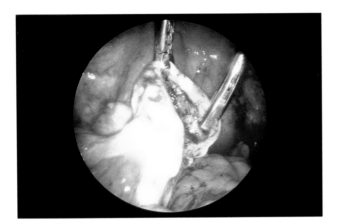

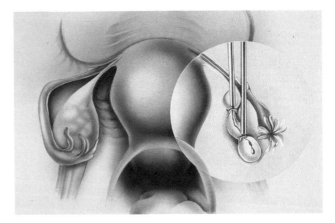

Figure 11(c)   *See legend above*

Figure 11(d)   *See legend above*

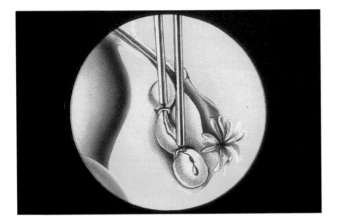

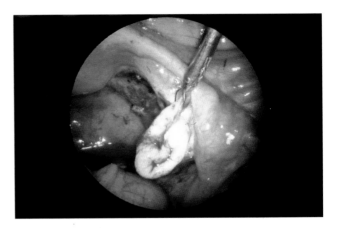

Figure 11(e)   *See legend above*

Figure 11(f)   *See legend above*

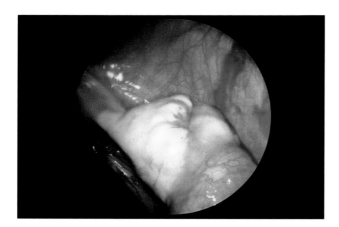

Figure 11(g)   *See legend on opposite page*

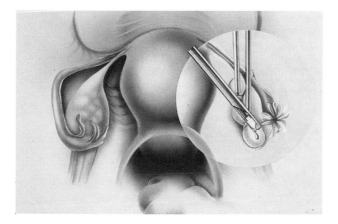

Figure 12(a)–(d)   Ovarian closure with titanium clips

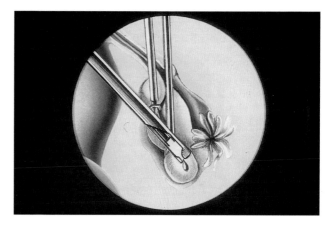

Figure 12(b)   *See legend opposite*

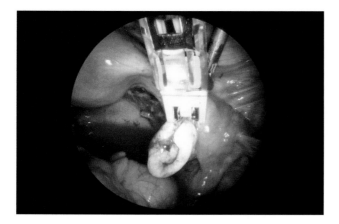

Figure 12(c)   *See legend above*

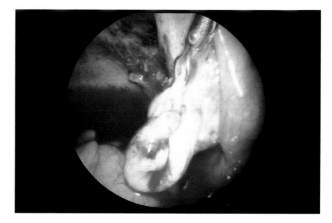

Figure 12(d)   *See legend above*

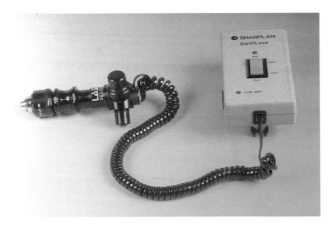

Figure 13 The SwiftLase (Sharplan Model 757) is a miniature optomechanical scanner compatible with any CO_2 laser

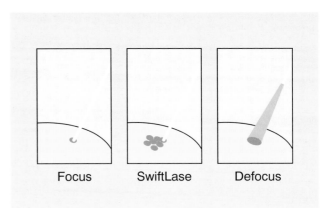

Figure 14 The CO_2 laser generates a focal spot which rapidly and homogeneously covers a 2.5-mm round area in about 100 ms

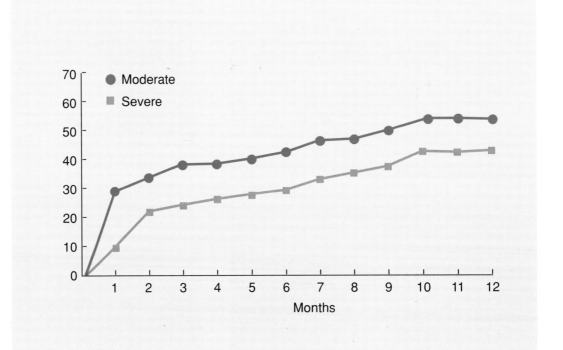

Figure 15 The cumulative pregnancy rate in cases of moderate and severe ovarian endometriosis

the ovarian closure was well accomplished. There was no inflammation.

So far, the technique has been used sucessfully in a series of 482 patients with endometriomas > 3 cm in diameter.

SwiftLase

The SwiftLase enables very rapid, homogeneous, single-layer char-free ablation even at low power levels. A first series of 20 patients were treated with the SwiftLase connected to the direct coupler and the laparoscope. A layer-by-layer ablation was possible and performed easily in all cases. Indeed, by moving the laparoscope smoothly, the surgeon can ablate a tissue layer as thin as 0.05–1 mm. For peritoneal endometriosis, the SwiftLase made the vaporization procedure easier. The char-free ablation allows the surgeon to check when the endometriotic lesion has been totally vaporized by easily visualizing the retroperitoneal fat, and there is a decreased risk of thermal injury to the bowel and ureter.

In cases of ovarian endometriotic cysts more than 3 cm in diameter, GnRH agonist is used for 3 months after the cyst has been punctured and washed out. After a 3-month course of GnRH agonist therapy, the thickness of the endometrial cyst is dramatically reduced and the epithelial lining is atrophic and white. Vaporization with the SwiftLase permits a very easy and fast vaporization of the internal wall with minimal thermal damage to the normal ovarian cortex. Indeed, histological studies have shown, in experimental studies, a char-free residual damage 0.1 mm deep[10]. Moreover, because the time required for the SwiftLase to homogeneously cover a 2.5-mm round area is about 100 ms, vaporization of large areas of peritoneal endometriosis as well as the endometrial ovarian cyst wall is performed very fast and it reduces the operating time. When compared to the conventional laser technique, the operating time needed to vaporize the internal wall of a 5-cm diameter cyst was significantly ($p < 0.01$) reduced (SwiftLase: 7.5 ± 3 min ($n = 8$); conventional laser: 14.3 ± 4.2 ($n = 8$)).

The reduced operating time, the better visual control (absence of carbonized particles), the reduced thermal damage (layer-by-layer ablation) and the possibility of using low-power operating lasers are the most significant advantages of this new technology.

Pregnancy rates

The cumulative pregnancy rates were analyzed (Figure 15) in a consecutive series of 407 patients with ovarian endometriosis (American Fertility Society (AFS) moderate, $n = 305$; AFS severe, $n = 102$).

A pregnancy rate of more than 55% was achieved in moderate endometriosis and 44% in severe

endometriosis. The majority of pregnancies occurred during the first 10 months after surgery.

OVARIAN CYSTECTOMY

Ovarian cystectomy, a frequently performed procedure, can be accomplished laparoscopically in most cases (see Chapter 9). The procedure begins with adhesiolysis. Once the cyst is mobilized, the cortex is grasped with a forceps introduced through a second trocar. The cortex is incised using laser or scissors. The cyst wall is then exposed. The incision is enlarged with scissors, and aquadissection can be used to separate the cyst wall from the ovarian stroma. If the cyst is opened and spillage occurs, peritoneal irrigation must be performed in order to remove the chocolate-colored fluid. Sometimes, ovarioscopy and careful evaluation of the internal cyst wall allow the surgeon to exclude the presence of malignant lesions. The ovary usually does not require suturing.

CONCLUSION

CO_2 laser laparoscopy offers several advantages over cautery. With the CO_2 laser, the laparoscopist is able to control the process of vaporization by seeing the three-dimensional boundaries of the lesion.

In a previous study[9], significantly different pregnancy rates according to the stage of endometriosis were found. Severe endometriosis had the poorest prognosis in terms of pregnancy rates. For this reason, a preoperative hormonal (gonadotropin releasing hormone agonist) therapy was given to patients with very large ovarian endometriomas (> 3 cm). The release of a GnRH agonist by a biodegradable implant is effective in reducing endometriotic size to a greater extent than other drugs, and permits a decrease in pelvic inflammation. Treatment by sustained release is an effective alternative to using steroid hormones before laser laparoscopy. A subcutaneous GnRH agonist implant permits a substantial reduction of large ovarian cyst diameter and a decrease in pelvic inflammation so that a second-look laser laparoscopy can be carried out for laser vaporization of residual endometriomas. During the ovarian cystoscopy, the interior ovarian wall was found to be atrophic. The cyst vascularity was decreased, and the vaporization was thus facilitated.

In cases of vaporization of very large cysts (> 3 cm), the risk of postoperative adhesions was found to be high in our study if the ovary was left open. Dense and fibrous periovarian adhesions between the vaporized area and other pelvic structures were diagnosed in eight out of nine patients who underwent a laparoscopy in the 3 months after the vaporization, although periovarian adhesions were not frequently observed after vaporization of small endometriotic implants. Our results were thus not in accordance with those of Nezhat and associates[2,6].

To decrease the risk of postoperative adhesions between the ovary and other pelvic structures, a fibrin glue (a two-component) was used. It was injected transabdominally through a catheter. A third look laparoscopy proved the absence of periovarian adhesions.

Recently, the SwiftLase has been used in our department; the SwiftLase is a miniature optomechanical scanner compatible with any CO_2 laser. It enables a very rapid, homogeneous, single-layer char-free ablation even at low power levels. It increases the visual control of tissue destruction and permits a layer-by-layer ablation, reducing the carbonization and the presence of carbonized particles in the tissue.

REFERENCES

1. Donnez, J., Fernandez, C., Willems, T. and Casanas-Roux, F. (1987). Experimental ovarian CO_2 laser surgery. In Donnez, J. (ed.) *CO_2 Laser in Intraepithelial Neoplasia and in Infertility*, p.25. (Leuven, Belgium: Nauwelaerts Printing)
2. Nezhat, C., Crowgey, S.R. and Garrison, C.P. (1986). Surgical treatment of endometriosis via laser laparoscopy. *Fertil. Seril.*, **45**, 778–83
3. Donnez, J. (1987). CO_2 laser laparoscopy in infertile women with adhesions or endometriosis. *Fertil. Steril.*, **48**, 390–4
4. Donnez, J., Nisolle, M. and Casanas-Roux, F. (1989). CO_2 laser laparoscopy in infertile women with adnexal adhesions and women with tubal occlusion. *J. Gynecol. Surg.*, **5**, 47–53
5. Donnez, J. and Nisolle, M. (1991). Laparoscopic management of large ovarian endometrial cyst: use of fibrin sealant. *J. Gynecol. Surg.*, **7**, 163–7
6. Nezhat, C., Nezhat, F. and Silfen, S.L. (1991). Video laseroscopy: the CO_2 laser for advanced operative laparoscopy. *Obstet. Gynecol. Clin. N. Am.*, **18**, 585–604
7. Donnez, J., Nisolle, M. and Casanas-Roux, F. (1989). Adminstration of nasal buserelin as compared with subcutaneous buserelin implant for endometriosis. *Fertil. Steril.*, **52**, 27–30
8. Nisolle, M., Casanas-Roux, F. and Donnez, J. (1988). Histologic study of ovarian endometriosis after hormonal therapy. *Fertil. Steril.*, **49**, 423–6
9. Donnez, J., Nisolle, M. and Casanas-Roux, F. (1990). Endometriosis-assocated infertility: evaluation of preoperative use of danazol, gestrinone and buserelin. *Int. J. Fertil.*, **42**, 128
10. Donnez, J., Zair, E., Reich, H., Nisolle, M. and Slatkine, M. (1994). SwiftLase: a new technology for endometriosis management. *Fertil. Steril.*, submitted for publication

Laparoscopic treatment of rectovaginal septum endometriosis

J. Donnez, M. Nisolle, F. Casanas-Roux, V. Anaf and M. Smets

INTRODUCTION

It is generally believed that endometriosis is caused by the implantation of retrograde menstrual endometrial cells, or by metaplasia. In the pelvis, three different forms of endometriosis must be considered:

(1) Peritoneal;

(2) Ovarian;

(3) Rectovaginal septum.

The early manifestations of the disease are believed to be subtle or non-colored lesions such as white lesions (white opacification, yellow-brown patches or hemosiderin patches). The presence of a lower mitotic activity in white lesions[1] suggests that this type of lesion is a patent form of the disease. The presence of a scanty stroma and poor stromal vascularization are two other arguments. Red lesions (red vesicles, polypoid lesions, flame-like lesions, hypervascularized areas or even peritoneal petechiae)[1-4] are more active forms of the disease. Recent experimental studies in the baboon[5] have suggested that these lesions undergo active remodelling, some disappearing while other new lesions are formed.

In women, our hypothesis is that red lesions are more aggressive and progress to the so-called typical or black lesions which must be considered as an enclosed implant surrounded by fibrosis. Red lesions have recently been proved to be a very active form of the disease[1].

Ovarian chocolate-colored fluid cysts are, according to the hypothesis of Hughesdon[6], the consequence of the invagination of superficial implants into the ovary. Endometriomas can also develop in the ovaries and this type of cystic ovarian endometriosis must be considered another severe form of endometriosis, often related to infertility.

A third form of the disease is deep-infiltrating endometriosis of the rectovaginal septum. Sampson[7] defined cul-de-sac obliteration as 'extensive adhesions in the cul-de-sac, obliterating its lower portion and uniting the cervix or the lower portion of the uterus to the rectum; with adenoma of the endometrial type invading the cervical and the uterine tissue and probably also (but to a lesser degree) the anterior wall of the rectum' (Figure 1). Cul-de-sac obliteration secondary to endometriosis implies the presence of deep fibrotic retrocervical endometriosis beneath the peritoneum. Treatment options for pain or infertility secondary to cul-de-sac obliteration include ovarian suppression therapy with danazol or gonadotropin releasing hormone agonists, or surgery[5,8,9].

For existing infertility or the preservation of fertility, reconstructive surgery can be considered either via laparotomy, microsurgery or laparoscopy, depending on the skill and experience of the surgeon.

At laparotomy, deep fibrotic retrocervical endometriosis is commonly managed by bowel resection, assuming that the major portion of the lesion infiltrates the anterior rectum. In such cases, the deep fibrotic lesion is mobilized, starting with the posterior uterus and progressing downward to the rectum where it appears to be attached. Recently, however, the endoscopic technique has been developed[8,10-12].

MATERIALS AND METHODS

Our series of 103 cases of rectovaginal septum endometriosis is presented here. The main symptom was pelvic pain in 79 women. The other 24 suffered pelvic pain and infertility. In all cases of infertility, an evaluation of ovulation, cervical mucus–sperm interaction (post-coital test) and male factor (defined as < 15 million sperm/ml using a Makler counting chamber) was undertaken. Preoperative radiography of the colon was carried out in order to evaluate the involvement of the rectal surface. Profile radiography offers the best evaluation of infiltration of the anterior rectal wall (Figure 2).

The surgical techniques have evolved gradually but all of them involve the separation of the anterior rectum from the posterior vagina and the excision or ablation of the endometriosis in that area. Aquadissection, scissor dissection and electrosurgery with an unmodulated (cutting) current are used by some authors[8], while others[10,12] prefer the use of the CO_2 laser.

CO_2 laser dissection is currently used in our department (103 cases). At present, all treatment modes have been used to some extent in most cases. Whenever extensive endometriotic involvement of the cul-de-sac was suspected preoperatively, either because of the clinical presentation or from another physician's operative record, a mechanical bowel preparation was administered orally on the afternoon before surgery to induce brisk, self-limiting diarrhea that rapidly cleanses the bowel without disrupting the electrolyte balance. In cases of endometriotic lesions of the anterior rectal wall

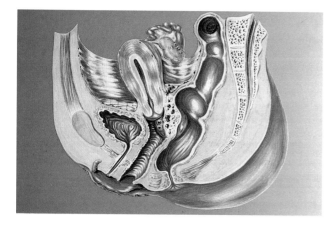

Figure 1(a) and (b)   Deep retrocervical endometriosis beneath the peritoneum

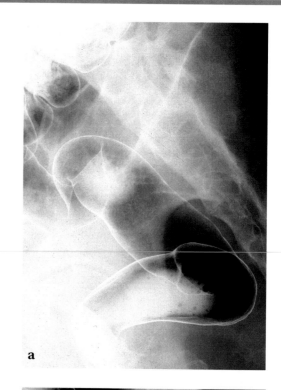

a

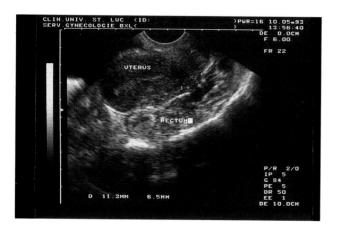

Figure 1(b)   *See legend above*

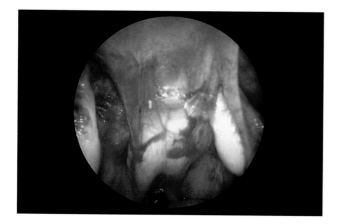

Figure 2(c)   *See legend opposite*

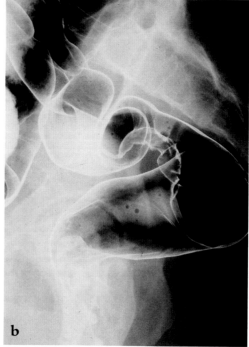

b

Figure 2   Profile radiography offers the best evaluation of the infiltration of the anterior rectal wall; (a) no signs of infiltration; (b) typical 'endometriotic' infiltration of the anterior rectal wall; (c) same patient showing evaluation of the rectal infiltration by vaginal echography

(diagnosed by colonic radiography – Figure 2(b)), a bowel preparation was proposed as for conventional bowel resection.

All the laparoscopic procedures were performed using general anesthesia. A 12-mm operative laparoscope was inserted through a vertical intraumbilical incision. Three other puncture sites were made: 2–3 cm above the pubis in the midline, and in the areas adjacent to the deep inferior epigastric vessels, which were visualized directly.

Preoperatively a GnRH agonist was used in the cases which required a second-look laparoscopy because of inflammatory disease or in cases of anterior rectal wall infiltration of more than 4–5 cm in length[12]. GnRH agonist can reduce the hypervascularization and the inflammation which are often present around endometriotic lesions[1-3, 9-12]. The reduced vascularization facilitates the surgical procedure.

CLINICAL AND LAPAROSCOPIC ASPECTS

Clinical aspects and diagnosis

Examination with a speculum reveals either a normal vaginal mucosa or a protruded endometriotic nodule in the posterior fornix (Figure 3). By palpation, the diameter of the lesion can be evaluated. Palpation is very often painful and the presence of the nodule accounts for symptoms like deep dyspareunia and dysmenorrhea.

Laparoscopic aspects

To determine the diagnosis of cul-de-sac obliteration, a sponge on a ring forceps was inserted into the posterior vaginal fornix. A dilator (Hegar 25) was systematically inserted into the rectum (Figure 4). Complete obliteration was diagnosed when the outline of the posterior fornix could not be seen through the laparoscope.

Cul-de-sac obliteration was partial when rectal tenting was visible but a protrusion of the sponge in the posterior vaginal fornix was identified between the rectum and the inverted U of the uterosacral ligaments. However, sometimes a deeply-infiltrating lesion of the rectovaginal septum is only barely visible by laparoscopy – this has been described by Koninckx[5] as type III infiltrating endometriosis. We believe that this type of lesion is not actually endometriosis, but a specific disease called adenomyosis, which is characterized by the presence of abundant muscular tissue invaded by glandular epithelium covered with a scanty stroma (see below). This type of 'adenomyosis' must be clearly differentiated in the new classification.

HISTOLOGY

Deep vaginal endometriosis associated with pelvic endometriosis can take the form of nodular or polypoid masses involving the posterior vaginal fornix. The differential diagnosis of vaginal endometriosis, particularly of the superficial type, includes vaginal adenosis of the tuboendometrial variety, but the latter lacks endometrial stroma and the characteristic inflammatory response of endometriosis[13]. In the body of the uterus, adenomyosis is a common condition characterized pathologically by the presence of endometrial glands and stroma within the myometrium. Microscopically, there are endometrial glands and stroma within the myometrium. The lower border of the endometrium is irregular and dips into the superficial myometrium.

In order to avoid misclassifying a normal histological finding as adenomyosis, some pathologists make the diagnosis only when the distance between the lower border of the endometrium and the adenomyosis exceeds one-half of a low-power field (about 2.5 mm).

Adenomyosis exhibits a varied functional response to ovarian hormones. Proliferative glands and stroma are generally observed in the first half of the menstrual cycle. Adenomyosis may not respond to physiological levels of progesterone, and secretory changes are frequently absent or incomplete during the second half of the cycle. Similar histological observations are made at the level of 'endometriotic' rectovaginal nodules. An adenomyoma is a circumscribed, nodular aggregate of smooth muscle, endometrial glands and, usually, endometrial stroma.

Histologically, scanty endometrial-type stroma and glandular epithelium are disseminated in muscular tissue (Figures 5 and 6). These very similar histological descriptions have led to the suggestion that the so-called endometriotic nodule of the rectovaginal septum is, in fact, just like an adenomyoma or an adenomyotic nodule. By three-dimensional evaluation (Figures 7–11), the reconstructed endometriotic lesion has the appearance of a unique 'gland' with multiple ramifications. Here also, as in the peritoneal 'red' lesion, the apparent multifocal aspect of the glands is not confirmed by three-dimensional evaluation. Sometimes the invasion of the muscle by a very active glandular epithelium (Figure 12) proved that the stroma is not necessary for invasion in this particular type of pathology called adenomyosis. Invasion of the vaginal musculature by the glandular epithelium is not rare (Figure 13).

SURGICAL TECHNIQUE

Deep fibrotic nodular endometriosis involving the cul-de-sac required an excision of the nodular fibrotic tissue from the posterior vagina, rectum, posterior cervix and uterosacral ligaments. As described by Reich and

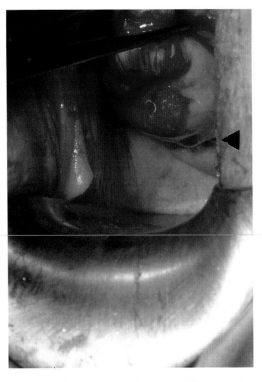

Figure 3(a) and (b) Protruding endometriotic nodule in the posterior fornix

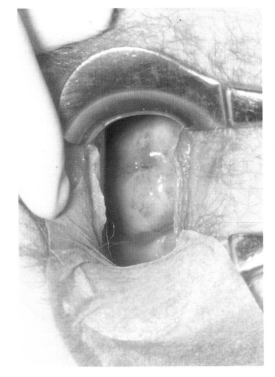

Figure 3(b)   *See legend above*

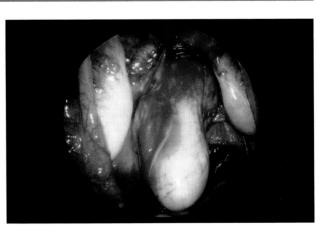

Figure 4 A dilator (Hegar 25) is inserted into the rectum while a sponge is inserted into the posterior vaginal fornix in order to determine the obliteration of the cul-de-sac

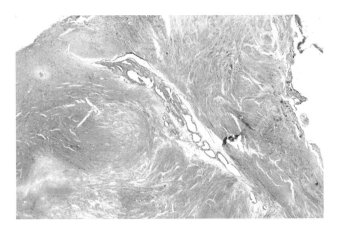

Figure 5 Rectovaginal septum adenomyosis (Gomori's trichrome, × 25); scanty endometrial type stroma and glandular epithelium are disseminated in muscular tissue

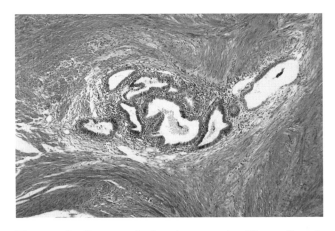

Figure 6 Rectovaginal adenomyosis (Gomori's trichrome × 56); the stroma is scanty

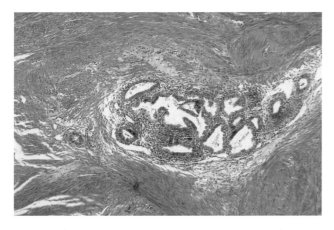

Figure 7(a) and (b) Histological structures (stroma, glandular epithelium and lumen) were drawn moving a cursor

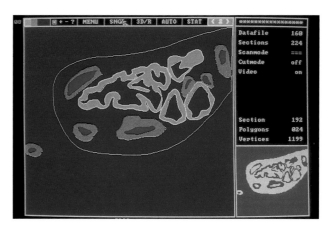

Figure 7(b)   *See legend opposite*

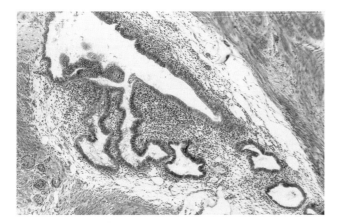

Figure 8(a) and (b)   By serial sections, each histological structure was transferred and stored at the end of an existing database

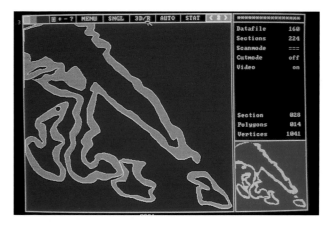

Figure 8(b)   *See legend opposite*

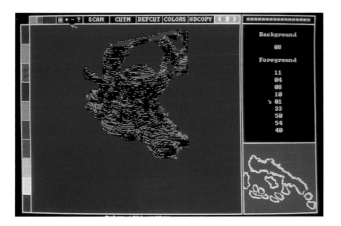

Figure 9 By a three-dimensional evaluation, the reconstructed endometriotic lesion has the appearance of a unique 'gland' with multiple ramifications

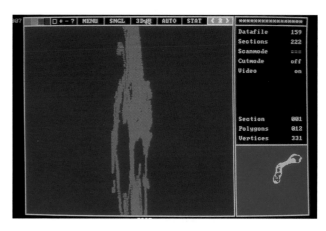

Figure 10 Another example of multiple ramifications diagnosed by the three-dimensional evaluation

colleagues[8], attention was first directed toward a complete dissection of the anterior rectum throughout its area of involvement until the loose tissue of the rectovaginal space was reached. A sponge on a ring forceps was inserted into the posterior vaginal fornix and a dilator (Hegar 25) was placed in the rectum (Figures 14 and 15). In addition, a cannula was inserted into the endometrial cavity to markedly antevert the uterus. The peritoneum covering the cul-de-sac of Douglas was opened between the 'adenomyotic' lesion (Figure 16) and the rectum.

We used a technique of first freeing the anterior rectum from the loose areolar tissue of the rectovaginal septum, prior to excising and/or vaporizing visible and palpable deep fibrotic endometriosis. This approach was possible even when anterior rectal muscle infiltration was present. Careful dissection was then carried out using the aquadissector, and the CO_2 laser for sharp dissection, until the rectum was completely freed and identifiable below the lesion (Figure 17).

Excision of the fibrotic tissue on the side of the rectum was attempted only after the rectal dissection was complete (Figure 18). A partial rectal resection was never performed in our series. In cases of deeply infiltrating lesions, the vaginal wall was more or less penetrated by the adenomyosis and excision of a part of the vagina was essential (Figure 19).

Dissection was performed accordingly, not only with the removal of all visible endometriotic lesions, but also the vaginal mucosa with at least a 0.5-cm disease-free margin. Lesions extending totally through the vagina were treated with *en bloc* laparoscopic resection from the cul-de-sac to the posterior vaginal wall (Figure 20); the pneumoperitoneum was maintained and the posterior vaginal wall was closed vaginally.

The anterior rectum can be reperitonealized by plicating the uterosacral ligaments and lateral rectal peritoneum across the midline using 4-0 Polydiox-anone[8], Tissucol or Interceed (Figure 21) (Donnez and Nisolle, personal communication). Deep rectal muscle defects can be closed with suture. Three full-thickness rectal lesion excisons were successfully repaired with suture in the series of Reich and associates[8].

In cases of full-thickness rectal lesions provoking menstrual rectorrhagia, translaparoscopic rectal resection can also be performed according to the technique of Nezhat and collegues[10]. In our series of 103 cases, laparoscopic dissection was performed successfully in all cases, even when the radiography of the colon showed bowel involvement (Figure 2(b)). Bowel resection is usually unnecessary, except in cases of bowel occlusion and rectal bleeding. Then, resection of the rectosigmoid junction must be carried out. In our series of 103 cases, laparoscopic rectal perforation occurred in two cases. Both perforations were diagnosed at the time of the laparoscopy. In one case, the rectum was repaired by laparotomy and in the other, by colpotomy.

During the same period, two patients who had rectal endometriosis with stenosis and rectal bleeding were operated on by laparotomy. A bowel resection with anastomosis was then carried out.

When a ureter is close to the lesion, its course can be traced starting at the pelvic brim. The peritoneum overlying the ureter can be opened to confirm the ureteral position deep in the pelvis.

Bipolar forceps were used to control arterial and venous bleeding. A final copious irrigation with saline solution was carried out and all clots were aspirated directly. Reich and co-workers[8] suggest leaving at least 2 l of Ringer's solution in the abdomen to separate the raw surfaces during early healing. In our department, Interceed was employed as an antiadhesion agent (Figure 21). All the women were discharged either the next day or 2 days after surgery.

The surgical objectives of laparoscopic treatment are similar: to remove all evident endometriosis by excising large superficial and deep lesions and vaporizing smaller deposits. With our approach, first the anterior rectum was freed; this was possible even when anterior rectal infiltration was present.

DISCUSSION

Deeply infiltrating endometriosis was defined as endometriosis infiltrating deeper than 5 mm[5]. Morphologically, superficial endometriosis (mostly subtle lesions) looks very active in some 50% of lesions, whereas lesions of intermediate depth (3–5 mm, mostly typical lesions) frequently have a burnt-out aspect[5]. Deeply infiltrating endometriosis, on the other hand, has the most active lesions and morphologically the transition zone is estimated to be at approximately 5–6 mm in depth.

Koninckx[5] recently described three types of deeply infiltrating endometriosis. Deeply infiltrating endometriosis of type I is a rather large lesion in the peritoneal cavity which infiltrates conically, with the deeper parts becoming progressively smaller. It has been suggested that this type of endometriosis is caused by infiltration.

In type II lesions, the main feature is a bowel which is retracted over the lesion, which thus becomes deeply situated in the rectovaginal septum although not really infiltrating it. The type III lesion is the deepest and most severe. It is spherically shaped, situated deep in the rectovaginal septum, and is often visible only as a small typical lesion at laparoscopy. This lesion is often more palpable than visible.

For us, there are two different types of deeply infiltrating endometriosis:

(1) True deeply infiltrating endometriosis causes the invasion of a very active peritoneal lesion deep in the

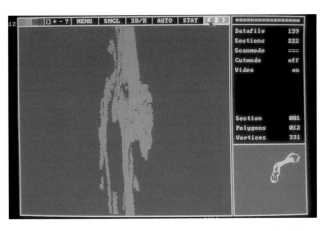

Figure 11 Another example of multiple ramifications diagnosed by the three-dimensional evaluation

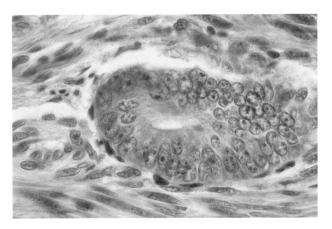

Figure 12 Very active glandular epithelium invading the muscle; the stroma is absent (Gomori's trichrome, × 440)

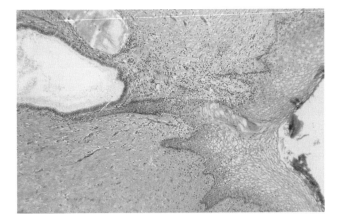

Figure 13 Invasion of the vaginal mucosa by the glandular epithelium (Gomori's trichrome, × 56)

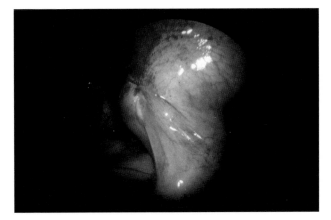

Figure 14 A sponge is inserted into the posterior vaginal fornix

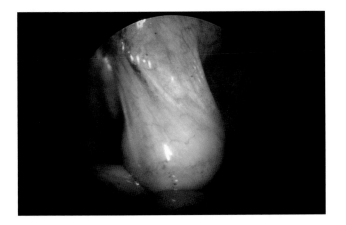

Figure 15 The dilator is placed in the rectum

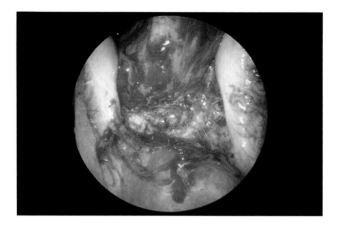

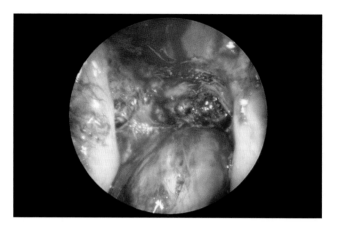

Figure 16(a) and (b) Opening of the peritoneum between the rectum and the adenomyotic lesion

Figure 16(b) *See legend opposite*

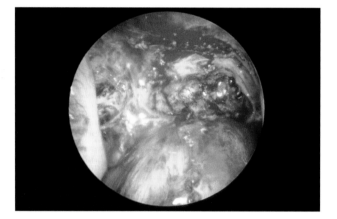

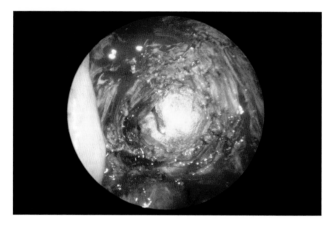

Figure 17(a) and (b) Dissection with the CO_2 laser until the rectum is completely freed and identifiable below the lesion. The vaginal sponge is visible

Figure 17(b) *See legend opposite*

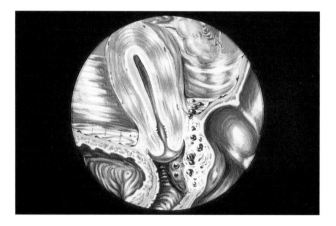

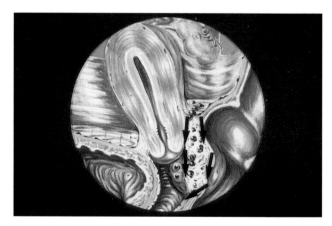

Figure 18(a) and (b) Excision of the fibrotic tissue only after the rectal dissection is complete

Figure 18(b) *See legend opposite*

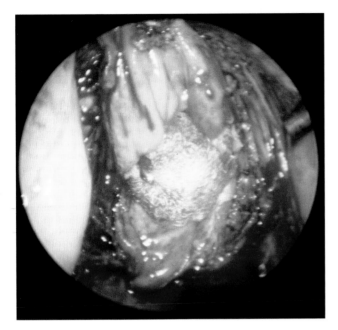

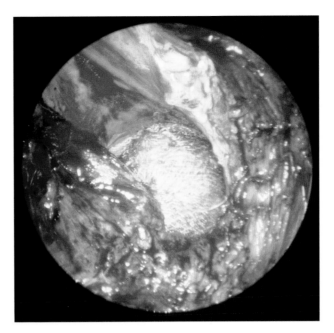

Figure 19(a) and (b)   The vaginal wall is more or less penetrated by the adenomyosis and excision of a part of the vagina is carried out

Figure 19(b)   *See legend opposite*

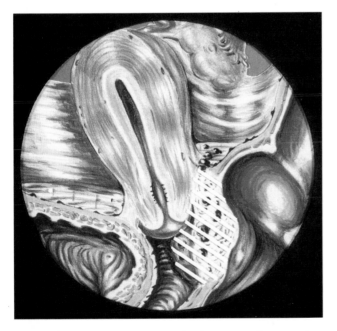

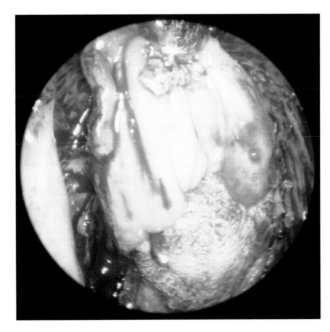

Figure 20(a) and (b)   *En bloc* laparoscopic resection from the cul-de-sac to the posterior vaginal wall

Figure 20(b)   *See legend opposite*

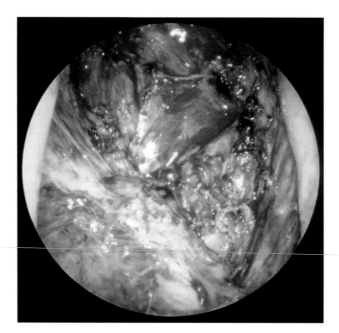

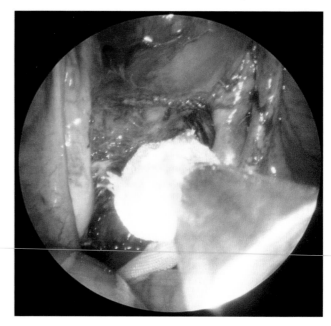

Figure 21 Interceed is used to cover the deperitonealized area. (a) Deperitonealized area after vaginal closure; (b) Interceed is introduced through the operative channel of the laparoscope; (c) the deperitonealized area is covered by Interceed

Figure 21(b)   *See legend opposite*

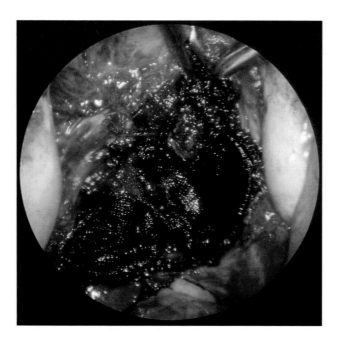

Figure 21(c)   *See legend above*

retroperitoneal space. In cases of lateral peritoneal invasion, the uterosacral ligaments can be involved as well as the anterior wall of the rectosigmoid junction, resulting in a retraction, adhesions and secondary obliteration of the cul-de-sac.

(2) Pseudo-deeply infiltrating endometriosis or adenomyosis of the rectovaginal septum originates from the tissue of the rectovaginal septum and consists essentially of smooth muscle with active glandular epithelium and scanty stroma.

Kelly and Diamond[14], reporting on a series of 68 women who underwent laparotomy for endometriosis, found that it was rarely necessary to penetrate the bowel lumen to excise the endometriosis; colonic endometriosis was vaporized down to normal tissue, as proved by palpation and viewing with magnification.

In our series, deep fibrotic tissue assumed to contain endometriosis was excised or vaporized from the anterior rectum with the aid of multiple rectovaginal examinations. Cul-de-sac dissection was followed by excision of deep fibrotic endometriosis, with or without cul-de-sac reconstruction. In two cases, the bowel lumen was entered.

A comprehensive laparoscopic procedure, while not eradicating all the endometriosis, may result in considerable pain relief or a desired pregnancy. While we recognize that bowel resection may be necessary in rare cases, it seems prudent to curtail, rather than encourage, the widespread use of an aggressive, potentially morbid procedure.

In conclusion, deeply infiltrating endometriosis should be considered as a specific disease, different from mild or minimal endometriosis and ovarian cystic endometriosis. We suggest that this disease be called 'rectovaginal adenomyosis'.

REFERENCES

1. Nisolle, M., Casanas-Roux, F., Anaf, V., Mine, J.M. and Donnez, J. (1993). Morphometric study of the stromal vascularization in peritoneal endometriosis. *Fertil. Steril.*, **59**, 681

2. Donnez, J. and Nisolle, M. (1988). Appearances of peritoneal endometriosis. In *Proceedings of the IIIrd International Laser Surgery Symposium*, Brussels

3. Donnez, J., Nisolle, M. and Casanas-Roux, F. (1992). Three-dimensional architectures of peritoneal endometriosis. *Fertil. Steril.*, **57**, 980–3

4. Nisolle, M., Paindaveine, B., Bourdon, A., Berliere, M., Casanas-Roux, F. and Donnez, J. (1990). Histologic study of peritoneal endometriosis in infertile women. *Fertil. Steril.*, **53**, 984–8

5. Koninckx, P.D. (1993). Deeply infiltrating endometriosis. In Brosens, I. and Donnez, J. (eds.) *Endometriosis: Research and Management*, pp.437–46. (Carnforth, UK: Parthenon Publishing)

6. Hughesdon, P.E. (1957). The structure of endometrial cysts of the ovary. *J. Obstet. Gynaecol. Br. Empire*, **64**, 481–7

7. Sampson, J.A. (1922). Intestinal adenomas of endometrial type. *Arch. Surg.*, **5**, 217

8. Reich, H., McGlynn, F. and Salvat, J. (1991). Laparoscopic treatment of cul-de-sac obliteration secondary to retrocervical deep fibrotic endometriosis. *J. Reprod. Med.*, **36**, 516

9. Donnez, J., Nisolle, M. and Casanas-Roux, F. (1990). Endometriosis-associated infertility: evaluation of preoperative use of danazol gestrinone and buserelin. *Int. J. Fertil.*, **42**, 128

10. Nezhat, C., Nezhat, F. and Pennington, E. (1992). Laparoscopic treatment of lower colorectal and infiltrative rectovaginal septum endometriosis by the technique of video laparoscopy. *Br. J. Obstet. Gynaecol.*, **99**, 664–7

11. Canis, M., Wattiez, A., Pouly, J.L., Bassil, S., Bouquet de Joliniere, J., Chapron, C., Manhes, H., Mage, G. and Bruhat, M.A. (1993). Laparoscopic treatment of endometriosis. In Brosens, I. and Donnez, J. (eds.) *Endometriosis: Research and Management*, pp.407–17. (Carnforth, UK: Parthenon Publishing)

12. Donnez J., Nisolle, M., Casanas-Roux, F., and Clerckx, F. (1993). Endometriosis: rationale for surgery. In Brosens, I. and Donnez, J. (eds.) *Endometriosis: Research and Management*, pp.385–95. (Carnforth, UK: Parthenon Publishing)

13. Zaloudek, C. and Norris, H.J. (1987). Mesenchymal tumors of the uterus. In Kurman, R. (ed.) *Blaustein's Pathology of the Female Genital Tract*, p.373. (New York)

14. Kelly, R. and Diamond, M.P. (1989). Laparotomy in infertile patients (use of CO_2 laser). *J. Reprod. Med.*, **34**, 25

Bowel endometriosis

C. Nezhat, F. Nezhat, C.H. Nezhat and D. Admon

9

INTRODUCTION

As with other organs, the etiology of bowel endometriosis is unknown. Its occurrence was reported as early as 1922 by Sampson[1]. Following his investigation of 19 cases, he proposed that 'implantation adenoma of endometrial type of some portion of the intestinal tract may be present in at least one-half of the cases of perforated ovarian hematoma of endometrial type with peritoneal implantations'[1].

Intestinal endometriosis has been reported to affect between 3 and 37% of women with endometriosis[2-6]. In a series of 1573 women treated consecutively for endometriosis, 5.4% had gastrointestinal involvement; of these, 65% had endometriosis of the rectum and rectosigmoid colon[2]. In another series of 1000 celiotomies, Williams and Pratt found that 485 women had endometriosis, of which 181 (37%) had gastrointestinal involvement. Of these, 172 (95%) had rectosigmoid involvement, nine (5%) had ileal involvement, and 19 (10%) had appendiceal involvement[7]. Bowel resection with or without castration has been suggested to treat symptomatic patients[2,6]. Coronado and colleagues[8] have reported satisfactory pain relief and pregnancy rates following anterior wall resection of the colon by laparotomy for deeply infiltrating lower colorectal endometriosis.

Bowel involvement is suggested by palpable tumor in the rectovaginal septum, gastrointestinal symptoms such as rectal bleeding, constipation or diarrhea associated with menses, or pain that persists after surgical removal of all recognizable lesions.

Endometriotic nodularity of the bowel and rectovaginal septum is one of the most difficult aspects of this disease to approach surgically. Because gynecologists are uncomfortable operating on the bowel, and general surgeons may not be familiar with endometriosis, these cases have frequently required bowel resection or temporary colostomy. Some have shown that when full-thickness bowel resection and immediate reanastomosis are performed by a surgical team familiar with the disease, low morbidity and good long-term relief of symptoms can be expected[8].

Because colorectal endometriosis is generally superficial, we feel that bowel resection should remain the last resort. We have been able to treat most cases involving the rectum and rectovaginal septum laparoscopically.

Women with endometriosis of the lower colon, rectum, uterosacral ligaments or rectovaginal septum often present with chronic pelvic pain; and dysmenorrhea, dyspareunia, back pain, dyschezia, constipation or diarrhea; or infertility with pelvic pain. Most women with small bowel or appendiceal endometriosis are asymptomatic, and rarely experience bowel obstruction.

PREOPERATIVE PREPARATION

To prepare a patient for laparoscopic treatment of bowel endometriosis, the surgeon should follow a protocol similar to that for laparotomy, including thorough clinical and laboratory evaluation. We have treated gastrointestinal endometriosis with different laparoscopic techniques and believe that an experienced laparoscopic surgeon who is familiar with this condition can treat most women completely endoscopically, or in combination with an abdominal minilaparotomy or anal approach. Additionally, the procedure is explained to the patient and proper consent obtained. The evening before surgery, patients are given a bowel preparation of 4 liters polyethylene glycol-3350 (Go-LYTELY, Braintree Laboratories, Braintree, MA) and take 1 g metronidazole at 23:00. Cefoxitin is administered prophylactically, both preoperatively and postoperatively. Preoperative sigmoidoscopy, barium enema or intravenous pyelogram should be performed when indicated.

The room set-up has been described before[9,10]. Trocar placement includes one subumbilical incision to introduce the video laparoscope, and two to three suprapubic incisions to pass the suction irrigator probe, grasping forceps, bipolar electrocoagulator, and needle holder. The CO_2 laser is placed through the operative channel of the laparoscope and used as a long knife. Videolaparoscopy is performed under general endotracheal anesthesia, with the patients in a modified dorsolithotomy and Trendelenburg position (Figure 1).

PRELIMINARY TREATMENT OF ENDOMETRIOSIS AND ADHESIONS

Although we prefer the CO_2 laser (Ultrapulse 5000L, Coherent, Palo Alto, California) set at 40–80 W to vaporize or excise the endometriosis, any cutting modality such as scissors or unipolar electrocautery may be used. An assistant stands between the patient's legs,

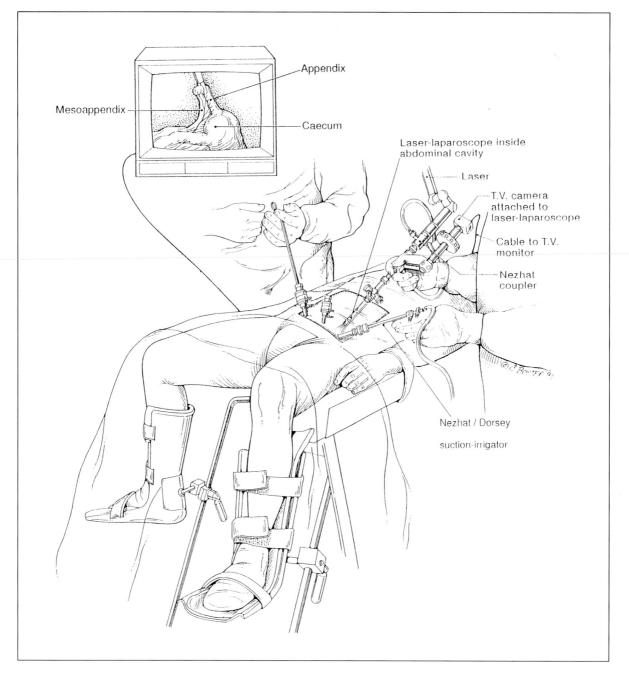

Mesoappendix

Appendix

Caecum

Laser-laparoscope inside abdominal cavity

Laser

T.V. camera attached to laser-laparoscope

Cable to T.V. monitor

Nezhat coupler

Nezhat / Dorsey

suction-irrigator

Figure 1 Patient in position for videolaparoscopy

performing rectovaginal examination with one hand. The other hand holds the uterus up with a rigid uterine elevator while both the assistant and the surgeon observe the monitor. The ureters are identified, and if they are involved with the endometriosis, an opening is made between the uterosacral ligaments and the ureter using hydrodissection and the CO_2 laser, they are pushed laterally. For rectovaginal septum and uterosacral ligament endometriosis, 5–8 ml of diluted vasopressin (10 U in 100–200 ml of lactated Ringer's) are injected in an uninvolved area with a 16-gauge laparoscopic needle. Using the CO_2 laser and hydrodissection[11], the peritoneum is opened to further dissect the diseased area.

While an assistant examines the rectum, the involved area is completely excised or vaporized until the loose areolar tissue of the rectovaginal space or normal muscularis layers of the rectum are reached. Due to the proximity of the uterine vessels and the vascularity of nodular uterosacral ligaments, caution is necessary to avoid injuring these vessels. The operator must be prepared to control bleeding. We prefer bipolar electrodesiccation (20–25 W). In patients whose rectum is pulled up and attached behind the cervix between the uterosacral ligaments, the uterus is first antiflexed sharply, and an incision is made at the right or left pararectal area and extended to the junction of the cervix and the rectum. The rectum is completely separated from the uterosacral ligaments. When the uterosacral ligament is adherent to the rectum, an incision is made on the side of the rectum and uterosacral ligament, separating them from the cervix. If the uterosacral ligaments are not fused with the rectum, the endometriosis is dissected from the rectum as much as possible. Any remaining endometriosis is vaporized. After the rectum is separated, an assistant performs a rectal examination of the lesion as it is vaporized or excised. If the rectal involvement is more extensive and higher up, or if the assistant's finger is not long enough, a sigmoidoscope, a sponge on forceps or a rectal probe is used. The sigmoidoscope not only helps the surgeon identify the rectum, but also aids in detecting bowel perforation by visualizing air bubbles as they pass from the air-inflated rectum into the posterior cul-de-sac which has been filled with irrigation fluid. With the assistant guiding the surgeon by rectovaginal examination, the rectum is completely freed from the back of the cervix. Any generalized oozing and bleeding may be controlled with an injection of 3–5 ml diluted vasopressin solution (1 ampule in 100 ml lactated Ringer's), laser or bipolar electrocoagulator. Occasional bleeding from the stalk vessels caused by dissection or vaporization of the fibrotic uterosacral ligaments and pararectal areas is controlled with bipolar electrodesiccation.

Because the ureters are lateral to the uterosacral ligaments, one should try to stay between the ligaments as much as possible. Using hydrodissection and making a relaxing incision lateral to the uterosacral ligament allows the ureters to retract laterally, helping to protect them. Different degrees of ureterolysis may be necessary to free the ureters from the surrounding fibrotic, endometriotic tissue and large or small endometriomas[12,13]. Endometriomas and ovaries may be severely attached to the bowel and ureter. Hydrodissection[11] along with the CO_2 laser and blunt dissection are used for ureterolysis, enterolysis and ovarian cystectomy.

For cases in which posterior cul-de-sac nodularity and endometriosis infiltration towards the vagina are present, vaporization and dissection of the nodularity are continued as an assistant evaluates the nodule by palpation until it is eliminated[14]. This may require a partial vaginectomy. Should a small vaginal perforation occur, it can be left alone as long as the perforation is less than 1.0 cm.

Endometriosis rarely penetrates the mucosa of the colon; however, endometriosis of the lower colorectal area commonly involves the serosa, subserosa and muscularis of the bowel. This disease can be excised or vaporized by an experienced videolaparoscopist. The procedure is very demanding and requires maximal cooperation between the assistant and the surgeon.

To detect possible rectal perforations, we use the sigmoidoscope, as described before, or inject indigo carmine into the rectum with a Foley catheter.

Perforations can be repaired laparoscopically with three to four interrupted 3-0 silk, or 4-0 polydioxanone sutures (Ethicon)[12,15,16].

Patients may be discharged within 24 h, except those who had bowel perforations or underwent bowel resection. Patients are instructed to have nothing by mouth for 24 h, except for sips of water, and if no complications are noted, the diet is gradually increased. Patients with bowel perforation or resection are allowed nothing by mouth until they pass flatus and then are instructed to avoid constipation by eating a high fiber diet. The patients should be examined at 1 and 6 weeks postoperatively[12].

BOWEL RESECTION – TECHNIQUE I

Several methods of laparoscopic and laparoscopically assisted bowel resection have been reported by our group and others[11,17–20]. To treat certain infiltrative symptomatic intestinal endometriosis, we have developed a new technique which eliminates stapling devices and much of the complex and time-consuming dissection. This total laparoscopic bowel resection and reanastomosis was devised for severe disease of the anterior wall of the colon. In select cases, preoperative hormonal suppressive therapy may be indicated.

A 10-mm incision is placed infraumbilically and three 5-mm incisions are made in the lower abdomen. The CO_2 laser is used via the operative channel of the video laparoscope to dissect and vaporize endometriosis and fibrosis. Grasping forceps, a suction–irrigator probe and a needle holder are placed via the three suprapubic incisions. Bipolar electrocoagulation is used to achieve hemostasis[21].

First, the severity of the pelvic pathology is evaluated and any gynecological procedures, such as salpingo-ovariolysis, ovarian cystectomy, and vaporization or excision of endometriosis are performed. Next, the extent of bowel involvement is evaluated. Women whose disease can be resected or vaporized completely without entering the lumen are not candidates for this procedure[12].

A sigmoidoscope is used to completely clean the rectum, further delineate the lesion and guide the surgeon. The extent of the lesion can be evaluated visually and by palpation, using the tip of the suction–irrigator probe. If the lesion is low enough, an assistant can identify it by performing a rectal examination. The ureters are identified on each side. The lower colon must usually be mobilized[16] in all aspects except posteriorly. Depending on the location of the lesion, the right pararectal area, left pararectal area or both may be entered using the CO_2 laser and hydrodissection, to separate the colon from adjacent organs. In contrast to previously reported techniques[14,19,20], it is not necessary to separate the

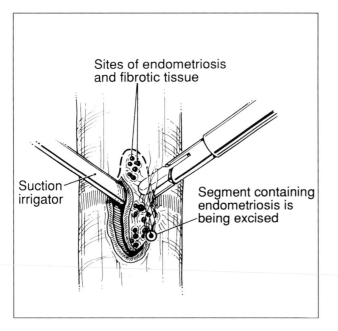

Figure 2 Lesion is held with the grasper and excised

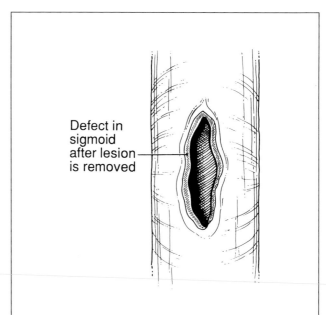

Figure 3 Defect in sigmoid colon after lesion is removed

rectum posteriorly. Any bleeding which is not controlled by the CO_2 laser may be managed with bipolar electrodesiccation.

Full-thickness excision is carried out, beginning above the area of visible disease as follows. After identifying the normal tissue, the lesion is held at its proximal end with grasping forceps (inserted via the right lower quadrant trocar). An incision is made using the CO_2 laser (50–80 W ultrapulse) through the bowel serosa and muscularis, and the lumen entered (Figure 2). The lesion is completely excised from the anterior rectal wall (Figure 3). The suction–irrigator probe serves as a backstop for the CO_2 laser and evacuates the laser plume. Following complete excision of the lesion, the pelvic cavity is thoroughly irrigated and suctioned. The removed lesion is extracted from the abdomen through the operative channel of the laparoscope using a long grasping forceps, or from the anus using polyp forceps, and submitted for pathology.

The bowel is repaired transversely in one layer[14]. Two traction sutures are applied to each side of the bowel defect, transforming it to a transverse opening (Figure 4). The stay sutures are brought out via the right and left lower quadrant trocar sleeves. The sleeves are removed, replaced in the peritoneal cavity next to the stay sutures, and the sutures are secured outside the abdomen. The bowel is then repaired by placing several interrupted through-and-through sutures in 0.3–0.6-cm increments until it is completely reanastomosed (Figures 5 and 6). We use 0 Vicryl laparoscopic sutures and a straight needle (Ethicon) with extracorporeal knot tying.

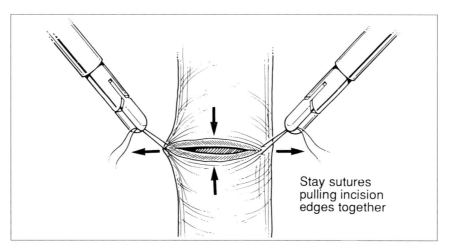

Figure 4 Stay sutures are applied on each side of the defect; the arrows indicate the transformation of the defect to a transverse incision

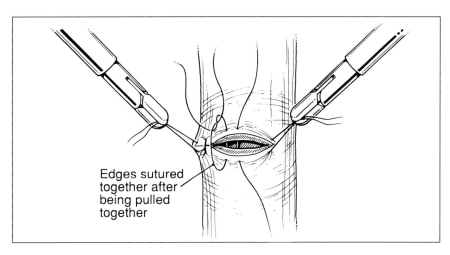

Figure 5 The sigmoid colon is repaired and reanastomosed using interrupted sutures

At the end of the procedure, the pelvic cavity is filled with lactated Ringer's and the rectosigmoid colon is insufflated with the sigmoidoscope to confirm by the absence of air bubbles that the closure is watertight. The sigmoidoscope is also used to ensure that there is no bowel stricture. Small air leaks may be repaired with additional interrupted 1-0 Vicryl sutures.

We do not use a Jackson–Pratt drain or a nasogastric tube. The Foley catheter is usually removed the day of surgery. Oral feeding may resume after the spontaneous release of flatus, usually the 1st or 2nd postoperative day. Patients are released from the hospital when they are able to tolerate clear liquids well. A low residual diet begins after the patient has a bowel movement. All women are instructed to monitor their fluid intake, urine output and temperature for 2 weeks following discharge from the hospital. The patients are contacted daily by one of the surgeons until they resume a normal diet. They are then contacted weekly by a nurse until their 4-week postoperative visit. Unless a woman is trying to conceive, we recommend oral contraceptives as hormonal suppressive therapy postoperatively.

Eight women, ages 29 to 38 years, with extensive symptomatic pelvic endometriosis underwent bowel resection using this technique. All were diagnosed to have severe pelvic endometriosis and had not responded to previous conservative surgical and hormonal therapy. In a 3–15-month follow-up, six women have reported complete relief of the symptoms. Two have right lower quadrant pain and menstrual cramping. Second-look laparoscopy was offered to all patients and so far, two have accepted. These procedures were performed 6 weeks postoperatively. At that surgery, we found that the anastomotic site had healed completely with filmy adhesions between the posterior aspect of the uterus and the rectosigmoid colon in one patient. The second woman had undergone extensive adhesiolysis at the first surgery, and these adhesions recurred; however, the anastomotic site had healed completely. One woman has

achieved pregnancy. The only complication was one patient with ecchymosis of the anterior abdominal wall. Sigmoidoscopy was performed 6 weeks postoperatively, to be repeated at 6 months postoperatively. To date, all anastomotic sites have healed well with no sign of stricture. Our results with this technique in a small series were positive.

BOWEL RESECTION – TECHNIQUE 2

When it is necessary to resect a longer portion of the bowel, the following technique may be used. The rectum is completely mobilized to allow prolapse of the lesion transanally. An assistant performs simultaneous digital examinations of the rectum and vagina to delineate the

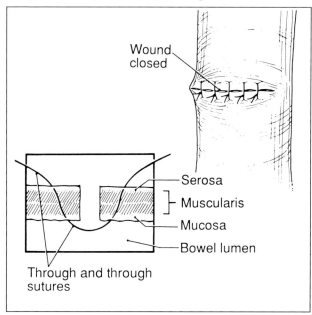

Figure 6 The sigmoid colon has been repaired; inset – layers of the bowel and placement of through-and-through sutures

rectovaginal septum[12]. The CO_2 laser is used to mobilize the rectum down to the pelvic floor. In a similar fashion, the rectal mesentery is dissected laterally with the CO_2 laser[12,14]. This dissection requires division of the lateral stalks. Hemostasis may be obtained using bipolar electrodesiccation. Posteriorly, the avascular space is dissected down to the level of the levator ani muscles.

The bowel is divided proximal to the lesion and prepared for anastomosis. The mesentery is divided with the CO_2 laser and bipolar electrodesiccation is used to coagulate major blood vessels. Vascular clips or suture may also be used[15].

In patients with anterior rectal lesions, the rectum is prolapsed via the anal canal and transected using two applications of an RL30 or RL60 stapler (Ethicon), then interrupted 2-0 vicryl sutures are used for reinforcement. In patients with circumferential lesions, the rectum is transected distal to the lesion and the proximal limb prolapsed into the distal limb, using Babcock clamps. A 2-0 polypropylene (Ethicon) purse-string suture is inserted into the end of the proximal bowel to secure the opposing anvil of a #33 ILS stapler (Ethicon). The anvil is separated from the gun, secured with the purse-string suture and replaced transanally into the pelvis along with the proximal bowel.

The rectal stump containing the endometrial lesion and fibrosis is then prolapsed out of the anus by grasping the transected end of the rectal stump with Babcock clamps (Baxter Mueller, Chicago, IL) and pulling it through the anal canal. The rectum is stapled shut with a RL60 linear stapler (Ethicon) and the rectal specimen is resected and sent to surgical pathology.

The rectal stump is reduced inside the pelvis and an end-to-end double-stapled anastomosis is performed with the #33 ILS stapler (Ethicon). The trocar in the gun is passed through the stapled end of the rectum. The laparoscope is used to attach the opposing anvil in the proximal bowel. Approximating the bowel ends and firing the stapler completes the anastomosis. The presence of intact 'donut' margins is verified.

Using a proctoscope, the anastomosis is inspected. The pelvis is filled with saline through the laparoscope and visualized as air is insufflated into the rectum from the proctoscope. An absence of air bubbles in the pelvis indicates anastomotic integrity.

The laparoscopic bowel resection is identical to a laparotomy except that bipolar electrocoagulator and laser replace sutures and scissors[14,19,20].

SMALL BOWEL AND CECUM RESECTION

In cases of gastrointestinal endometriosis, the small bowel and cecum are the areas least often involved[2,7]. We have treated three such cases laparoscopically. In the first, the patient had cecal and appendiceal endometriosis. Following laparoscopic mobilization of the bowel, the cecum was resected and reanastomosed through a McBurney incision. An appendectomy was then performed. The other two women had small bowel endometriosis which was causing partial stricture. The mesentery was desiccated and cut, and the bowel exteriorized through a small Pfannenstiel incision in one case and through a posterior colpotomy in the other. Resection and reanastomosis were then completed and the bowel replaced. All three procedures were completed with no intraoperative or postoperative complications, and the women are doing well.

With these modifications, we believe that all bowel endometriosis can be treated laparoscopically, decreasing the need for laparotomy.

APPENDECTOMY

During laparoscopic treatment of diverse pelvic pathologies, incidental appendectomy is often performed[22]. We use the following technique to remove the appendix when indicated.

The current procedure evolved from efforts initiated in 1983 using video-augmented instrumentation at hand to develop optimal techniques for laparoscopic surgery including appendectomy. The trocar punctures allow the introduction of ancillary instruments such as grasping forceps, endoloop suture applicators, a suction–irrigator probe (American Hydro-Surgical Instruments, Delray Beach, FL) and bipolar electrocoagulator. Hemostasis is accomplished with the bipolar electrocoagulator.

Frequently an incidental procedure, appendectomy may be concomitant with surgeries for pelvic endometriosis and/or adhesions, including CO_2 laser ablation or excision of peritoneal and ovarian endometriosis, ovarian cystectomy, salpingo-ovariolysis, salpingectomy, salpingo-oophorectomy, salpingoneostomy, adnexectomy, myomectomy, enterolysis and ureterolysis.

Upon completing thorough treatment of pelvic pathology, the appendix is mobilized and examined following lysis of periappendiceal or pericecal adhesions as necessary, proceeding carefully in cases of attachment to the lateral pelvic wall or retrocecal appendix. Then, the bipolar electrocoagulator and the CO_2 laser (Coherent) are used sequentially to coagulate and cut the mesoappendix 0.2–0.5 cm from the ileocecal area. When using the bipolar electrocoagulator in this area, caution should be exercised to prevent thermal damage to the cecum. Additionally, a backstop is required when using the CO_2 laser to avoid injury to the major blood vessels in this area (external iliac artery and vein).

At this point, the bipolar electrocoagulator is withdrawn and the Endoloop applicator (Ethicon) inserted through the suprapubic midline puncture. Two chromic Endoloop sutures (Ethicon) or polydioxanone sutures (Ethicon) are passed to the base of the appendix

2–5 mm from the cecum and then tied, one on top of the other. Both suture ends are cut with the CO_2 laser or scissors. A third Endoloop suture is applied, < 1 cm distal to the other sutures and then cut long, leaving a 15-cm 'tail' to facilitate retrieval should the appendix inadvertently fall into the pelvic well. Using the CO_2 laser, the appendix is cut between the second and third sutures placed. Luminal portions of the appendiceal stump and the removed appendix are seared with the CO_2 laser, and the tissues copiously irrigated with lactated Ringer's.

The appendix is removed from the abdomen with a long grasping forceps passed through the operating channel of the laparoscope, suprapubically with the short grasper or with an Endopouch tissue removal bag (Ethicon). If appropriate, an appendix extractor may be placed via the sleeve of a 10-mm trocar, replacing the central 5-mm one. Instruments, which may be contaminated, are removed from the surgical area. No adjunctive therapy is added to the pelvic cavity. Lastly, the appendiceal and other operative sites are inspected for hemostasis and then irrigated with lactated Ringer's[23].

Appendectomies may last from 4 to 21 minutes. Postoperative instructions should include avoiding solid food for 24 h; otherwise, they are routine for gynecological procedures, including an outpatient evaluation the day following surgery.

In a series of 254 appendectomies, no major intraoperative complications were noted. Postoperatively, one woman had a small pelvic abscess which required surgical intervention. All patients were discharged from the hospital within 24 h of surgery[22].

Semm[24] has described a technique which uses sutures and crocodile forceps. After the appendix is freed from any adhesions, two sutures are placed at the base and the area between the sutures is electrocoagulated using the crocodile forceps. The appendix is separated using hooked scissors and removed.

In a series of 356 women who underwent laparoscopic treatment of bowel endometriosis using different techniques, two patients required intraoperative laparotomy early in our experience. The first patient underwent laparotomy for repair of enterotomy after treatment of infiltrative rectal endometriosis. The other patient required laparotomy for anastomosis due to an unsuccessful attempt to place a purse-string suture around the patulous rectal ampulla. Significant postoperative complications occurred in 1.7% of patients. Two women developed leaks and pelvic infections. One required a temporary colostomy with subsequent take-down and repair, and one was managed by prolonged drainage. One woman had bowel stricture requiring resection and reanastomosis by laparotomy. One developed a pelvic abscess and subsequently underwent laparoscopic right salpingo-oophorectomy. One had an immediate rectal prolapse which was reduced without surgical management. Her bowel symptoms persisted, and she finally had an ileostomy.

Minor complications included skin ecchymosis, temporary urinary retention, temporary diarrhea or constipation, and dyschezia.

REFERENCES

1. Sampson, J.A. (1922). Intestinal adenomas of endometrial type. *Arch. Surg.*, **5**, 217–80
2. Prystowsky, J.B., Stryker, S.J., Ujiki, G.T. *et al.* (1988). Gastrointestinal endometriosis. *Arch.Surg.*, **123**, 855–8
3. Samper, E.R., Slagle, G.W. and Hand, A.M. (1984). Colonic endometriosis: its clinical spectrum. *South Med. J.*, **77**, 912–14
4. Cattell, R.B. (1987). Endometriosis of the colon and rectum with intestinal obstruction. *N. Engl. J. Med.*, **217**, 9–16
5. Forsgren, H., Lindhagen, J., Melander, S. *et al.* (1983). Colorectal endometriosis. *Acta Chir. Scand.*, **149**, 431–5
6. Meyers, W.C., Kelvin, F.M. and Jones, R.S. (1979). Diagnosis and surgical treatment of colonic endometriosis. *Arch. Surg.*, **114**, 169–75
7. Williams, T.J. and Pratt, J.H. (1977). Endometriosis in 1000 consecutive celiotomies: incidence and management. *Am. J. Obstet. Gynecol.*, **129**, 245–50
8. Coronado, C., Franklin, R.R., Lotze, E.C., Bailey, H.R. and Valdes, C.T. (1990). Surgical treatment of symptomatic colorectal endometriosis. *Fertil. Steril.*, **53**, 411–16
9. Nezhat, C., Nezhat, F. and Silfen, S.L. (1991). Videolaseroscopy: the CO_2 laser for advanced operative laparoscopy. *Obstet. Gynecol. Clin. N. Am.*, **18**, 585–604
10. Nezhat, F. and Nezhat, C. (1992). Setup for operative laparoscopy and videolaseroscopy. *Contemp. Obstet. Gynecol.*, **36**, 50–64
11. Nezhat, C. and Nezhat, F. (1989). Safe laser excision or vaporization of peritoneal endometriosis. *Fertil. Steril.*, **52**, 149–51
12. Nezhat, C., Nezhat, F. and Pennington, E. (1992). Laparoscopic treatment of lower colorectal and infiltrative rectovaginal septum endometriosis by the technique of videolaseroscopy. *Br. J. Obstet. Gynaecol.*, **99**, 664–7
13. Nezhat, C., Nezhat, F. and Green, B. (1992). Laparoscopic treatment of obstructed ureter due to endometriosis by resection and uretero-ureterostomy. A case report. *J. Urol.*, **148**, 865–8
14. Nezhat, C., Pennington, E., Nezhat, F. and Silfen, S.L. (1991). Laparoscopically assisted anterior rectal wall resection and reanastomosis for deeply infiltrating endometriosis. *Surg. Laparosc. Endosc.*, **1**, 106–8
15. Nezhat, C., Nezhat, S.L., Nezhat, F. and Martin,

D. (1991). Surgery for endometriosis. *Curr. Op. Obstet. Gynecol.*, **3**, 385–93

16. Nezhat, C., Nezhat, F., Ambroze, W. and Pennington, E. (1993). Laparoscopic repair of small bowel, colon, and rectal enterotomies: a report of twenty-six cases. *Surg. Endosc.*, **7**, 88–9

17. Redwine, D.B. and Sharpe, D.R. (1991). Laparoscopic segmental resection of the sigmoid colon for endometriosis. *J. Laparoendosc. Surg.*, **1**, 217–20

18. Sharpe, D.R. and Redwine, D.B. (1992). Laparoscopic segmental resection of the sigmoid and rectosigmoid colon for endometriosis. *Surg. Laparosc. Endosc.*, **2**, 120–4

19. Nezhat, F., Nezhat, C. and Pennington, E. (1992). Laparoscopic proctectomy for infiltrating endometriosis of the rectum. *Fertil. Steril.*, **57**, 1129–32

20. Nezhat, F., Nezhat, C., Pennington, E. and Ambroze, W. (1992). Laparoscopic segmental resection for infiltrating endometriosis of the rectosigmoid colon: a preliminary report. *Surg. Laparosc. Endosc.*, **2**, 212–16

21. Nezhat, C., Nezhat, F. and Nezhat, C. (1992). Operative laparoscopy (minimally invasive surgery): state of the art. *J. Gynecol. Surg.*, **8**, 111–41

22. Nezhat, C. and Nezhat, F. (1991). Incidental appendectomy during videolaseroscopy. *Am. J. Obstet. Gynecol.*, **165**, 559–64

23. Nezhat, C., Nezhat, F. and Winer, W. (1991) Salpingectomy via laparoscopy: a new surgical approach. *J. Laparosc. Surg.*, **1**, 91–5

24. Semm, K. (1987) *Operative Manual for Endoscopic Abdominal Surgery*. (Chicago: Year Book Medical Publishers)

Part 2

Tubal pathology

CO₂ laser laparoscopic surgery: adhesiolysis, salpingostomy and fimbrioplasty

10

J. Donnez, M. Nisolle, F. Casanas-Roux, V. Anaf and S. Bassil

Laser endoscopy has been in established use in otolaryngology, gastroenterology and gynecology for some years. Prototype instruments for CO_2 laser laparoscopy were developed independently on three continents[1-4]. With the development of new laparoscopic instrumentation for CO_2 laser use (Donnez and colleagues, unpublished report), the majority of technical problems have now been overcome.

Several procedures have been carried out with the CO_2 laser laparoscope. The most frequent procedures include the following:

(1) Vaporization of peritoneal and ovarian endometriosis;

(2) Pelvic adhesiolysis, salpingolysis and ovariolysis;

(3) Uterosacral ligament ablation;

(4) Fimbrioplasty and salpingostomy;

(5) Salpingostomy in cases of tubal pregnancy;

(6) Vaporization of small uterine fibroids.

From 1982 to 1991, more than 5500 CO_2 laser laparoscopies were carried out in our department. The most frequent indication was endometriosis[5] (Table 1), which can be vaporized by means of CO_2 laser laparoscopy with a good postoperative pregnancy rate[4,6,7]. Peritubal adhesions ($n = 1113$) and/or tubal occlusion ($n = 612$) (occlusion degree I to IV according to the classification of Donnez and Casanas-Roux[8,9]) represent an important factor in infertility.

Table 1 Indications for CO_2 laser laparoscopy, 1982–1991 ($n = 5500$)

Indication	Number of procedures performed
Tuboplasty	612
fimbrioplasty	501
salpingostomy	111
Pelvic adhesions (salpingolysis or salpingo-ovariolysis)	1113
Endometriosis	2214
LUNA	780
Other	781

LUNA = laser uterine nerve ablation

INSTRUMENTATION AND OPERATIONAL INSTRUCTIONS

Single puncture laser laparoscopy and instrumentation

The operating laparoscope for laser laparoscopy is 12 mm in diameter with a 7.3-mm operating channel (Storz, Germany). To use the CO_2 laser through the laparoscope, the operator simply attaches the articulated arm of the laser to the direct coupler containing the alignment mirror and focusing lens, which transmits the laser beam through the operating channel of the laparoscope. The hook for fimbrioplasty and the probe with a backstop for use in vaporizing adhesions near the blood vessels are two essential instruments for this type of endoscopic surgery.

ADHESIONS

Three types of adhesions must be defined:

(1) Type I (Figure 1(a)–(c)): filmy and avascular adhesions;

(2) Type II (Figure 1(d)–(f)): filmy and vascular adhesions; and

(3) Type III (Figure 1(g)–(i)): dense, fibrous and vascular adhesions.

Adhesiolysis

In many patients, postoperative or postinfectious adhesions are amenable to vaporization by laser laparoscopy. When compared to the standard technique with cautery and the use of laparoscopic scissors or blunt dissection, there is probably no difference in the outcome when the adhesions are small and avascular. With more vascular adhesions or particularly thick tubo-ovarian adhesions, however, the CO_2 laser allows more precise destruction of the adhesions with minimal injury to the adjacent normal tissue. Filmy peritubal and periovarian adhesions are easily vaporized with the operative laser laparoscope. The adhesiolysis probe with its backstop should be used to make the procedure safer. Traction to adhesions must be applied by two atraumatic forceps.

The adhesion is positioned across the 'firing' platform when the laser is activated to prevent damage to any tissue distal to the adhesion.

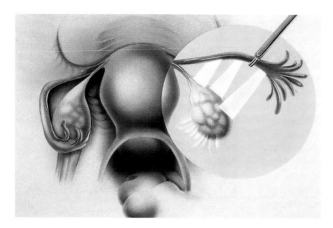

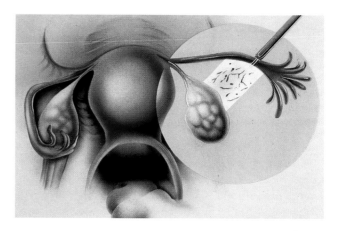

Figure 1 Three types of adhesions are distinguished: (a)–(c) type I, filmy and avascular adhesions; (d)–(f) type II, filmy and vascular adhesions; (g)–(i) type III, dense, fibrous and vascular adhesions

Figure 1(d)   *See legend opposite*

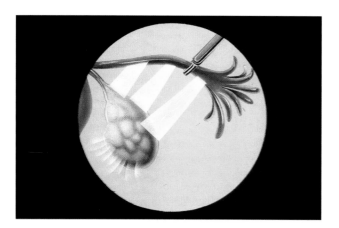

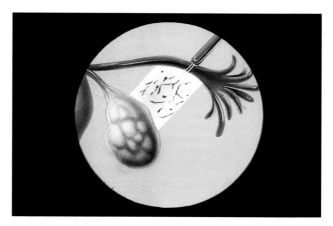

Figure 1(b)   *See legend above*

Figure 1(e)   *See legend above*

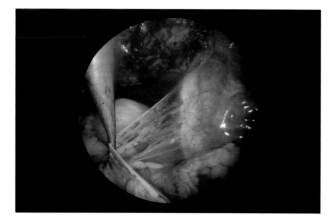

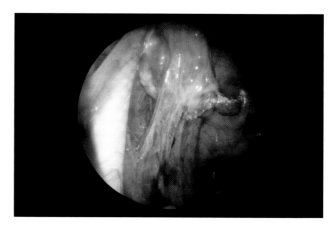

Figure 1(c)   *See legend above*

Figure 1(f)   *See legend above*

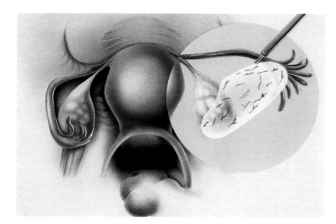

Figure 1(g)   *See legend on opposite page*

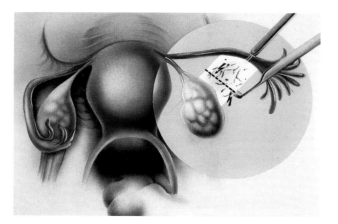

Figure 2(a)–(d)   Salpingolysis is usually performed by applying traction to adhesions by a suprapubic atraumatic grasping forceps and by one or two other probes (probe with the hook or with the backstop)

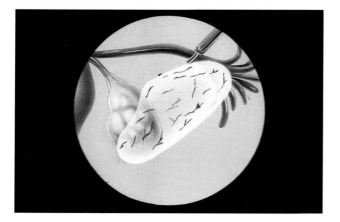

Figure 1(h)   *See legend on opposite page*

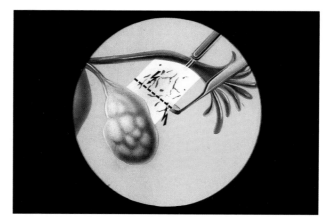

Figure 2(b)   *See legend above*

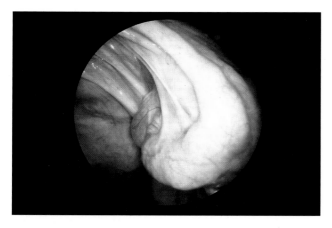

Figure 1(i)   *See legend on opposite page*

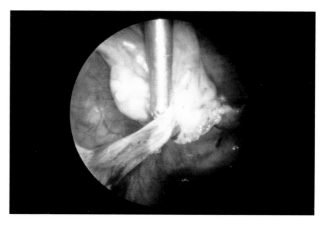

Figure 2(c)   *See legend above*

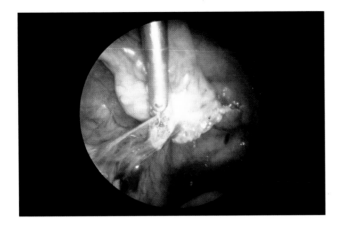

Figure 2(d) *See legend on previous page*

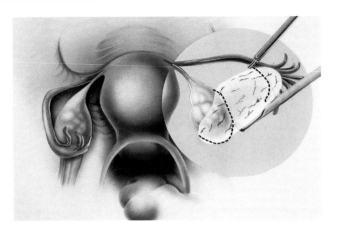

Figure 2(e)–(j) In cases of adhesions of degree III, CO_2 laser is useful to cut dense and fibrous adhesions

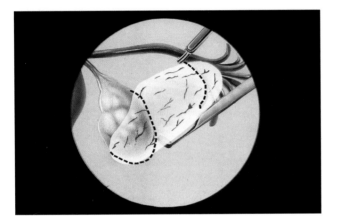

Figure 2(f) *See legend above*

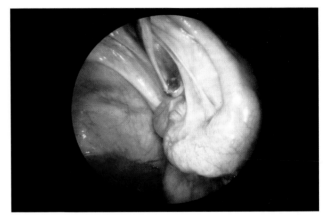

Figure 2(g) *See legend above*

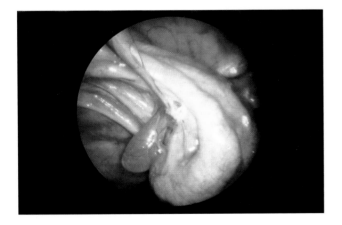

Figure 2(h) *See legend above*

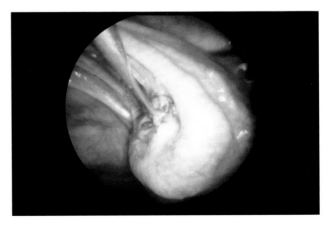

Figure 2(i) *See legend above*

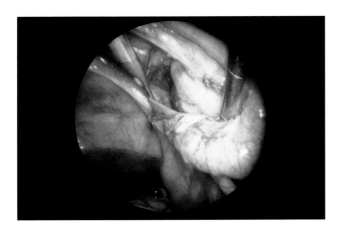

Figure 2(j)   *See legend on opposite page*

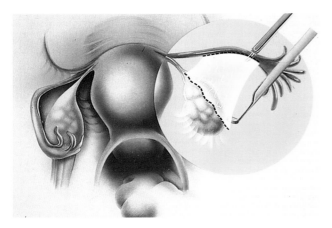

Figure 3(a)–(d)   Ovariolysis is performed by applying traction. Elevation and rotation of the ovary are performed while continuing traction and torsion. A probe with a backstop is used to avoid damage behind the adhesion

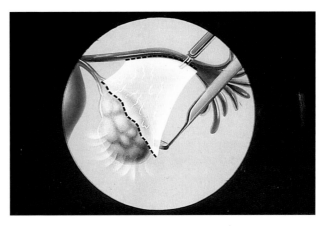

Figure 3(b)   *See legend opposite*

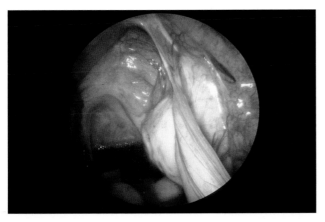

Figure 3(c)   *See legend above*

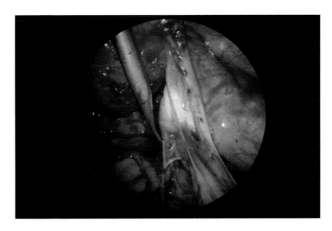

Figure 3(d)   *See legend above*

Using a power output of 40 W, adhesions can be both coagulated and incised. For beginners, single or repeat pulse modes should be used for laser vaporization of the adhesions until confidence in the technique is gained. Great care should be taken when dividing adhesions between the tube and the ovary because this area is very vascular.

Adhesions of degree I (filmy and avascular) and II (dense and vascular, but not very thick) are easily vaporized with the operative laser laparoscope.

Salpingolysis is performed by applying traction to the adhesions by a suprapubic atraumatic grasping forceps and by another probe (smooth manipulating probe, hook, probe with its backstop) (Figure 2). The probe with a backstop can be used to make it easier. When this probe is used, the adhesion is placed across the 'firing' platform and the laser is fired to vaporize the band. The use of the probe with a backstop eliminates the risk of inadvertent injury to intraperitoneal structures.

Using a power output of 40 W, the adhesions are coagulated and incised. Short exposure times are adequate to vaporize the adhesions around the Fallopian tubes and ovaries, and will prevent the laser beam from penetrating more than 100–200 μm. In the hands of more experienced laparoscopists, continuous mode is easily used.

Ovariolysis is performed by applying torsion to the utero-ovarian ligaments with atraumatic tubal forceps (Figure 3). Elevation and rotation of the ovary are performed while continuing traction and torsion. Adhesions can easily be dissected from the ovarian surface by superficial vaporization. Care must also be taken not to apply too much traction for fear of tearing the ovarian ligament from its attachment, which can result in copious bleeding that can only be stopped by hemostatic clips or coagulation.

During adhesiolysis, the use of the probe with a backstop eliminates the risk of inadvertent injury to other intraperitoneal structures, particularly the bowel. Irrigation fluid can be introduced into the pelvis as an aquatic backstop to protect the bowel from any damage from the scatter of the laser beam.

TUBAL OCCLUSION

According to the prognostic factors of functional microsurgery, five degrees must be defined (Figure 4):

(1) Degree 1: phymotic ostium with preserved tubal patency;

(2) Degree 2: total distal occlusion without ampullary dilatation;

(3) Degree 3: ampullary dilatation < 2.5 cm; ampullary folds well-preserved;

(4) Degree 4: hydrosalpinx simplex; dilatation more than 2.5 cm; well-preserved ampullary folds;

(5) Degree 5: thick-walled hydrosalpinx; absence of ampullary folds.

For us[9], the degree of dilatation and the presence of ampullary folds represent the main factors in infertility. Hysterosalpingography permits the evaluation of both the dilatation and the ampullary folds and allows the surgeon to classify preoperatively the tubal pathology.

Tubal occlusion: degree 1

Fimbrioplasty is also carried out during laparoscopy. When fimbrial adhesions are found as the blue dye begins to spill through the open tube, these adhesions between the fimbrial folds are carefully grasped by means of the probe with a hook passed through a third-puncture trocar, and cut in a bloodless fashion with the finely focused CO_2 beam set at 40 W (Figure 5). Thereafter, a defocused beam (10 W) is used in order to cause blanching of the serosa (Figure 6). The SwiftLase (see Chapter 2) is useful for this purpose. This allows adequate eversion of the mucosa and prevents any recurrence of adhesions.

Tubal occlusion: degrees 2, 3 and 4

Salpingostomy (Figure 7) can be performed with the CO_2 laser and is indicated in cases of thin-walled hydrosalpinx where both proximal tubal patency and the presence of ampullary folds have been confirmed by a hysterosalpingogram. In our department, in cases of thick-walled hydrosalpinx without ampullary folds, a salpingectomy is carried out. Two grasping forceps are introduced for traction and manipulation at the ampullary–fimbrial segment. The blocked tube is held so that the focused laser beam can be aligned at a 90° angle to the dimple (Figure 7). The laser is set on continuous mode (40 W) and two linear incisions are made (Figure 8), cutting from anterior to posterior along blood vessels. As soon as the lumen is entered, the tube collapses; continuous dye injection keeps it distended. Only then is the incision enlarged. At this point, the probes and grasping forceps gently hold the incision edges and a reduced-power (10–15 W), defocused beam (SwiftLase) is used to evert the serosal aspect of the incised edge (Figure 9).

The final aspect (Figure 10) of the tube reveals a well everted fimbria. At the end of the procedure, the peritoneal cavity is irrigated with Ringer's solution to remove carbonized particles.

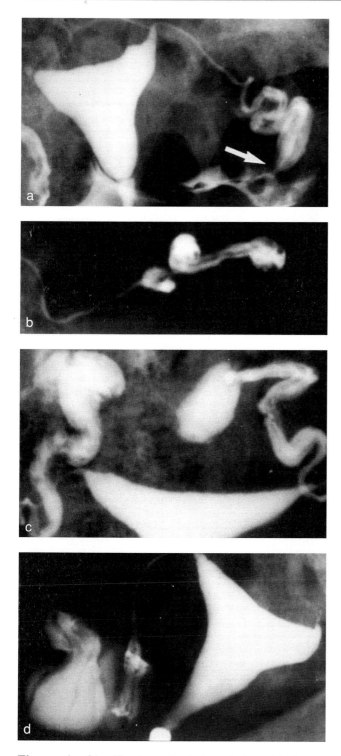

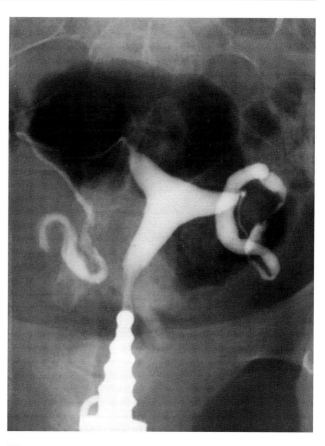

Figure 4(e)   *See legend opposite*

Figure 4   Classification of tubal occlusion: (a) degree 1: phymotic ostium with preserved tubal patency; (b) degree 2: total distal occlusion without ampullary dilatation; (c) degree 3: ampullary dilatation < 2.5 cm, ampullary folds well-preserved; (d) degree 4: hydrosalpinx simplex dilatation more than 2.5 cm, well-preserved ampullary folds; (e) degree 5: thick-walled hydrosalpinx, absence of ampullary folds

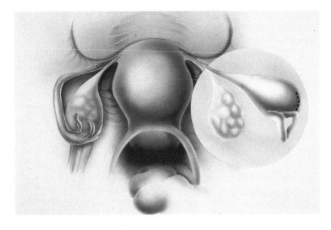

Figure 5(a)–(d)   Fimbrioplasty: the peritoneum covering the ostium is cut by means of the hook

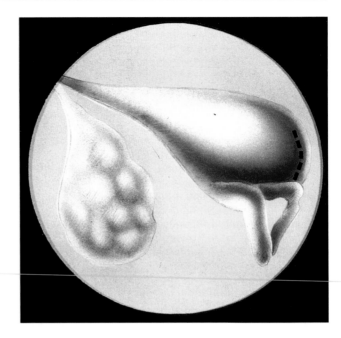

Figure 5(b)   *See legend opposite*

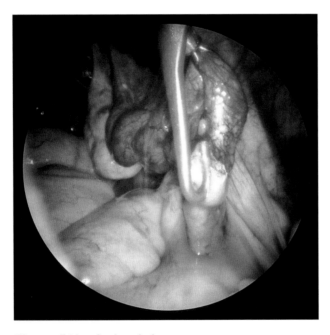

Figure 5(c)   *See legend above*

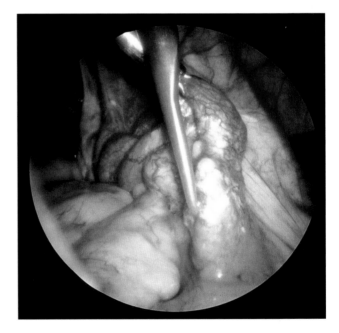

Figure 5(d)   *See legend above*

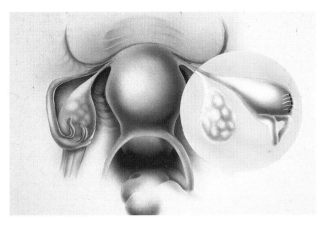

Figure 6(a)–(d) Fimbrioplasty: adequate eversion of the mucosa is allowed by causing blanching of the serosa. The SwiftLase is useful for this purpose

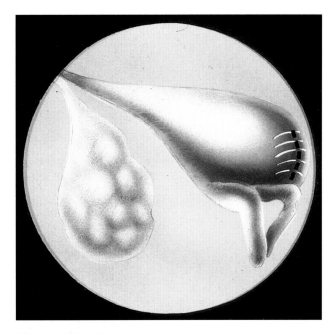

Figure 6(b) *See legend opposite*

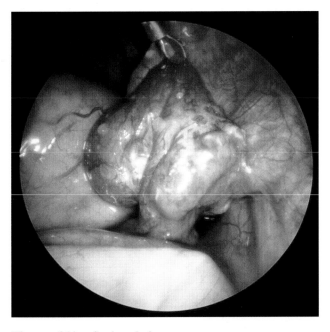

Figure 6(c) *See legend above*

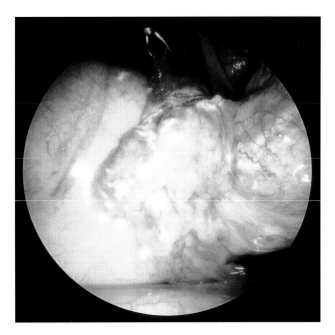

Figure 6(d) *See legend above*

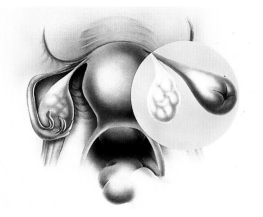

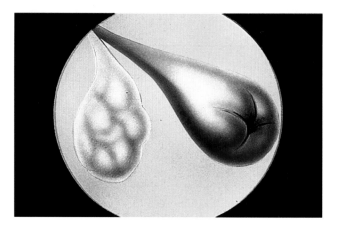

Figure 7(a)–(c) Hydrosalpinx: tubal occlusion of degree 4; hysterography (d) and preoperative vaginal echography (e) reveal the presence of well-preserved ampullary folds

Figure 7(b)   *See legend opposite*

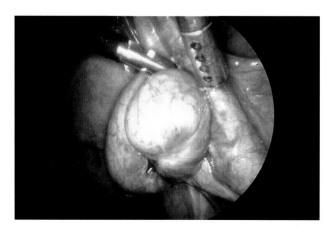

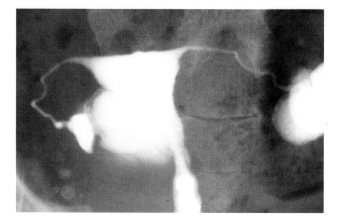

Figure 7(c)   *See legend above*

Figure 7(d)   *See legend above*

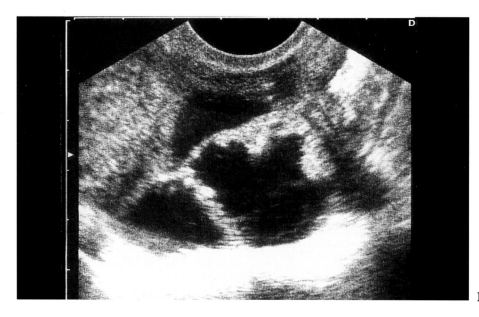

Figure 7(e)   *See legend above*

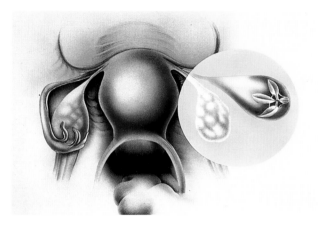

Figure 8(a)–(d) Two linear incisions are made with focused beam

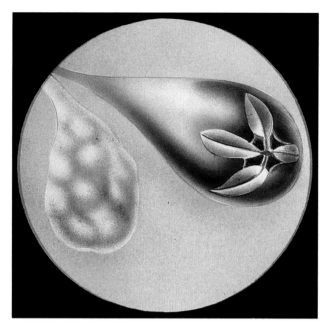

Figure 8(b)   *See legend opposite*

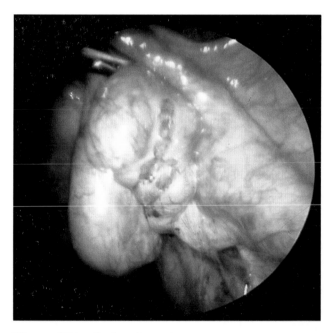

Figure 8(c)   *See legend opposite*

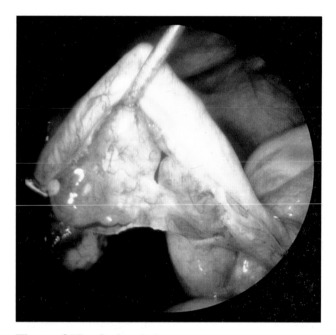

Figure 8(d)   *See legend above*

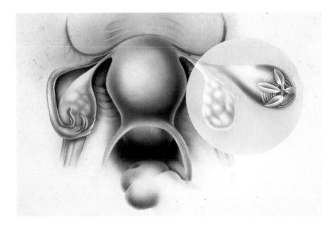

Figure 9(a)–(d)   When the incision is enlarged, defocused beam (with the SwiftLase on) is used to evert the serosal aspect of the incised edge

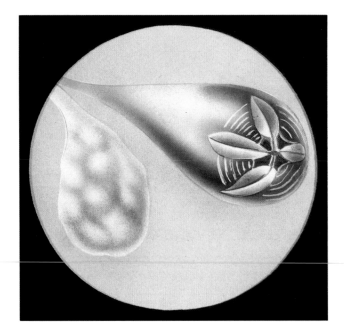

Figure 9(b)   *See legend opposite*

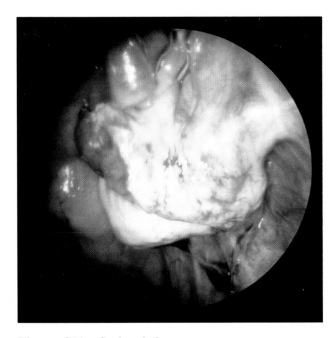

Figure 9(c)   *See legend above*

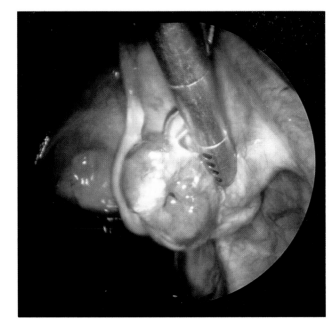

Figure 9(d)   *See legend above*

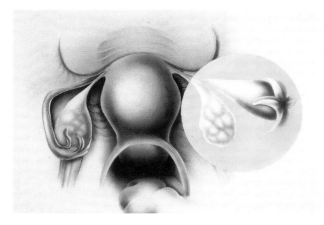

Figure 10(a)–(d) At the end of the procedure, a tuboscopy is not systematically performed, but when performed, as in this case, ampulloscopy reveals the presence of well-vascularized ampullary folds

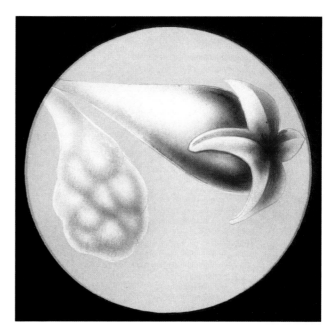

Figure 10(b) *See legend opposite*

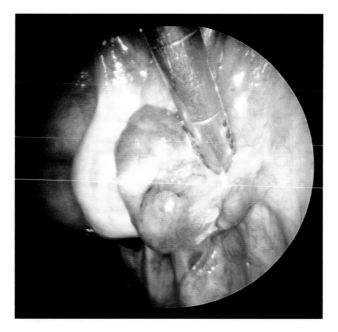

Figure 10(c) *See legend above*

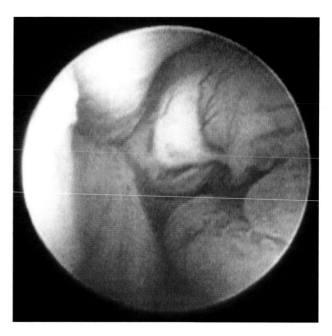

Figure 10(d) *See legend above*

Tubal occlusion: degree 5

In cases of thick-walled hydrosalpinx, the ampullary folds are absent. The pregnancy rate after microsurgery[9] is 0%; for this reason, there is no indication for salpingostomy. We propose a laparoscopic salpingectomy to the patient before an *in vitro* fertilization procedure, in order to avoid the risk of tubal pregnancy after embryo transfer. The technique of endoscopic salpingectomy will be described further in Chapter 11.

RESULTS

Results are shown in Table 2. The pregnancy rate was evaluated for a follow-up period of 18 months. In our series of adhesiolysis, pregnancy rates of 62% and 51% were obtained, respectively, after adhesiolysis for adhesions of degree I (filmy and avascular) and II (dense and vascular but not very thick).

Table 2 Viable pregnancy rate in 1184 patients for a follow-up period of 18 months

	Number of patients	Pregnancies	
		Number	%
Adhesiolysis			
degree I	412	255	62
degree II	307	157	51
Fimbrioplasty	380	228	60
Salpingostomy	85	23	27

After fimbrioplasty, the postoperative pregnancy rate was 60% in a series of 380 patients. This rate was similar to that obtained in a series of 142 fimbrioplasties carried out by microsurgery.

In our department, hysterosalpingography was performed systematically 3 months after laparoscopic salpingostomy. Recovery of a normal tubal pattern was found (Figure 11) when postoperative patency was achieved. A postoperative patency rate of 80% was achieved, with an intrauterine pregnancy rate of 27%.

The operating time varied from 30 to 60 min. All patients were released in good condition the following day. Typical post-laparoscopic pain, such as pelvic discomfort and signs of diaphragmatic irritation, was the most common postoperative complaint. None of the patients experienced any postoperative infection. No patient sustained any urinary bladder damage.

In patients requiring salpingo-ovariolysis, the incision of vascular adhesions was infrequently followed by intraoperative bleeding that required electrocautery. No patient required laparotomy for control of bleeding.

DISCUSSION

Conservative microsurgical procedures for pelvic adhesions and tubal occlusion are efficacious[8-10] (also Donnez and colleagues, unpublished report). Pregnancy rates depend on pre-existent lesions of the tubal mucosa[9]. In this study, surgical treatment via laser laparoscopy was evaluated.

In cases of laser adhesiolysis, the pregnancy rate (58%) was similar to that obtained after microsurgical salpingolysis by laparotomy (56%). In many patients, postoperative or postinfectious adhesions are amenable to vaporization by laser laparoscopy. When compared to the standard technique with cautery and the use of the laparoscopic scissors or blunt dissection, there is probably no difference in the outcome when the adhesions are small and avascular. With more vascular adhesions or particularly thick tubo-ovarian adhesions, however, the CO_2 laser allows more precise destruction of the adhesions with minimal injury to the adjacent normal tissue. The precision of the CO_2 laser allows the experienced operator to vaporize adhesions near the ureter or on the bowel. The magnification obtained with the laparoscope and the precision of the CO_2 laser beam allow precise removal of diseased tissue in many sites often unapproachable by electrocautery.

Laser procedures permit the incision of numerous adhesions by laparoscopy, but adhesiolysis of very dense and fibrous adhesions (degree III) between the fimbria and the ovary is quite difficult. It is well known that adhesions recur very often after adhesiolysis for degree III adhesions. Sometimes the CO_2 laser allows the surgeon to find the plane of dissection more easily than with scissors or electrocautery. However, if the adhesions of degree III are too numerous (frozen pelvis), *in vitro* fertilization must be proposed. In our series of 719 infertile women with pelvic adhesions operated on with the CO_2 laser laparoscope, none required laparotomy for bleeding and no bladder or bowel injury was reported. Investigating clinical gynecological surgical applications with great care, we are able to conclude that, for selected patients, CO_2 laser laparoscopy will become the preferred procedure for the resection of postoperative or postinfectious adhesions.

Results of fimbrioplasty carried out by laparotomy and laparoscopy are similar. Vaporizing fimbrial adhesions is easily done with the CO_2 laser and the operating time is not greater than 20 min. The high pregnancy rate obtained in our study confirms that laser laparoscopic fimbrioplasty must be considered as the procedure of choice in cases of phymotic ostium.

The results of microsurgical salpingostomy for hydrosalpinx are poor[11]. Indeed, a 20–30% term pregnancy rate is generally reported. A classification of distal tubal occlusion has been proposed, according to the ampullary dilatation and the presence of well-preserved ampullary folds[9]. The rate obtained in our

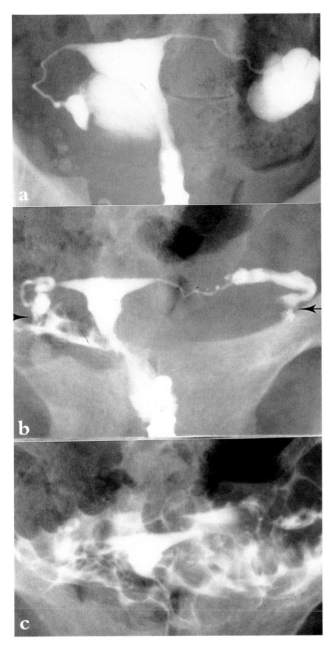

Figure 11 Hysterosalpingography: (a) hydrosalpinx: preoperative evaluation; (b) and (c) 3 months after laparoscopic salpingostomy, bilateral tubal patency is proved

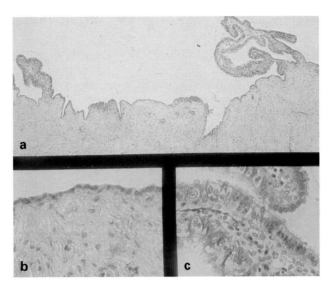

Figure 12 Hydrosalpinx: (a) flattened epithelium between the ampullary folds; (b) a normal percentage of ciliated cells is observed in the ampullary folds; (c) between the ampullary folds, ciliated cells are mostly absent

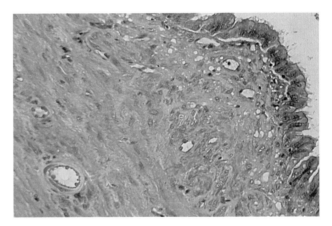

Figure 13 Hydrosalpinx: fibrosis of the tubal muscularis due to connective tissue

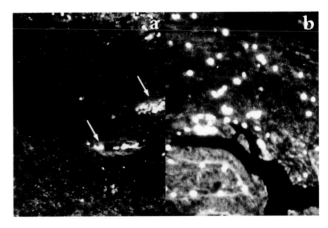

Figure 14 Hydrosalpinx: adrenegic denervation is observed in dilated tubal wall (a) when compared to the normal tube (b)

series is similar to that obtained by laparotomy and microsurgery. Laser salpingostomy by laparoscopy is the ideal procedure for the management of the large hydrosalpinx.

As for microsurgery, the prognosis of endoscopic surgery is related to pre-existent tubal pathology: the percentage of ciliated cells (Figure 12), muscularis fibrosis (Figure 13) and adrenergic denervation (Figure 14).

Other advantages found in the study were:

(1) The precision achieved by the CO_2 laser allows the experienced operator to vaporize adhesions close to the ureter or even on the bowel;

(2) The magnification obtained with the laparoscope and the precision of the CO_2 laser allow precise removal of diseased tissue in many sites often unapproachable by electrocautery[12].

In conclusion, by reducing the hospitalization time and the morbidity rate, CO_2 laser laparoscopy offers several advantages over other operative techniques for the treatment of adhesions and tubal occlusion.

REFERENCES

1. Bruhat, M., Mage, G. and Manhes, M. (1979). Use of the CO_2 laser in laparoscopy. In Kaplan, I. (ed.) *Proceedings of the Third International Society for Laser Surgery*, pp.235–8. September 24–28, 1979, Tel Aviv

2. Tadir, Y., Kaplan, I., Zuckerman, Z., Edelstein, T. and Ovadia, J. (1984). New instrumentation and technique for laparoscopic carbon dioxide laser operations: a preliminary report. *Obstet. Gynecol.*, **63**, 582

3. Daniell, J.F. and Brown, D.H. (1982). Carbon dioxide laser laparoscopy: initial experience in experimental animals and humans. *Obstet. Gynecol.*, **59**, 761

4. Kelly, R.W. and Roberts, D.K. (1983). Experience with the CO_2 laser in gynecologic microsurgery. *Am. J. Obstet. Gynecol.*, **146**, 585

5. Donnez, J. (1987). CO_2 laser laparoscopy in infertile women with endometriosis and women with adnexal adhesions. *Fertil. Steril.*, **48**, 390

6. Nezhat, C., Crowgey, S.R. and Garrison, C.P. (1986). Surgical treatment of endometriosis via laser laparoscopy. *Fertil. Steril.*, **45**, 778

7. Donnez, J. (1987). CO_2 laser laparoscopy in tubal infertility. In Donnez, J. (ed.) *CO_2 Laser in Intraepithelial Neoplasia and in Infertility*. (Leuven: Nauwelaerts Printing)

8. Donnez, J. (1984). In Donnez, J. (ed.) *La Trompe de Fallope: Histophysiologie normale et Pathologique*, p.105. (Leuven: Nauwelaerts Printing Publisher)

9. Donnez, J. and Casanas-Roux, F. (1986). Prognostic factors of fimbrial microsurgery. *Fertil. Steril.*, **46**, 200

10. Donnez, J. (1985). Microchirurgie et fécondation *in vitro*: méthodes concurrentes ou complémentaires? *Rev. Med. Brux.*, **6**, 627

11. Daniell, J.F. and Feste, J.R. (1985). Laser laparoscopy. In Keye, W.R. Jr (ed.) *Laser Surgery in Gynecology and Obstetrics*, pp.147–63 (Boston)

12. Donnez, J., Fernandez, C., Willems, T. and Casanas-Roux, F. (1987). Experimental ovarian CO_2 laser surgery. In Donnez, J. (ed.) *CO_2 Laser in Intraepithelial Neoplasia and in Infertility*, p.25. (Leuven: Nauwelaerts Printing)

Surgical and non-surgical techniques in the management of ectopic pregnancy

11

J. Donnez and M. Nisolle

Ectopic gestation affects a large segment of the fertile population, and its incidence has been steadily increasing in recent years. The aim of this chapter is to describe the surgical and non-surgical techniques in the management of ectopic pregnancy.

NON-CONSERVATIVE SURGICAL TECHNIQUES: SALPINGECTOMY

Salpingectomy, the traditional treatment for tubal gestation, results in a significant reduction in fertility without a parallel decrease in the rate of recurrent ectopic pregnancy. Classically, treatment of tubal ectopic pregnancy has involved salpingectomy. However, by 1989, salpingectomy was being carried out for only a few indications and was no longer considered as the primary approach of therapy.

Indications for salpingectomy

Indications for salpingectomy can be classified as in Table 1.

Table 1 Indications for salpingectomy

Absolute indications:

A ruptured ectopic gestation with irreparable damage
An ectopic gestation occurring after an *in vitro* fertilization (IVF) procedure in thick-walled hydrosalpinx
In hemodynamically unstable patients, to control the bleeding site as soon as possible

Relative indications:

A severely scarred tube with a high risk of subsequent ectopic pregnancy
Uncontrollable bleeding during attempted conservative management
The occurrence of a repeat ectopic pregnancy in a tube previously treated conservatively
In women planning to be or already involved in attempts at *in vitro* fertilization; in this group, salpingectomy reduces the risk of development of an ectopic gestation following an IVF attempt
In women who no longer desire fertility
In women with ectopic pregnancy who had previously undergone a sterilization procedure

---

Salpingectomy for the treatment of an ectopic pregnancy is performed at the time of laparoscopy. This can be done using one of these three techniques:

(1) The suture ligatures of Semm[1];

(2) Coagulation of the vessels underlying the Fallopian tube and the mesosalpinx either by electrocautery or by thermocoagulation or with the CO_2 laser (Figure 1). After the vessels have been coagulated, the tissue can be excised with scissors or with the CO_2 laser (Figure 2). The tube is then removed from the abdominal cavity through the channel of the operative laparoscope;

(3) Stapling: this method is too expensive and does not offer any advantage.

CONSERVATIVE SURGICAL TECHNIQUES

In 1953, Stromme[2] described for the first time a conservative surgical approach to the treatment of tubal gestation. The improvement of diagnostic modalities and microsurgical instrumentation has enabled a widespread use of conservative techniques. The rationale for conservative management is the preservation of reproductive potential. Therefore, a conservative therapeutic approach should be attempted.

The objective of the conservative treatment of ectopic gestation is the removal of the products of conception, while inflicting as little damage as possible to the involved tube. The 'appropriate' management of ectopic pregnancy will potentially vary according to the desires of the patient, the location of the ectopic gestation and the anatomical status of the pelvis.

Ectopic gestations can be present in any one of the four portions of the Fallopian tube: infundibular or fimbrial portion, ampullary segment, isthmic segment or the cornua. The methods of treatment, while partially overlapping, will vary with the location of the ectopic gestation.

Diagnostic laparoscopy should always be considered when the diagnosis of ectopic gestation is contemplated, except when the patient is hemodynamically unstable. At the time of laparoscopy, a definitive diagnosis of tubal gestation is usually possible. In a patient who desires future fertility, the most conservative procedure should be attempted whenever possible.

The choice of surgical technique will be determined by various considerations:

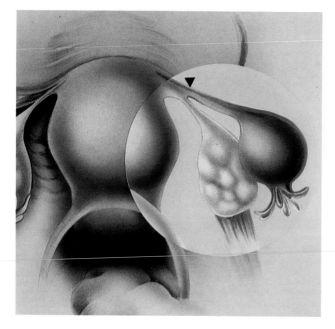

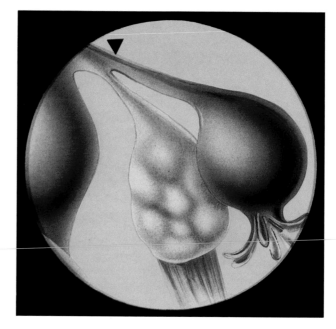

Figure 1(a)–(d) Salpingectomy: coagulation of the isthmic portion of the Fallopian tube

Figure 1(b) *See legend opposite*

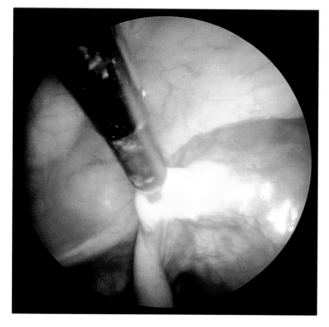

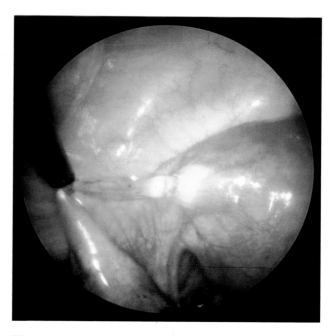

Figure 1(c) *See legend above*

Figure 1(d) *See legend above*

(1) The condition of the tube (ruptured, unruptured);

(2) The location of the gestation within the tube (interstitium, isthmus, ampulla);

(3) The size of the gestation (≤ 5 cm, > 5 cm);

(4) The accessibility (presence of adhesions);

(5) The occurrence of complications (uncontrollable bleeding).

Ampullary (and infundibular) pregnancy

The most common site for a tubal ectopic gestation is the ampullary segment of the Fallopian tube (Figure 3).

Linear salpingotomy by laparoscopy

Two trocars are inserted:

(1) The grasping forceps is inserted on the side contralateral to the site of tubal pregnancy. It is used for the introduction of atraumatic grasping forceps for stabilization of the tube.

(2) The operative instruments are inserted through the lateral puncture site. The lateral trocar can then be replaced with a 10-mm sleeve for evacuation of tissue.

First, a linear salpingotomy is performed over the proximal portion of the dilated segment of the tube. The salpingotomy incision should be made along the anti-mesenteric tubal border over the ectopic gestation. The linear salpingotomy can be achieved with a monopolar needle (TRITON®)[3] or with the CO_2 laser (Figure 4).

A second, more recent addition is the use of the laser to make the salpingotomy incision. This can be accomplished with a CO_2, argon, KTP-532, or Nd : YAG laser. The CO_2 laser has the shallowest depth of penetration into the target tissue and results in minimal damage to adjacent structures; however, its hemostatic properties are poorer than those of the other lasers. The properties reflect the effect of the CO_2 laser beam on tissue surfaces, which is primarily a vaporization action. In contrast, the other three types of laser exert their effect by coagulating protein and possessing more efficacious hemostatic properties.

Compared to the depth of penetration of the CO_2 laser of approximately 0.1 mm, the argon and KTP-532 laser beams penetrate approximately 1–2 mm and the Nd : YAG laser, 4–5 mm. Moreover, the greater lateral dispersion of the laser beam observed with the argon, KTP-532 and Nd : YAG laser may also result in greater damage to the tubal lumen or other pelvic structures.

The incision made along the antimesenteric border of the Fallopian tube should extend over a sufficient length to allow the removal of the products of conception (Figure 4).

Since the products of conception are under pressure, they will usually extrude spontaneously, or can be removed easily by suction through the operative probe (Triton, large suction cannula, Figure 5) after copious irrigation with saline solution (Figure 6). The Triton is also successfully used to perform the incision (Figure 7).

The ectopic site should be irrigated carefully with either saline solution or Ringer's lactate and any remaining tissue should be removed gently from the ectopic bed.

Pitressin and hemostasis

In an attempt to minimize bleeding from the operative site or the ectopic site, some surgeons routinely inject a diluted pitressin solution along the operative site before performing the salpingotomy incision. This has the advantage of decreasing blood flow to the operative area.

However, this might reduce the bleeding only temporarily, so that clinically significant bleeding could occur after completion of the operative procedure. We prefer to perform the salpingotomy incision without an injection of pitressin, but if bleeding persists, vasopressin 5 IU in 20 ml of saline solution can be injected into the mesosalpinx of the tubal wall. This occurred in less than 10% of cases in our series of 500 (Figure 8).

Our data proved that an injection of pitressin before salpingotomy was unnecessary in more than 90% of cases. If these measures fail to provide hemostasis, hemostasis can be accomplished with careful coagulation by electrocautery or laser.

Removal of products of conception from the peritoneal cavity

The removal of a large bulk of tissue through a small trocar sleeve can be a frustrating experience. Various techniques can be used to facilitate this process:

(1) Retrieval of the tissue with grasping forceps introduced through the operating channel of the laparoscope, and removal of the grasping forceps and laparoscope as one unit;

(2) Insertion of long Kocher forceps instead of a trocar through the suprapubic incision;

(3) Division of the tissue intra-abdominally and its removal in pieces;

(4) Insertion of a trocar (12 mm in diameter) and removal through a large probe (12 mm in diameter) for irrigation and suction.

Closure or non-closure of the tubal incision

Bruhat and colleagues[3], DeCherney and co-workers[4], and Donnez[5] leave the operative site open after laparoscopic salpingotomy.

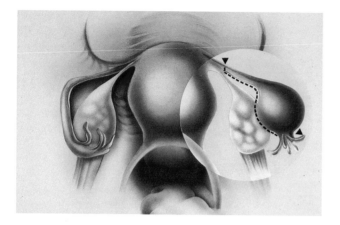

Figure 2(a) and (b) After the proximal and distal vessels are coagulated, the tissue may be excised with scissors or with CO_2 laser

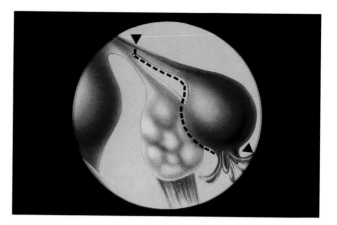

Figure 2(b) *See legend opposite*

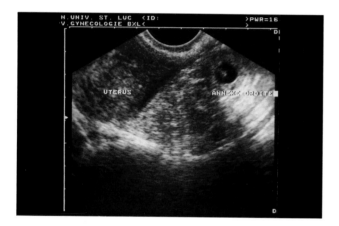

Figure 3 Vaginal echography rarely reveals the presence of an embryo in the Fallopian tube

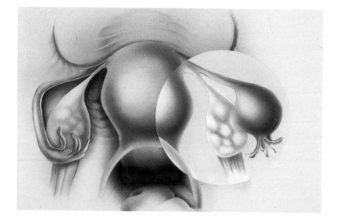

Figure 4(a) and (b) Laparoscopic view; (c)–(i) a linear salpingotomy is carried out along the antimesenteric tubal border over the ectopic gestation with the CO_2 laser. Note that the incision must be carried over the proximal portion of the dilated tubal portion

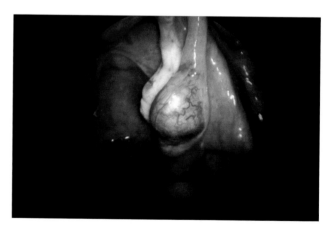

Figure 4(b) *See legend opposite*

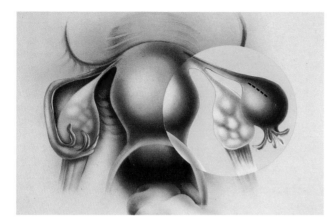

Figure 4(c)   *See legend on opposite page*

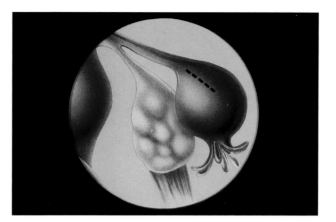

Figure 4(d)   *See legend on opposite page*

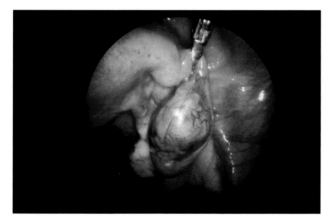

Figure 4(e)   *See legend on opposite page*

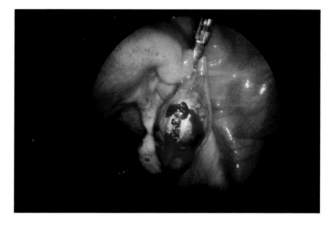

Figure 4(f)   *See legend on opposite page*

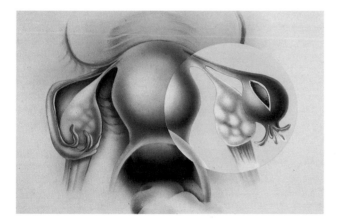

Figure 4(g)   *See legend on opposite page*

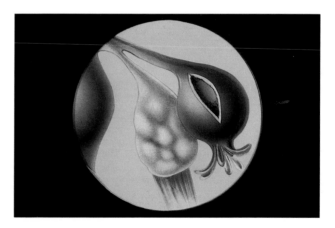

Figure 4(h)   *See legend on opposite page*

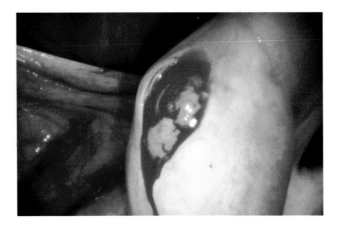

Figure 4(i)   *See legend on p.116*

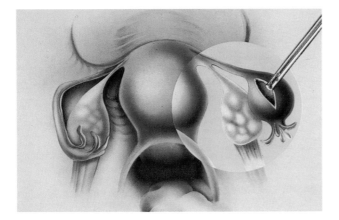

Figure 5(a)–(d)   The products of conception are removed by suction through the operative probe

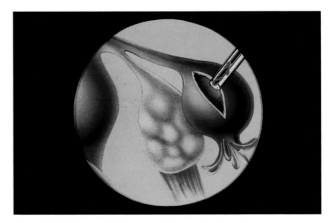

Figure 5(b)   *See legend opposite*

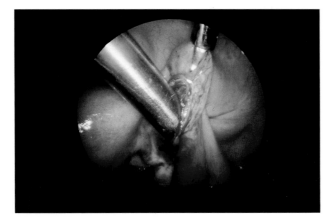

Figure 5(c)   *See legend above*

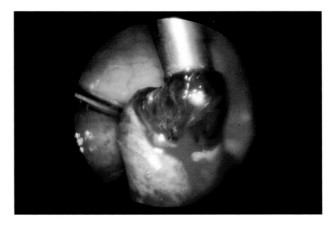

Figure 5(d)   *See legend above*

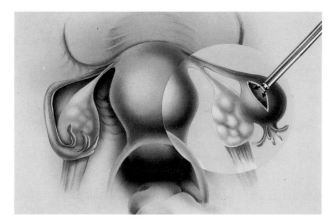

Figure 6(a)–(c)   Copious irrigation with saline solution

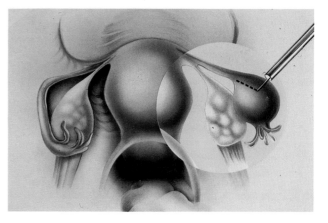

Figure 7(a)–(c)   The Triton® can also be used for the salpingotomy incision

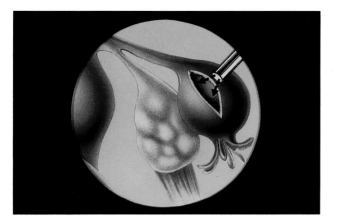

Figure 6(b)   *See legend above*

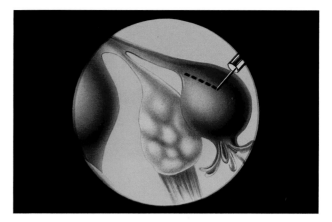

Figure 7(b)   *See legend above*

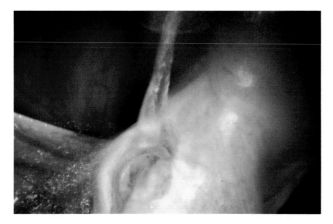

Figure 6(c)   *See legend above*

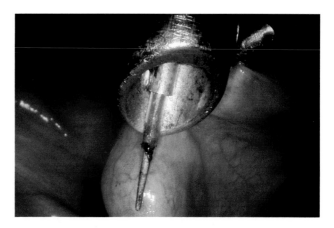

Figure 7(c)   *See legend above*

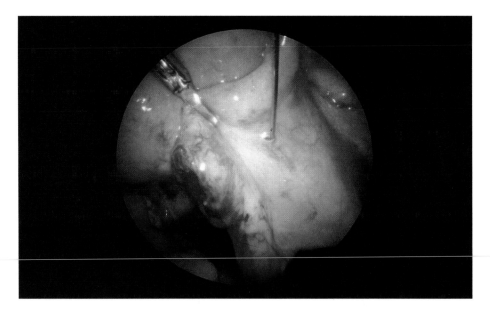

Figure 8 Vasopressin (5 IU in 20 ml of saline solution) is injected into the mesosalpinx beneath the tubal pregnancy site *only* if bleeding persists. It occurs in less than 10% of cases

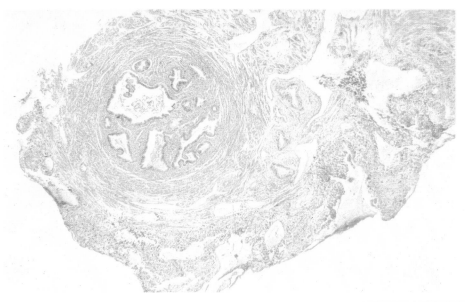

Figure 9 Tubal isthmus: microscopic aspect of the isthmic portion proximal to the implantation site. The tubal lumen is divided by fusion of the fimbriae folds. This represents the causal factor. (Gomori's trichrome × 25)

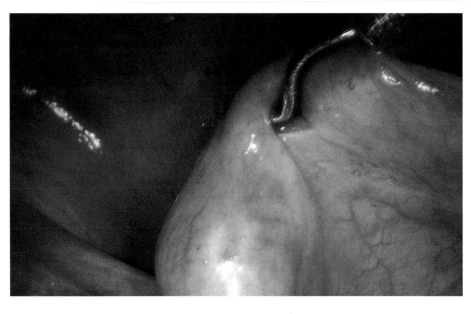

Figure 10 Isthmic tubal pregnancy

Semm[1] described a laparoscopic method of reapproximation with the Ethiendosuture using the extracorporeal knot. Reich and associates[6] initially used bipolar forceps to pinch the edges together; however, they later abandoned this technique.

Nelson and colleagues[7] compared the primary and secondary closure of ampullary salpingotomy in the rabbit and found no statistically significant difference in subsequent pregnancy rates, nidation index, or percentages of adhesions. According to these data, it seems reasonable to conclude that primary closure of the tubal wall is unnecessary.

Regardless of whether or not the linear salpingotomy incision is closed, postoperative assessment by hysterosalpingogram will routinely demonstrate a patent tube. Observations at subsequent operative procedures have demonstrated that the incision will heal even if not primarily closed[8,9].

Isthmic tubal pregnancy

Isthmic tubal pregnancy can also be treated by laparoscopy.

Segmental resection (partial salpingectomy)

Segmental resection is the most appropriate technique for a ruptured, but also for an unruptured isthmic gestation. In such cases, it may be preferable to a linear salpingotomy, since the site of ectopic gestation represents an area of pre-existent tubal pathology (Figure 9). Furthermore, it has been shown that the developing trophoblast infiltrates into the tubal wall, between the muscularis and serosa, and is not confined solely to the lumen[10].

After aspiration of the hemoperitoneum, the part of the tube containing the gestation product is grasped and elevated (Figure 10). The tube proximal and distal to the ectopic pregnancy is coagulated with bipolar forceps and then cut with scissors or the laser. The mesosalpinx is then coagulated and cut in a similar fashion. The segment is removed entirely or in pieces through a 10-mm sleeve, as previously described.

Linear salpingotomy

In such cases, linear salpingotomy is a less attractive option because of the potential for profuse bleeding and because of poor subsequent postoperative patency rates.

Cornual tubal pregnancy

Cornual tubal pregnancy is, in our opinion, the only indication for laparotomy in some cases.

Laparotomy

The cornual ectopic pregnancy is the least common of the four tubal sites for an ectopic gestation to be located. These ectopic gestations are most often treated by surgical excision, which at times necessitates the removal of a portion of the myometrium as well. This raises concern for possible uterine rupture if a subsequent pregnancy is achieved; thus, the mass of tissue excised must be kept to a minimum.

After a cornual ectopic pregnancy, anastomosis is usually not possible, and an implantation procedure is required for restoration of tubal patency with a poor postoperative intrauterine pregnancy rate.

Laparoscopy

Sometimes, after copious irrigation and suction, the removal of the products of conception can be carried out by laparoscopy. Cornual injection of diluted vasopressin (5 IU/20 ml saline solution) and coagulation of the implantation site are often necessary to stop the bleeding. An injection of methotrexate (20 mg) in the site of implantation can be useful. Laparoscopic techniques must be used only in cases of cornual pregnancy where the site of implantation is the distal portion of the intramural tube.

CONSERVATIVE NON-SURGICAL TREATMENT

Recently, several non-surgical methods have been employed, with varying degrees of success, in the treatment of small, unruptured tubal gestations. The development of sensitive and rapid assays for human chorionic gonadotropin (hCG) and improved ultrasound technology facilitate early diagnosis. These modalities include:

(1) Expectant management;

(2) Methotrexate;

(3) RU 486; and

(4) Prostaglandins.

Expectant management

Expectant management was practised as early as 1955 by Lund[11]. However, out of 119 patients thus treated, 51 subsequently required surgical intervention. Two patients died in a series of women treated by Wone[12]. In this series, 90% of 800 cases of possible ectopic pregnancy were treated with Chinese medicinal plants.

More recent reports[13-15] of the spontaneous resolution of ectopic gestation have suggested that surgery may not be necessary in certain cases. However, tubal occlusion occurs in about 30% of cases.

Fernandez and co-workers[15] treated expectantly 14 women with a laparoscopically confirmed diagnosis of ectopic gestation. The inclusion criteria included a hematosalpinx < 2 cm in diameter in the ampulla, and a hemoperitoneum < 50 ml. Among the 14 women, 4 required reoperation.

Gomel and Filmar[16] demonstrated that chorionic villi are capable of surviving and causing tubal destruction for at least 15 months after the termination of a pregnancy. Expectant management may also be associated with an inflammatory reaction at the site of the ectopic gestation. Moreover, intra-abdominal bleeding can occur. For these reasons, expectant management is not the treatment of choice for patients desiring future fertility.

Methotrexate

Methotrexate has been known for years to be effective in the treatment of trophoblastic disease. The first reports of methotrexate therapy for extrauterine gestations were in cases of abdominal pregnancies.

The treatment of unruptured tubal gestations with this folinic acid antagonist was suggested in 1982 by Tanaka and colleagues[17], who treated an unruptured interstitial gestation with intramuscular methotrexate, with the subsequent preservation of tubal patency.

Ory and associates[18] reported the complete resolution of seven unruptured ectopic gestations within 5–50 days of a single course of methotrexate (1.0 mg/kg intramuscularly) and citrovorumfactor (0.1 mg/kg). The same group of investigators reported the results of 21 patients treated by the same protocol. All, except one with intra-abdominal bleeding, resolved without surgery. They concluded that methotrexate may be used safely to treat selected (≤ 3 cm) unruptured ectopic gestations.

Ichinoe and colleagues[19] treated 23 patients with intramuscular injections of methotrexate (0.4 mg/kg/day for 5 days) every other week. Resolution of the ectopic gestation was obtained by 22 patients (95.7%) within 6–47 days (mean, 29.7 days). Oviduct patency was confirmed by hysterosalpingography or laparoscopy in 10 out of 19 patients (52.6%). Severe side-effects were not observed.

Pansky and colleagues[20] completed the treatment of more than 100 such patients with unruptured tubal pregnancy with very favorable results and only a 17% failure rate.

Mottla and co-workers[21] recently reported preliminary results of a randomized trial for treatment of ectopic pregnancy. This trial comparing surgical laparoscopic treatment to medical treatment via laparoscopy was stopped because of poor results in the medical group.

Fernandez and associates[22] comparing two regimens (methotrexate 0.5 and 1 mg/kg), demonstrated that the more appropriate dose was 1 mg/kg, and the best way of administration was by transvaginal injection under sonographic control. They found by using a 0.5 mg/kg dose, that an additional intramuscular injection of methotrexate was frequently needed because hCG titers failed to decrease. They demonstrated in a series of 95 medically treated patients that hCG titers returned to pretreatment values only on day 8 after the injection of methotrexate, whereas an initial rise was always observed. This initial increase in the hCG level could be explained by two phenomena: the acceleration of hCG metabolism under the methotrexate effect, and the necrosis of trophoblastic cells with the release of free hCG into the circulation. Moreover, the return of hCG titers to < 10 mIU/ml occurs within a mean of 28 days[23]. Kooi and Kock[24] considered that the comparison of future fertility rates is possible only in large patient groups because of the need for stratification of other fertility-influencing factors.

Further studies are needed to determine whether or not treatment with methotrexate is a safer option than laparoscopic surgery and to compare the subsequent intrauterine and recurrent ectopic pregnancy rates. In our opinion, methotrexate must be considered only as an adjuvant medical therapy in cases of incomplete removal of trophoblast and not as the primary approach.

RU 486

This antiprogesterone has been shown recently to be an effective abortifacient. In the process of demonstrating the effectiveness of this agent as an abortifacient, however, there have been some failed attempts wherein tubal gestation was later discovered[25,26]. In addition, a single attempt at treating a patient with residual ectopic pregnancy also met with failure.

Prostaglandins

There have been no randomized clinical studies of the treatment of ectopic pregnancy with prostaglandins. However, in vitro administration of prostaglandin $F_{2\alpha}$ ($PGF_{2\alpha}$) has been shown to induce a marked increase in the activity of tubal musculature, and a reduction of the hCG-induced increase in prostesterone production by the corpus luteum[27]. These results suggest that $PGF_{2\alpha}$ may be useful in the medical treatment of ectopic pregnancy.

CONCLUSION

Conservative treatment of ectopic pregnancy is increasingly common. A recent review by Maruri and Azziz[28] clearly demonstrated that laparoscopic surgery was not only a safe procedure, but also resulted in a saving of direct medical costs, including reduced hospitalization time, decreased nursing care and decreased drug usage.

REFERENCES

1. Semm, K. and Mettler, L. (1980). Technical progress in pelvic surgery via operative laparoscopy. *Am. J. Obstet. Gynecol.*, **138**, 121–7
2. Stromme, W.B. (1953). Salpingostomy for tubal pregnancy: report of a successful case. *Obstet. Gynecol.*, **87**, 757
3. Bruhat, M.A., Mahnes, H., Mage, G. and Pouly, J.L. (1980). Treatment of ectopic pregnancy by means of laparoscopy. *Fertil. Steril.*, **33**, 411
4. Decherney, A.H., Romero, R. and Naftolin, F. (1981). Surgical management of unruptured ectopic pregnancy. *Fertil. Steril.*, **35**, 21
5. Donnez, J. (1982). Conservative treatment of ectopic pregnancy. A first series of 50 cases. *Acta Endosc.*, **4**, 62
6. Reich, H., Freifeld, M.L., McGlynn, F. and Reich, E. (1987). Laparoscopic treatment of tubal pregnancy. *Obstet. Gynecol.*, **69**, 275
7. Nelson, L.M., Margara, R.A. and Winston, R.M.L. (1986). Primary and secondary closure of ampullary salpingotomy compared in the rabbit. *Fertil. Steril.*, **45**, 292
8. Donnez, J. and Nisolle, M. (1989). Laparoscopic treatment of amupullary tubal pregnancy. *J. Gynecol. Surg.*, **5**, 19
9. Pouly, J.L., Manhes, H., Mage, G., Canis, M. and Bruhat, M.A. (1986). Conservative laparoscopic treatment of 321 ectopic pregnancies. *Fertil. Steril.*, **46**, 1093
10. Donnez, J. (1984). La trope de Fallope. In Donnez, J. (ed.) *Histophysiologie Normale et Pathologique.* (Leuven: Nauwelaerts Printing)
11. Lund, J. (1955). Early ectopic pregnancy. Comments on conservative treatment. *J. Obstet. Gynecol. Br. Commonw.*, **62**, 395
12. Wone, I. (1979). Traitement de la grossesse extra-utérine par la combinaison de la médecine traditionnelle chinoise et de la médecine moderne. *Dakar Med.*, **24**, 119
13. Mashiach, S., Carp, J.H.A. and Serr, D.M. (1982). Nonoperative management of ectopic pregnancy. *J. Reprod. Med.*, **27**, 127
14. Garcia, A.J., Aubert, J.M., Sama, J. and Josimovich, J.B. (1987). Expectant management of presumed ectopic pregnancies. *Fertil. Steril.*, **48**, 395
15. Fernadez, J., Rainhorn, J.D., Papiernik, E., Bellet, D. and Frydman, R. (1988). Spontaneous resolution of ectopic pregnancy. *Obstet. Gynecol.*, **71**, 171
16. Gomel, V. and Filmar, S. (1987). Arrested tubal pregnancy. *Fertil. Steril.*, **48**, 1043
17. Tanaka, T., Hayashi, H., Kutsuzawa, T., Fujimoto, S. and Ichinoe, K. (1982). Treatment of interstitial ectopic pregnancy with methotrexate: report of a successful case. *Fertil. Steril.*, **37**, 851
18. Ory, S.J., Villanueva, A.L., Sand, P.K. and Tamura, R.K. (1986). Conservative treatment of ectopic pregnancy with methotrexate. *Am. J. Obstet. Gynecol.*, **154**, 1299
19. Ichinoe, K., Wake, N., Shinkai, N., Shiina, Y., Miyazaki, Y. and Tanaka, T. (1987). Nonsurgical therapy to preserve oviduct function in patients with tubal pregnancies. *Am. J. Obstet. Gynecol.*, **156**, 484
20. Pansky, M., Golan, A., Bukovsky, I. and Caspi, E. (1993). Critical comparisons of alternative therapies for ectopic pregnancy. *Fertil. Steril.*, **59**, 244
21. Mottla, G.L., Rulin, M.C. and Guzick, D.S. (1992). Lack of resolution of ectopic pregnancy by intra-tubal injection of methotrexate. *Fertil. Steril.*, **57**, 685
22. Fernandez, H., Baton, C., Lelaidier, C. and Frydman, R. (1991). Conservative management of ectopic pregnancy: prospective randomized clinical trial of methotrexate versus prostaglandin sulfrostone by combined transvaginal and systemic administration. *Fertil. Steril.*, **55**, 746–50
23. Fernandez, H. and Lelaidier, C. (1993). Critical comparison of alternative therapies for ectopic pregnancy. *Fertil. Steril.*, **59**, 246
24. Kooi, S. and Kock, H.C.L.V. (1991). Treatment of tubal pregnancy by local injection of methotrexate after adrenaline injection into the mesosalpinx: a report of 25 patients. *Obstet. Gynecol. Surv.*, **3**, 185
25. Kovacs, L., Sa, S.M., Resch, B.A., Ugocsai, A. Swahn, M.L., Bydeman, M. and Rowe, P.J. (1981). Termination of very early pregnancy by RU 486-antiprogestatio compound. *Contraception*, **29**, 399
26. Keningsberg, D., Porte, J., Hull, M. and Spitz, I.M. (1987). Medical treatment of residual ectopic pregnancy: RU 486 and methotrexate. *Fertil. Steril.*, **47**, 702
27. Croxatto, H.B., Ortiz, M.E., Guiloff, E., Ibarra, A., Salvatierra, A.M., Croxatto, H.D. and Spilman, C.H. (1978). Effect of 15(s)-15-methyl prostaglandin F2α on human oviductual motility and ovum transport. *Fertil. Steril.*, **30**, 408
28. Maruri, F. and Azziz, R. (1993). Laparoscopic surgery for ectopic pregnancy: technology assessment and public health implications. *Fertil. Steril.*, **59**, 487

Laparoscopic management of ectopic pregnancy: a 500-case evaluation

12

G. Mage, J.L. Pouly, M. Canis, A. Wattiez, C. Chapron and M.A. Bruhat

The combination of sensitive human chorionic gonado-tropin (hCG) assays and ultrasonography makes an early diagnosis of ectopic pregnancy possible. Progress in operative laparoscopy allows an endoscopic manage-ment of ectopic pregnancy[1-3]. From 1974 to 1987, 500 cases of ectopic pregnancy were treated by laparoscopic procedures by our team.

MATERIALS AND METHODS

Patients

A total of 500 cases were managed by a laparoscopic approach: 427 were treated conservatively and 73 were treated by salpingectomy. The average age of the patients was 25.4 ± 4.9 years (in the first 321 cases). The absolute and relative contraindications to the laparoscopic treatment of ectopic pregnancy, reported in Table 1 were respected.

Table 1 Contraindications to the laparoscopic treatment of ectopic pregnancy

Absolute contraindications
Interstitial pregnancy
Retrouterine hematocela
Shock

Relative contraindications
Hemoperitoneum over 1500 ml
Obesity
Large adhesions

Laparoscopic treatment

The laparoscopic management of ectopic pregnancy requires the following equipment:

(1) An 11-mm laparoscope with its trocar (Storz France, Paris, France) introduced through the umbilicus;

(2) Two operating trocars (5 and 7 mm) inserted by means of two small lateral suprapubic incisions;

(3) A 5-mm atraumatic forceps (Microfrance, Bourbon l'Archambault, France);

(4) The 7-mm Triton (Microfrance), an instrument with three functions: potential aspiration through a 6-mm diameter channel, injection of saline solution under pressure and electrocoagulation with a retractable monopolar needle electrode;

(5) A 19-gauge needle;

(6) 5 IU of Vasopressin (POR 8, Sandoz Laboratories, Basel, Switzerland);

(7) In cases of radical treatment, bipolar cautery forceps and laparoscopic scissors; and

(8) Since 1984, we have been using a video system, which gives us more precision and comfort and allows better teaching.

Methods

After diagnosis of ectopic pregnancy, two suprapubic operative trocars are inserted: a 5-mm trocar at the end of an imaginary Pfannenstiel at the site of ectopic pregnancy and a 7-mm one on the opposite side. The first stages of conservative or radical laparoscopic management are the same:

(1) Aspiration of the hemoperitoneum with the triton;

(2) Washing of the pelvis with saline solution under pressure;

(3) Evaluation of the ectopic pregnancy for location and operability.

The factors reported in Table 2 determine the choice between conservative and radical treatment.

Conservative treatment

In the case of conservative treatment, the different stages of the treatment are:

(1) Preventive hemostasis: vasopressin is diluted in 20 ml of serum saline and injected into the mesosalpinx through a 19-gauge needle (Figure 1). Blanching of the tube and temporary ischemia provide a virtually bloodless operating field. The use of this drug must be carefully controlled due to the dramatic arterial hypertension in cases of intravascular injection. Extravascular injection induces a moderate increase

Table 2 Choosing between conservative and radical treatment of ectopic pregnancy: scoring system

History of the patient	
Infertility	2
Ectopic pregnancy	2 (+ for following ectopic pregnancies)
Tubal plasty	2
Location	
Isthmus	1
Ampulla	0
Fimbria	−1
In case of solitary tube	
Salpingectomy	2
Obstructed tube	1
Bilateral ectopic pregnancy	2
In case of rupture	1
Score 1–4	conservative treatment
Score 6 or more	radical treatment
Score = 5	?

in arterial pressure and a moderate bradycardia in some cases. The temporary ischemia does not affect tubal patency as was verified by a second-look laparoscopy (15 cases), and provides a similar intrauterine pregnancy rate in groups with or without vasopressin (Table 3).

(2) Salpingotomy: a 10–15-mm incision is made in the antimesenteric proximal portion of the hematosalpinx with the needle electrode of the triton (Figures 2 and 3). Salpingotomy must be the systematic approach whenever there is a hematosalpinx. The high incidence of residual trophoblastic tissue in women treated without salpingotomy led us to perform tubal

abortion only in cases of fimbrial ectopic pregnancies. The salpingotomy must be performed in the proximal portion of the hematosalpinx, which is the usual location of the trophoblast (Figure 2).

(3) Extraction of the trophoblast (Figure 4). The triton is introduced through the salpingotomy incision; clots and trophoblast are aspirated. In most cases, aspiration removes the product of conception entirely. In some cases, saline solution injected under pressure by the triton or grasping forceps, is used to separate the trophoblast from the tubal wall. In all cases, the salpingotomy is left open (Figure 5).

At the end of the procedure, it is necessary to:

(1) Check the tube vacuity;

(2) Wash the pelvis with saline solution under pressure (Figure 6);

(3) Remove all clots and products of conception with the triton;

(4) Assess the contralateral Fallopian tube.

It is not necessary to insert an intraperitoneal drain through the pouch of Douglas.

The postoperative follow-up includes weekly hCG assays from the 2nd day after the operation until the level is undetectable (less than 5 mIUml)[4].

Radical treatment

In the case of radical treatment[5], a salpingotomy is performed by bipolar coagulation and scissors after aspiration of the ectopic pregnancy from the tube as in conservative treatment. The proximal part of the isthmus is coagulated and sectioned. Then the mesosalpinx is progressively coagulated and sectioned until the tube can be removed with grasping forceps and extracted from the abdomen.

RESULTS

A total of 427 cases of ectopic pregnancy treated conservatively between 1974 and 1986 were studied. Failures occurred in 22 cases (5.15%) because of an incomplete removal of the trophoblast requiring a second laparoscopic procedure in ten cases and laparotomy in 12 cases. Of the 73 patients treated by salpingectomy, we had only one postsurgical complication (1.36%): a 10th postoperative day hemorrhage which was successfully resolved by laparotomy. Postectopic fertility was evaluated in 149 patients who wished to become pregnant, with a minimum follow-up of 1 year.

Fertility results are summarized in Table 4. Of the 149 women who desired fertility, 97 (65.1%) had a

Table 3 Postoperative fertility and ectopic pregnancy in relation to the status of the tubal wall, the location of ectopic pregnancy and the use of vasopressin

	n	*Intrauterine pregnancy* *n* (%)	*Extrauterine pregnancy* *n* (%)
Use of vasopressin			
no	54	33 (61.1)	12 (22.2)
yes	95	64 (67.4)	13 (13.7)
Tubal wall			
ruptured	55	35 (63.6)	8 (14.5)
unruptured	94	62 (66)	17 (18.1)
Location			
isthmus	27	16 (59.3)	8 (29.6)
ampulla	101	63 (62.4)	16 (15.8)
fimbria	21	18 (85.7)	1 (4.8)

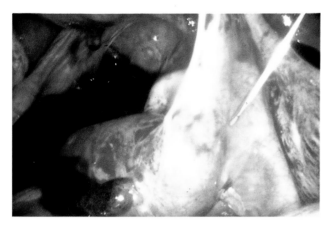

Figure 1 Injection of vasopressin into the mesosalpinx

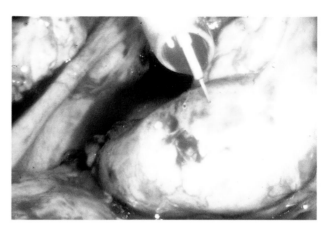

Figure 2 Salpingotomy in the antimesenteric proximal portion of the hematosalpinx with the needle electrode of the triton

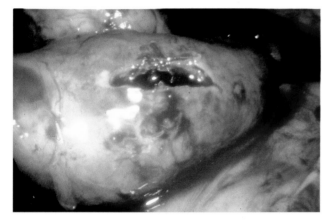

Figure 3 The incision

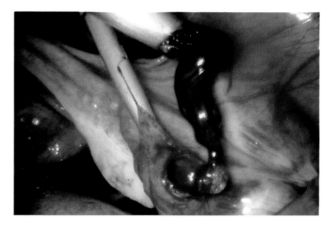

Figure 4 Aspiration of the trophoblast with the triton

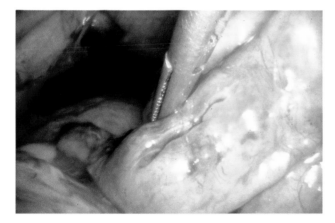

Figure 5 At the end of the procedure, the salpingotomy is left open

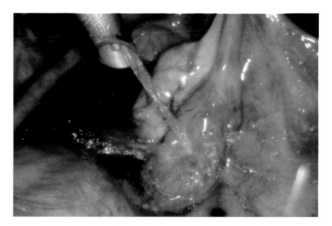

Figure 6 Washing of the pelvis

Table 4 Fertility results

Number of cases	Intrauterine pregnancy n (%)	Ectopic pregnancy n (%)	Sterility n (%)
149	97* (65.1)	25 (16.8)	49† (32.9)

*, five after a second ectopic pregnancy; †, 17 after a second ectopic pregnancy

subsequent intrauterine pregnancy. Five intrauterine pregnancies occurred after a second ectopic pregnancy which was also treated using a conservative laparoscopic procedure. The ectopic pregnancy rate was 16.8% (25 patients) and 49 patients (32.9%) suffered subsequent infertility (recurrent ectopic pregnancy + failure to conceive). (As can be seen in Table 6, our results compare favorably with those of other studies.)

According to their history, the 149 patients were divided into two groups: group I, 80 patients without any history of infertility or ectopic pregnancy; and group II, the other 69 patients. The results are summarized in Table 5. Statistical differences exist between the subsequent fertility rates of these two groups. An intrauterine pregnancy occurred in 68 patients in group I (85%) and in 29 patients (42%) in group II ($p < 0.001$). An ectopic pregnancy occurred in 12% of cases (ten patients) in group I and 22% of cases (15 patients) in group II. The postectopic infertility rate was 12% (ten cases) in group I and 56% (39 cases) in group II ($p < 0.001$).

Group III included 21 patients who had an ectopic pregnancy after microsurgical tuboplasty: four subsequently had an intrauterine pregnancy (19%), 17 remained sterile (81%) and six (29%) had a recurrence.

The 'solitary tube' group included patients who had undergone a previous salpingectomy, patients with a previously obstructed contralateral tube and patients who presented an ectopic pregnancy in each tube successively, both treated by laparoscopy.

Postoperative fertility and recurrence of ectopic pregnancy were studied in relation to the rupture of the tubal wall and location of the ectopic pregnancy (Table 3). The tube was ruptured in 55 patients. Among these women there were 35 intrauterine pregnancies (63.6%) and eight had a recurrence of ectopic pregnancy (14.5%). Of the 94 with an unruptured ectopic pregnancy 62 developed an intrauterine pregnancy (66%) and 17 a recurrence of ectopic pregnancy (18.1%).

The first ectopic pregnancy was located in the ampulla in 101 cases (67.8%), in the fimbria in 21 cases (44%) and in the isthmus in 27 cases (18.2%). The intrauterine pregnancy rates in these groups were 62.4%, 85.7% and 59.3%, respectively. The recurrence rates in these groups were 15.8%, 4.8% and 29.6%, respectively.

A simple scoring system (Table 2) allows the categorization of patients into two groups according to a high or poor chance of subsequent intrauterine pregnancy. This scoring system has been used by our team for 2 years now to choose between radical and conservative treatment.

CONCLUSION

Conservative laparoscopic treatment of ectopic pregnancy is a safe and effective laparoscopic procedure. In cases with contraindications to conservative management, a salpingectomy can be performed with a laparoscopic procedure. Failure due to residual trophoblastic tissue can occur. The failure necessitates a careful follow-up by monitoring of hCG levels.

Comparisons of postectopic pregnancy fertility results must be made critically. However, our postoperative rate of 65.1% intrauterine pregnancies compares favorably with previous studies (Table 6). The incidence of a previous history in relation to the success rate of the patient is emphasized in our series and must be taken into account when making the choice between radical and conservative treatment. Broad experience in

Table 5 Fertility according to history

	Number of patients	Intrauterine pregnancy n (%)	Ectopic pregnancy n (%)	Sterility n (%)
Group I: without history†	80	68* (85)	10** (12)	10* (12)
Group II: with history†	69	29* (42)	15** (22)	39* (56)
Group III: post-plasty	21	4 (19)	6 (29)	17 (81)
Solitary tube	27	11 (41)	6 (22)	15 (55)
Postectopic	38	7 (18)	15 (39)	29 (76)
Non-tubal infertility	38	23 (60)	6 (16)	15 (39)

*, $p < 0.001$; **, not significant; †, refers to history of infertility or ectopic pregnancy

operative laparoscopy is, however, required before management of ectopic pregnancy by laparoscopy is undertaken. Our techniques are, by and large, simple and easily feasible for most laparoscopic surgeons after adequate training. The advantages of laparoscopic procedures compared to laparotomy are evident in the reduction of hospital stay and patient trauma.

Table 6 Comparison of our postectopic pregnancy fertility results with other principal series

Author	Year	Number of patients	Intrauterine pregnancy n (%)	Ectopic pregnancy n (%)
Conservative treatment				
Ploman	(1960)[6]	31	16 (52)	1 (3)
Skjul	(1964)[7]	92	23 (25)	1 (1)
Timonen	(1967)[8]	185	46 (25)	21 (11)
Palmer	(1972)[9]	55	11 (20)	9 (16)
Swollin	(1972)[10]	40	10 (25)	7 (17)
Jarvinen	(1972)[11]	43	22 (51)	4 (9)
Stromme	(1973)[12]	37	20 (54)	7 (19)
Bukowski	(1979)[13]	20	14 (70)	1 (5)
DeCherney	(1979)[14]	48	19 (39)	4 (8)
Giana	(1979)[15]	51	17 (33)	4 (8)
Henri-Suchet	(1979)[16]	52	22 (42)	10 (19)
Sherman	(1982)[17]	47	39 (83)	7 (15)
Lalau	(1985)[18]	118	35 (30)	29 (25)
Microsurgery				
DeCherney	(1980)[19]	9	5 (55)	0 (0)
Janecek	(1980)[20]	10	6 (60)	2 (20)
Laparoscopic treatment				
Our results	(1987)	149	97 (65)	25 (17)

REFERENCES

1. Bruhat, M.A., Manhes, H., Mage, G. and Pouly, J.L. (1980). Treatment of ectopic pregnancy by means of laparoscopy. *Fertil. Steril.*, **33**, 411

2. Manhes, H., Mage, G., Pouly, J.L., Ropert, J.F. and Bruhat, M.A. (1983). Traitement coelioscopique de la grossesse extra utérine non rompue: améliorations techniques. *Nelle Presse Med.*, **12**, 1431

3. Pouly, J.L. Manhes, H., Mage, G., Canis, M. and Bruhat, M.A. (1986). Conservative laparoscopic treatment of 321 ectopic pregnancies. *Fertil. Steril.*, **46**, 1093

4. Pouly, J.L., Gachon, M., Gaillard, G., Mage, G. and Bruhat, M.A. (1987). La décroissance de l'HCG après traitement coelioscopique conservateur de la grossesse extra-utérine. *J. Gynecol. Obstet. Biol. Reprod.*, **16**, 195

5. Dubuisson, J.B. Aubriot, F.X. and Cardone, V., (1987) Laparoscopic salpingectomy for tubal pregnancy. *Fertil. Steril.*, **47**, 225

6. Ploman, L. and Wicksell, F. (1960). Fertility after conservative surgery in tubal pregnancy. *Acta Obstet. Gynecol. Scand.*, **39**, 143

7. Skjul, V., Palvic, Z., Stoiljkovic, C., Basic, G. and Drazancic, A. (1964). Conservative operative treatment of tubal pregnancy. *Fertil. Steril.*, **15**, 634

8. Timonen, S. and Nieminen, U., (1967). tubal pregnancy, choice of operative method of treament. *Acta Obstet. Gynecol. Scand.*, **46**, 327

9. Palmer, R., (1972). Résultats et indications de la chirurgie conservatrice au cours de la grossesse extra-utérine. *C. R. Soc. Fr. Gynecol.*, **42**, 317

10. Swollin, K. and Fall, M. (1972). Ectopic pregnancy. *Acta Eur. Fertil.*, **3**, 147

11. Jarvinen, P.A. (1972). Conservative operative treatment of tubal pregnancy with post-operative daily hydrotubation. *Acta Obstet. Gynecol. Scand.*, **51**, 169

12. Stromme, W.B. (1973). Conservative surgery for ectopic pregnancy. *Obstet. Gynecol.*, **41**, 251

13. Bukowsky, J., Langer, R., Sherman, A. and Caspi, E., (1979). Conservative surgery for ectopic pregnancy. *Obstet. Gynecol.*, **53**, 709

14. DeCherney, A. and Kase, N. (1979). The conservative surgical management of unruptured ectopic pregnancy. *Obstet. Gynecol.*, **54**, 541

15. Giana, M. (1979). Tratamento chirurgico conservativo in 51 caza digravidenza tubarica. *Minera Ginecol.*, **30**, 99

16. Henri-Suchet, J. (1979). Chirurgie conservatrice de la grossesse extra-utérine. In *Oviducte et Fertilité*, p.393 (Paris: Masson)

17. Sherman, D. Langer, R., Sadovsky, G. Bukovsky, I., and Caspi, E., (1982). Improved fertility following ectopic pregnancy. *Fertil. Steril.*, **37**, 497

18. Lalau Keraly, M. (1985). Récidives de grossesse extra-utérine. A propos d'une étude multicentrique de 470 cas de GEU. *Thèse Paris*

19. DeCherney, A.H., Polan, M.L., Kort, H. and Kase, N. (1980). Microsurgical technique in the management of tubal ectopic pregnancy. *Fertil. Steril.*, 34:324

20. Janecek, J. (1979). Resultats de la chirurgie reconstructrice dans les grossesses extra-utérines non rompues. *Rev. Méd. Suisse Romande*, **99**, 603

Postoperative management and reproductive outcome after conservative laparoscopic procedures

13

J. Donnez and M. Nisolle

POSTOPERATIVE MANAGEMENT

Complete removal of trophoblastic tissue is not always possible and functional residual trophoblast may remain in the affected tube and result in growth and delayed hemorrhage.

Incidence of residual trophoblast

In a series of 321 patients who had undergone conservative laparoscopic surgery, Pouly and colleagues[1] reported 15 cases with residual trophoblast. Of those patients, seven underwent a second laparoscopic procedure, and six required a salpingectomy via laparotomy[2] (Table 1).

Rivlin and co-workers[7,8] reviewed five case reports of persistent ectopic gestation, and recommended that salpingectomy be the standard procedure undertaken.

Recently, Di Marchi and colleagues[5] reported four cases (4.8%) of persistent ectopic pregnancy, out of 84 patients who had undergone a salpingotomy or fimbrial expression. Three patients required a repeated laparotomy and salpingectomy, and one was managed expectantly.

In a series of 20 patients undergoing linear salpingotomy[4,9], two patients (10%) demonstrated a postoperative rise in serum β-human chorionic gonadotropin (β-hCG) levels, suggesting the persistence of trophoblastic tissue. Both patients were asymptomatic and were managed expectantly.

In a first series of 300 patients[6] treated conservatively by laparoscopic salpingotomy (Tables 1 and 2), two cases in 1982 required a second-look laparotomy for recurrent bleeding due to persistent trophoblast. In 15 other cases, persistent trophoblast was observed. All were treated successfully with methotrexate. The incidence of persistent ectopic gestation following conservative surgery was 5%. This incidence is similar to that observed in the literature (Table 1).

In a second series of 320 patients who underwent conservative laparoscopic treatment, persistent trophoblastic tissue was observed in 41 cases (13%) (Table 3). Again, all patients were treated with methotrexate intramuscularly. However, in this second series, eight failures were encountered in spite of the administration of methotrexate (in the first series, the postoperative administration of methotrexate was successful in all 15 cases).

Diagnosis and management of persistent trophoblast

The diagnosis of persistent ectopic pregnancy is made by measuring hCG levels postoperatively. It has been shown and proved by one of our studies[6] that 2 days postoperatively, the hCG level should be less than 50% of the preoperative level, and after 4 days, less than 25% of the preoperative level. Figure 1 illustrates the

Table 1 Incidence of residual trophoblast after conservative management

Author	Number of patients	Failures n (%)
Donnez (1982)[3]	50	2 (4.0)
Pouly et al. (1986)[1]	321	15 (4.7)
Cartwright et al. (1986)[4]	20	2 (10.0)
Di Marchi et al. (1987)[5]	84	4 (4.8)
Donnez and Nisolle[6]	300	17 (5.7)
Total	775	40 (5.2)

Table 2 Tubal pregnancy: laparoscopic procedures ($n = 300$)

Failures ($n = 2$, < 1%)	bleeding due to persistent trophoblast occurred 8 and 12 days after the laparoscopic procedure treatment: laparotomy with conservative treatment
Relative failures ($n = 15$, 5%)	persistently high hCG levels treatment: methotrexate 40 mg

Table 3 Tubal pregnancy: laparoscopic procedures

	1980–1986 ($n = 300$)	1987–1990 ($n = 320$)
Persistent ectopic pregnancy	$n = 15$ (5%)	$n = 41$ (13%)
Therapy	methotrexate	methotrexate
Failure	0	8

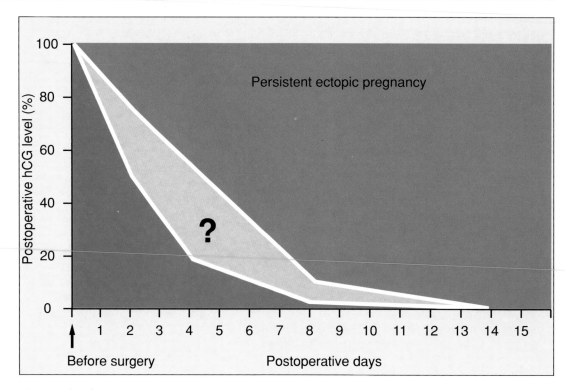

Figure 1 Graph illustrating the postoperative decrease in the hCG level: the purple area is the successful area; the dark blue area is the failed area; the intermediate light blue area is the repeated monitoring area

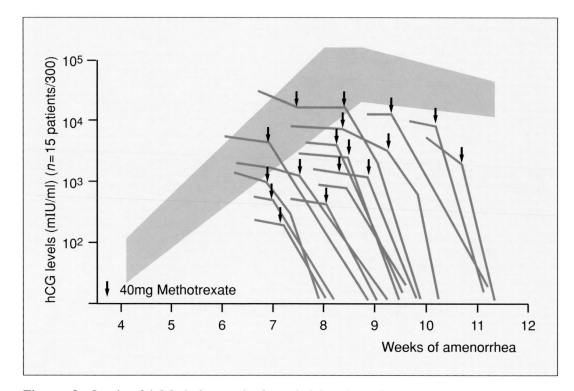

Figure 2 Levels of hCG before and after administration of 40 mg of methotrexate intramuscularly in 15 cases of persistent trophoblast (first series)

postoperative hCG decrease: if the postoperative hCG level is within the purple area, the laparoscopic treatment is considered to have been successful. If the postoperative hCG level is within the dark blue area, the diagnosis of persistent ectopic tissue is made. Indeed, the absence of any decrease proved the active secretion of hCG by persistent and well-vascularized trophoblastic tissue. However, if the hCG level falls within the light blue intermediate area (between the purple and dark blue), then a follow-up evaluation must be made by repeated hCG level monitoring 2 days later in order to evaluate the presence or absence of any significant decrease. Different procedures (Table 4) have been suggested for the management of persistent trophoblast.

In our department, if the 2-day postoperative hCG level remained higher than 50% of the initial (before laparoscopy) value, methotrexate (40 mg intramuscularly) was administered. The hCG level was evaluated 4 days postoperatively and if necessary, methotrexate was again given intramuscularly if hCG levels were > 25% of the initial value. In our first series of 300 patients undergoing laparoscopic treatment (Figure 2), an injection of methotrexate was necessary in 15 cases (5%); hCG levels were tested until the level was undetectable (< 5 mU/ml).

Since the hCG levels were systematically controlled, neither a second laparoscopic procedure nor a laparotomy was necessary to remove residual trophoblast in this first series of 300 cases.

In the second series, the same postoperative monitoring of the hCG levels was carried out and methotrexate was administered when required. Of the 320 cases, methotrexate was required in 41 (13%), and in eight cases this treatment failed.

Thus, two important questions remained to be answered, namely:

(1) Why was there an increased persistent ectopic pregnancy rate in the second series?

(2) Why, in this series, did the administration of methotrexate fail in eight cases?

Concerning the increased use of methotrexate, a distinction must be made between true and false failures. True failures can be explained by the fact that, in an academic and teaching hospital, residents are in the process of learning, when performing the laparoscopic procedure. The rate of such failures was 8.5%, higher than the rate observed in the first series of 300 patients treated by the same surgeons (i.e. the authors). In these cases, methotrexate was required because of the abnormal decrease in the hCG level. After an initial decrease, the hCG level increased into the dark blue area. The diagnosis of persistent trophoblast was made and methotrexate was administered intramuscularly twice or three times if needed (Figure 3). False failures can be accounted for by the inadequate use of methotrexate (4.5%). Indeed, in a few cases, methotrexate was given when it was not required, when the hCG level decrease was normal (Figure 4).

In conclusion, the failure rate of 8.5% observed in the second series was higher than that noted in the first series, as a result of necessary 'internship' in the department.

The second question to be addressed was why the administration of methotrexate failed in eight cases of the second series (Table 5). In patients receiving medication for ovulation, an ectopic pregnancy may be double. In one case, we observed a heterotubal pregnancy and another patient presented a double tubal implantation site. Both patients had received clomifene citrate and both underwent a second-look laparoscopy. In the case of the heterotubal pregnancy, a salpingotomy

Table 4 Management of persistent ectopic pregnancy

	Patients	Primary procedure	Management
Kelly et al. (1979)[10]	1	salpingotomy	salpingectomy
Johnson et al. (1980)[11]	1	fimbrial expression	salpingectomy
Kamrava et al. (1983)[12]	1	fimbrial expression	expectant
Richards (1984)[13]	1	salpingotomy	salpingectomy
Rivlin et al. (1985)[7]	1	salpingotomy	salpingectomy
Cowan et al. (1986)[14]	1	fimbrial expression	methotrexate
Higgins and Schwartz (1986)[15]	1	salpingectomy	methotrexate
Cartwright et al. (1986)[4]	2	salpingotomy	expectant
Pouly et al. (1986)[1]	11	salpingotomy	salpingotomy
	4	fimbrial expression	salpingectomy
Donnez (1982)[3]	2	salpingotomy	salpingotomy and coagulation
Keningsberg et al. (1987)[16]	1	salpingotomy	RU 486 and methotrexate
DiMarchi et al. (1987)[5]	3	salpingotomy	salpingectomy
	1	fimbrial expression	expectant
Bell et al. (1987)[17]	1	salpingotomy	partial salpingectomy
Donnez and Nisolle (1989)[6]	15	salpingotomy	methotrexate

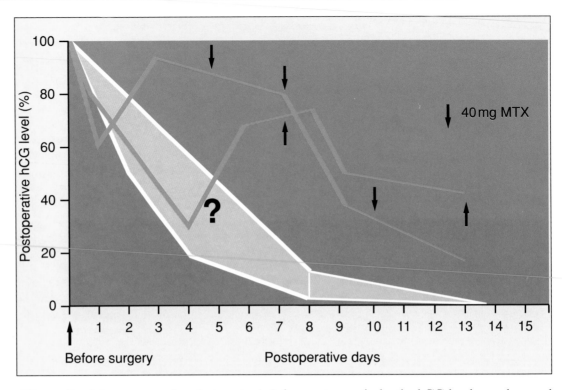

Figure 3 Adequate use of methotrexate: 4–5 days postoperatively, the hCG level was abnormal (dark blue area) and methotrexate was required

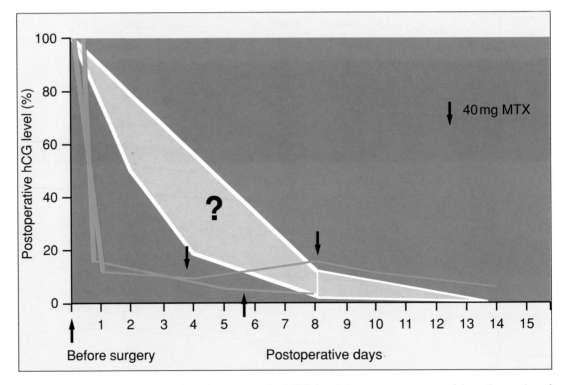

Figure 4 Inadequate use of methotrexate: the hCG level decrease was normal (purple area) and methotrexate was not required

Table 5 Failures of methotrexate used as therapy for persistent ectopic pregnancy ($n = 8$)

Problem	n	Post-methotrexate procedure
Heterotubal pregnancy (clomifene citrate)	1	salpingotomy (second-look)
Double tubal implantation site (clomifene citrate)	1	salpingotomy (second-look) salpingotomy (third-look)
(Too) early laparoscopic procedure	2	salpingotomy (second-look) echo-guided methotrexate injection
Imperfect laparoscopic procedure incorrect salpingotomy site insufficient trophoblastic aspiration	3 1	salpingotomy (second-look) salpingotomy and injection of methotrexate into the broad ligament (second-look)

was carried out and was successful. The second patient underwent a third laparoscopy because of recurrent bleeding after the second salpingotomy. Laparoscopic salpingectomy was then carried out. There was one implantation site in the ampulla (Figure 5) and another in the isthmus. In this case, the first procedure (ampullary salpingotomy) was well chosen, as proved by the anatomical aspect (Figure 5) observed at the time of the third laparoscopy. The recurrent bleeding was provoked by persistent trophoblast in the isthmic tubal portion.

In two cases, the laparoscopy was performed too early (< 6 weeks of amenorrhea) and the ectopic pregnancy was not visible (too small); no surgical therapy was administered. A salpingotomy was performed 2 weeks later in one case. In the second case, an echo-guided methotrexate injection was given: the hCG level decreased, but the hysterosalpingography performed 3 months later showed ampullary dilatation and occlusion at the ectopic pregnancy site (Figure 6).

In four cases, the laparoscopic procedure itself was imperfect. The salpingotomy site was incorrect in three cases, requiring a second salpingotomy. In one case, the trophoblastic aspiration was insufficient and a salpingotomy and injection of methotrexate into the broad ligament were required.

Reproductive outcome

Most patients undergoing conservative tubal surgery for an ectopic gestation will attempt to conceive soon after. A hysterosalpingogram and/or a second-look laparoscopy may be considered if conception has not occurred within 12 months of the procedure. In our department, hysterosalpingography is systematically carried out 3 months after a conservative procedure. The images (Figure 7) permit an evaluation of:

(1) The tubal patency;

(2) The quality of ampullary folds;

(3) The contralateral Fallopian tube;

(4) The presence of endosalpingiosis, often responsible for recurrent isthmic tubal pregnancy.

The reproductive outcome is largely dependent on the type of procedure carried out, but is also influenced by other factors including age, parity, tubal disease, and whether or not the ectopic gestation is ruptured.

Postoperative fertility after segmental resection and anastomosis

After segmental resection (Table 6), the intrauterine and recurrent ectopic pregnancy rates were, respectively, 39.5% and 9.2%[25,26,27]. These rates are not different from those observed following a total salpingectomy. The more conservative procedure, however, offers the distinct advantage of preserving the affected tube.

Different postoperative pregnancy rates were found when cases were selected according to the time of anastomosis. Higher postoperative pregnancy rates were found after elective (> 3 months) anastomosis (60%) than after intraoperative anastomosis (33%).

In our department, segmental resection was carried out only in cases of isthmic tubal pregnancy. Reanastomosis of the single remaining tube was carried out 3 months after the tubal pregnancy surgical procedure according to the principles of microsurgery. The results are found in Table 6.

Postoperative fertility after linear salpingotomy

In a series of 120 patients without any history of infertility who wished to become pregnant, an intrauterine pregnancy rate of 63% was achieved (Table 7). The recurrent tubal pregnancy rate after laparoscopy was similar to that obtained in another series of 148 patients who underwent conservative surgery (linear salpingotomy) by laparotomy (8% in both groups).

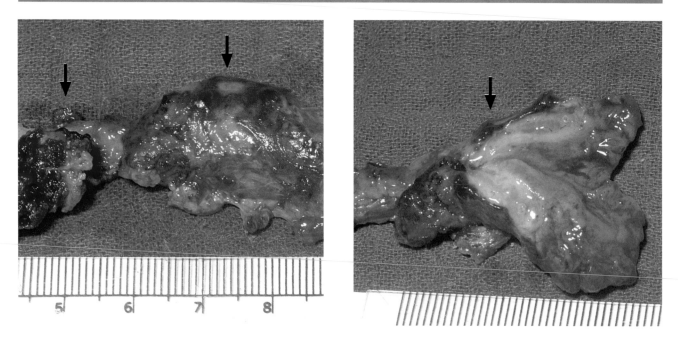

Figure 5 (a)   Macroscopical aspect of the tube 2 weeks after ampullary salpingotomy for ampullary tubal pregnancy (the tube was removed because of a ruptured isthmic pregnancy). Arrow (right) indicates the healing of the salpingotomy and the other arrow (on the left) indicates the second site of implantation (in the isthmic portion); (b) the site of salpingotomy was then opened. The process of tubal healing is clearly visible and the recovery of the ampullary folds is surprisingly excellent (arrow)

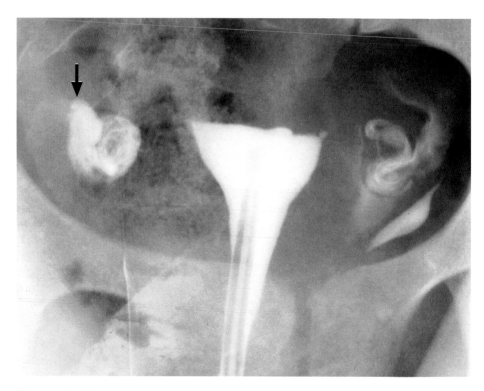

Figure 6   Hysterosalpingography 3 months after the echo-guided methotrexate injection. Occlusion and ampullary dilatation are see clearly at the site of the ectopic pregnancy (arrow)

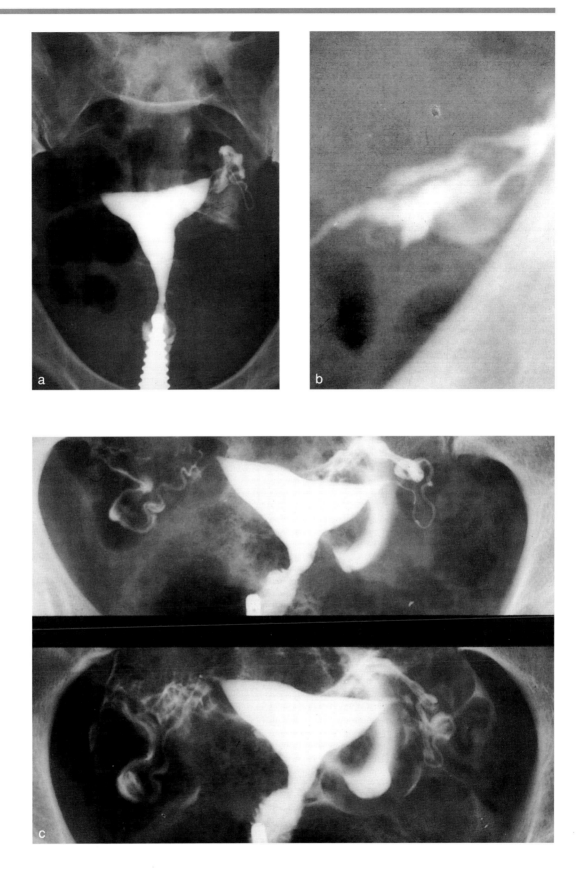

Figure 7 Hysterosalpingography: (a) normal ampullary folds and normal tubal patency after salpingotomy for tubal pregnancy in a 'solitary' tube; (b) fistula at the site of salpingotomy; this occurs in less than 2% of cases; (c) contralateral Fallopian tube; presence of endosalpingiosis

Table 6 Pregnancy rates following segmental resection for ectopic gestation according to the time of anastomosis

	Number of patients	Intrauterine pregnancy n (%)	Ectopic pregnancy n (%)
Intraoperative anastomosis			
Swolin (1972)[18]	42	10 (24)	6 (14)
Janecek and De Grandi (1978)[19]	6	3 (50)	0
Stangel and Gomel (1980)[20]	7	2 (28)	0
Siegler *et al.* (1981)[21]	8	6 (75)	0
Total	63	21 (33)	6 (9)
Elective anastomosis (> 3 months)			
Gomel (1980)[22]	6	4 (67)	0
DeCherney and Boyers (1985)[23]	6	4 (67)	0
Donnez (1984)[24]	14	8 (57)	1 (7)
Total	26	16 (62)	1 (4)

Among patients with a history of microsurgical tuboplasty, the postoperative intrauterine pregnancy rate was significantly ($p < 0.005$) lower than that obtained in the group of patients without any history of infertility (27% vs. 54%). When compared, the recurrent tubal pregnancy rates were also significantly ($p < 0.005$) different (22% vs. 8%). Similar data were obtained in the group of patients who underwent a conservative approach by laparotomy.

Among patients with a 'solitary' tube (Table 8), the intrauterine pregnancy rate was 52% (11/21) and the recurrent tubal pregnancy rate, 24% (5/21). Linear salpingotomy seems to result in a higher rate of subsequent intrauterine pregnancy than either total or partial salpingectomy. However, the more favorable reproductive outcome may, in part, reflect a selection bias, since linear salpingotomies were performed in cases of small unruptured gestations, whereas salpingectomies were usually performed in cases of ruptured ectopic gestations. The advantage of conservative surgery over radical surgery becomes more evident when treating ectopic gestations in solitary tubes. In these cases, a conservative approach is the only one that preserves reproductive potential.

DISCUSSION

Conservative treatment of ectopic pregnancy by laparoscopy is increasingly common. In very rare instances, the procedure cannot be completed by laparoscopy, and laparotomy may be required.

Relative contraindications to a laparoscopic approach to tubal pregnancy are the following:

(1) Shock;

(2) Ampullary diameter > 5 cm;

(3) Ruptured tubal wall;

(4) Inexperienced surgeon;

(5) Hematocelia.

Table 7 Postoperative fertility after conservative management of unruptured ampullary tubal pregnancy (Department of Gynecology, UCL, 1978–1987)

	Number of patients	Intrauterine pregnancy n (%)	Ectopic pregnancy n (%)
Laparotomy			
No history of infertility	148	92 (62)	12 (8)
After microsurgical tuboplasty	64	19 (30)	13 (20)
Total	212	111 (52)	25 (12)
Laparoscopy			
No history of infertility	120	65 (54)	10 (8)
After microsurgical tuboplasty	18	5 (27)*	4 (22)*
Total	138	70 (51)	14 (10)

*, $p < 0.005$; significantly different from the group of women without any history of infertility

Table 8 Results of conservative surgery for tubal pregnancy in women with a solitary tube desiring pregnancy

Author	Number of patients	Intrauterine pregnancy n (%)	Ectopic pregnancy n (%)
Henri-Suchet et al. (1979)[28]	14	8 (57)	2 (14)
DeCherney et al. (1982)[29]	12	6 (50)	2 (17)
Langer et al. (1982)[30]	8	5 (62)	2 (25)
Valle and Lifchez (1983)[31]	11	11 (100)	0
Oelsner et al. (1986)[32]	21	10 (48)	9 (43)
Pouly et al. (1986)[1]	24	11 (46)	7 (29)
Donnez and Nisolle (1989)[6]	21	11 (52)	5 (24)
Total	90	51 (57)	22 (24)

In our department, these five circumstances are no longer contraindications to laparoscopic surgery.

In our series, conservative laparoscopic treatment proved to be safe and effective. No serious intraoperative complications were encountered. There were two cases of delayed hemorrhage caused by the presence of residual trophoblastic tissue, confirmed by persistently high hCG levels. These two cases occurred in the first 50 cases of tubal pregnancy treated by laparoscopy.

In the remaining patients, hCG levels were then systematically monitored. Residual trophoblastic tissue was present in 15 patients as suggested by the failure of hCG levels to return to normal. Methotrexate (40 mg intramuscularly) was then given and hCG levels were monitored until the level was less than 5 mU/ml. If necessary, a second injection was administered.

In the second series, residual trophoblastic tissue was noted in 41 patients but eight cases failed to respond to methotrexate and other treatment was required. In another study[1], a second laparoscopic procedure or a laparotomy was performed in cases of incomplete removal of trophoblastic tissue.

In our department, incomplete removal of trophoblastic tissue required laparotomy in two cases out of the first 50 of our first series, and a second laparoscopic procedure (salpingotomy) in six cases of the second series. In one case, a salpingectomy was required during a third laparoscopy, and in another case, an echo-guided methotrexate injection was followed by a successful decrease in the hCG level, but complicated by tubal occlusion.

Other studies (Table 8) of conservative procedures for tubal pregnancy by laparotomy have shown a subsequent intrauterine pregnancy rate between 20 and 83% and recurrent ectopic gestations between 1.1 and 19%. Our results of a 63% postoperative intrauterine pregnancy rate after laparoscopic treatment in women without any history of tuboplasty are similar to those obtained by Pouly and colleagues[1]. In our comparative study, the intrauterine and recurrent tubal pregnancy rates were similar in the group of patients treated by laparotomy and those treated by laparoscopy.

The recurrent tubal pregnancy rate found in our study (8%) was lower than that obtained by Pouly and

Table 9 Pregnancy rates following linear salpingotomy for ectopic pregnancy

	Number of patients	Intrauterine pregnancy n (%)	Ectopic pregnancy n (%)
Laparotomy			
Vehaskari (1960)[33]	88	43 (49)	14 (16)
Timonen and Nieminen (1967)[34]	185	90 (49)	22 (12)
Jarvinen et al. (1972)[35]	43	26 (60)	4 (9)
Bukovsky et al. (1979)[36]	20	14 (70)	1 (5)
DeCherney and Kase (1979)[37]	48	19 (39)	4 (8)
DeCherney et al. (1981)[38]	16	8 (50)	0 (0)
Donnez and Nisolle (1989)[6]	212	111 (52)	25 (12)
Total	612	311 (51)	70 (11)
Laparoscopy			
Pouly et al. (1986)[1]	118	75 (64)	26 (22)
Donnez and Nisolle (1989)[6]	138	70 (51)	14 (10)
Total	256	145 (57)	40 (16)

co-workers[1]. As suggested in their study, the incidence of repeated tubal pregnancy was overestimated because their series began before *in vitro* fertilization (IVF) programs were widespread. At that time, the conservative procedure was the only one possible, even in severe cases, such as recurring tubal pregnancy in a solitary tube or after tuboplasty. Although postoperative results among patients with previous tuboplasty are inferior to those observed among patients without a history of tuboplasty, we nevertheless suggest, in cases of tubal pregnancy, a conservative treatment and not a salpingectomy for women with a history of tuboplasty. In our department, salpingectomy is indicated only in cases of tubal pregnancy occurring after IVF and embryo transfer, in patients with thick-walled hydrosalpinx.

The high intrauterine pregnancy rate occurring in women after the removal of trophoblast from a single functioning tube confirms the findings of other studies[1] and proves the efficacy of the laparoscopic approach.

The advantages of laparoscopic treatment are the reduced morbidity rate and a shorter hospitalization time. Because of these advantages and the good results in terms of postoperative intrauterine pregnancy rates (Table 9), we suggest that the laparoscopic approach should be the procedure of choice in cases of ampullary tubal pregnancy. However, patients need to be advised that they will require postoperative serial β-subunit check-ups to exclude the presence of any persistent trophoblastic tissue.

REFERENCES

1. Pouly, J.L., Manhes, H., Mage, G., Canis, M., Bruhat, M. A. (1986). Conservative laparoscopic treatment of 321 ectopic pregnancies. *Fertil. Steril.*, **46**, 1093
2. Bruhat, M.A., Manhes, H., Mage, G. and Pouly, J.L. (1980). Treatment of ectopic pregnancy by means of laparoscopy. *Fertil. Steril.*, **33**, 411
3. Donnez, J. (1982). Conservative treatment of ectopic pregnancy. A first series of 50 cases. *Acta Endosc.*, **4**, 62
4. Cartright, P.S., Herbert, C.M. and Maxson, W.S. (1986). Operative laparoscopy for the management of tubal pregnancy. *J. Reprod. Med.*, **31**, 589
5. DiMarchi, J.M., Losasa, T.S., Kobara, T.Y., and Hale, R. W. (1987). Persistent ectopic pregnancy. *Obstet. Gynecol.*, **70**, 555
6. Donnez, J. and Nisolle, M. (1989). Laparoscopic treatment of ampullary tubal pregnancy. *J. Gynecol. Surg.*, **5**, 19
7. Rivlin, M.E., Meeks, G.R., Cowan, B.D. and Bates, G.W. (1985). Persistent trophoblastic tissue following salpingostomy for unruptured ectopic pregnancy. *Fertil. Steril.*, **43**, 323
8. Rivlin, M.E. (1985). Persistent ectopic pregnancy: complication of conservative surgery. *Int. J. Fertil.*, **30**, 10
9. Cartwright, P.D. and Entman, S.S. (1984). Repeat ipsilateral tubal pregnancy following partial salpingectomy: a case report. *Fertil. Steril.*, **42**, 642.
10. Kelly, R.W., Martin, S.A. and Srickler, R.C. (1979). Delayed hemorrhage in conservative surgery for ectopic pregnancy. *Am. J. Obstet. Gynecol.*, **133**, 225
11. Johnson, T.R.B., Sanborn, J.R., Wagner, K.S. and Compton, A.A. (1980). Gonadotropin surveillance following conservative surgery for ectopic pregnancy. *Fertil. Steril.*, **33**, 207
12. Kamrava, M.M., Taymor, M.L., Berger, M.J., Thompson, I.E. and Seibel, M.M. (1983). Disappearance of human chorionic gonadotropin following removal of ectopic pregnancy. *Obstet. Gynecol.*, **62**, 484
13. Richards, B.C. (1984). Persistent trophoblast following conservative operation for ectopic pregnancy. *Am. J. Obstet. Gynecol.*, **150**, 100
14. Cowan, B.D., McGehee, R.P. and Bates, G.W. (1986). Treatment of persistent ectopic pregnancy with methotrexate and leukovorum rescue: a case report. *Obstet. Gynecol.*, **67**, 50
15. Higgins, K.A. and Schwartz, M.B. (1986). Treatment of persistent trophoblastic tissue after salpingostomy with methotrexate. *Fertil. Steril.*, **45**, 427
16. Keningsberg, D., Porte, J., Hull, M. and Spitz, I.M. (1987). Medical treatment of residual ectopic pregnancy: RU 486 and methotrexate. *Fertil. Steril.*, **47**, 702.
17. Bell, O.R., Awadalla, S.G. and Mattox, J.H. (1987). Persistent ectopic syndrome: a case report and literature review. *Obstet. Gynecol.*, **69**, 521
18. Swolin, K. and Fall, M. (1972). Ectopic pregnancy. *Acta Eur. Fertil.*, **3**, 147.
19. Janecek, P. and DeGrandi, P. (1978). Chirurgie restauratrice d'emblée dans le traitement des grossesses extrautérines. *J. Gynecol. Obstet. Biol. Reprod.*, **7**, 261.
20. Stangel, J.J. and Gomel, V. (1980). Techniques in conservative surgery for tubal gestation. *Clin. Obstet. Gynecol.*, **23**, 1221
21. Siegler, M., Wang, C.F. and Westoff, C. (1981). Management of unruptured tubal pregnancies. *Obstet. Gynecol. Surv.*, **36**, 599
22. Gomel, V. (1980). Clinical results of infertility microsurgery. In Crosignani, P.G. and Rubin, B.L. (eds.) *Microsurgery in Female Infertility*, p.7. (London: Academic Press)
23. DeCherney, A.H. and Boyers, S.P. (1985). Isthmic ectopic pregnancy: segmental resection as the treatment of choice. *Fertil. Steril.*, **44**, 307
24. Donnez, J. (1984). La trompe de Fallope. In Donnez, J. (ed.) *Histophysiologie Normale et Pathologique.* (Leuven: Nauwelaerts Printing)

25. Vermesh, M., Silva, P.D., Sauer, M.V., Vargyas, J.M. and Lobo, R.A. (1988). Persistent tubal ectopic gestation: patterns of circulating human chorionic gonadotropin and progesterone, and management options. *Fertil. Steril.*, **50**, 584

26. Vermesh, M., Silva, P.D., Rosen, G.F., Stein, A.L., Fossum, G.T. and Sauer, M.V. (1989). Management of unruptured ectopic gestation by linear salpingostomy: a prospective, randomized clinical trial of laparoscopy versus laparotomy. *Obstet. Gynecol.*, **73**, 400

27. DeCherney, A.H., Polan, P.L., Korth, H. and Kase, N. (1980). Microsurgical techniques in the management of tubal ectopic pregnancy. *Fertil. Steril.*, **34**, 324

28. Henri-Suchet, J., Tesquier, J. Loffredo, V., Loron, Y. and Debrux, J. (1979). La chirurgie conservative de la grossesse extrautérine. In Brosens, I. *et al.* (eds.) *Oviducte et Fetilité*, p.5, (Paris: Masson)

29. DeCherney, A.H., Maheux, R. and Naftolin, F. (1982). Salpingotomy for ectopic pregnancy for the sole patient oviduct: reproductive outcome. *Fertil. Steril.*, **37**, 619

30. Langer, R., Bukovski, I., Herman, A., Sherman, D., Sadovsky, G. and Caspi, E. (1982). Conservative surgery for tubal pregnancy. *Fertil. Steril.*, **38**, 427

31. Valle, J.A. and Lifchez, A.S. (1983). Reproductive outcome following conservative surgery for tubal pregnancy in women with a single fallopian tube. *Fertil. Steril.*, **39**, 316

32. Oelsner, G., Rabinovitch, O., Morad, J., Mashiach, S. and Serr, D.M. (1986). Reproductive outcome after microsurgical treatment of tubal pregnancy in women with a single fallopian tube. *J. Reprod. Med.*, **31**, 483

33. Vehaskari, A. (1960). The operation of choice for ectopic pregnancy with reference to subsequent fertility. *Acta Obstet. Gynecol. Scand.*, **39**, (Suppl. 13), 3

34. Timonen, S. and Nieminen, U. (1967). Tubal pregnancy: choice of operative method of treatment. *Acta Obstet. Gynecol. Scand.*, **46**, 327

35. Jarvinen, P.A., Nummi, S. and Pietila, K. (1972). Conservative operative treatment of tubal pregnancy with postoperative daily hydrotubations. *Acta Obstet. Gynecol. Scand.*, **51**, 169

36. Bukovsky, I., Langer, R., Herman, A. and Caspi, E. (1979). Conservative surgery for tubal pregnancy. *Obstet. Gynecol.*, **53**, 709

37. DeCherney, A.H. and Kase, N. (1979). The conservative surgical management of unruptured ectopic pregnancy. *Obstet. Gynecol.*, **54**, 451

38. DeCherney, A.H., Romero, R. and Naftolin, F. (1981). Surgical management of unruptured ectopic pregnancy. *Fertil. Steril.*, **35**, 21

Part 3

Ovarian pathology

Laparoscopic management of ovarian cysts

M. Nisolle, S. Bassil and J. Donnez

In most clinical circumstances, a unilocular ovarian cyst does not require aspiration, but does require medical therapy (such as oral contraceptives) for 3 months. If the cyst does not disappear after a 3-month course of therapy, it requires careful evaluation (echography, CA-125 level and, in some instances, computerized tomography (CT) and magnetic resonance imaging (MRI)), and finally laparoscopic diagnosis and management. The most frequent types of cysts found in young women are:

(1) The unilocular clear fluid cyst (mucous or serous);

(2) The dermoid cyst;

(3) The endometrial cyst (endometrioma).

Laparoscopic removal of benign ovarian cysts is an effective technique, involving little risk of complications[1,2]. Nevertheless, several criteria must be taken into account before performing this procedure. Various diagnostic methods have been used to discriminate between benign and malignant ovarian tumors: physical examination, transvaginal ultrasound color flow imaging and tumor markers such as CA-125.

PREOPERATIVE EVALUATION

Ultrasound examination

Using high-frequency transvaginal sonography it is possible to detect malignant ovarian tumors more efficiently than by transabdominal echography[3]. The vaginal approach produces greater image resolution than the abdominal, thus allowing a more detailed morphological assessment of ovarian masses (Figure 1(a) and (b)).

The following criteria must be assessed: size and location, borders of the mass and free pelvic fluid (ascites). The internal structure of a mass is considered to be the most important sonographic criterion for distinguishing benign from malignant disorders. The tumor can be purely cystic, complex (mainly cystic, or mainly solid) or purely solid. Loculations, thick septa, irregular solid parts within a mass, undefined margins, and the presence of ascites are considered as malignant patterns (Figure 1(c)). Such cases certainly require conventional surgery by laparotomy. A sonographic diagnosis of benign disease is generally accurate; indeed, a predictive non-malignant rate of 95.6% was found by Herrmann and colleagcs[4].

Transvaginal Doppler ultrasound with color flow imaging

Transvaginal Doppler ultrasound with color flow imaging is a new technique for the evaluation of ovarian masses[5-7]. It allows the positioning of the probe closer to the tumor and visually reflects the state of blood flow of the ovarian tumor (Figure 2(a) and (b)); it permits the detection of low-resistance intratumoral blood vessels, characteristic of malignant tumors (Figure 2(c)).

The pulsatility index (PI), defined as the difference between the peak-systolic and the end-diastolic flow velocity divided by the mean flow velocity, is calculated. Bourne and co-workers[5] reported that this method can be used to differentiate between primary ovarian cancer and other forms of benign pelvic masses. In their study, low impedance to ovarian blood flow was associated with malignant ovarian tumors (PI < 1).

Weiner and associates[8] made an attempt to compare transvaginal color flow imaging with conventional sonographic findings and other screening procedures to predict ovarian malignancy. They found that suspicious sonographic findings had low specificity and were inadequate in distinguishing between benign and malignant ovarian tumors. They concluded that transvaginal color flow imaging provided high sensitivity and specificity and was superior to the other methods used for preoperative evaluation of ovarian masses.

A simple measurement of the PI in the newly formed intratumoral blood vessels can discriminate accurately between malignant and non-malignant ovarian tumors. Moreover, because early development of neovascularity may precede tumor growth, screening for ovarian malignancy with transvaginal color flow imaging may detect early ovarian neoplasms before sonography. According to the results of Bourne and colleagues[5], Fleischer and co-workers[9], and Kurjak and associates[6], transvaginal color Doppler is a valuable method of differentiating benign from malignant ovarian tumors. However, others[10] have recently been unable to reproduce their results.

CA-125

The preoperative evaluation of serum CA-125 levels must be made before endoscopic surgery, especially in premenopausal and postmenopausal patients, in order to suspect malignant disease preoperatively. Values of

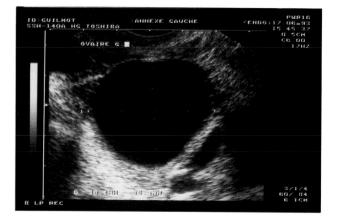

Figure 1 Transvaginal sonography: (a) unilocular cyst, without solid structures; (b) multilocular cyst; (c) cyst with thick septa and irregular solid parts suspected to be malignant

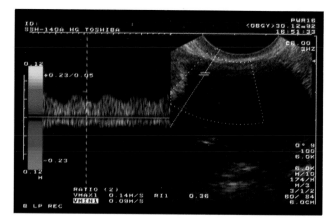

Figure 2 Transvaginal Doppler ultrasound with color flow imaging (corresponding to the cysts shown in Figure 1): (a) unilocular cyst: normal pulsatility index

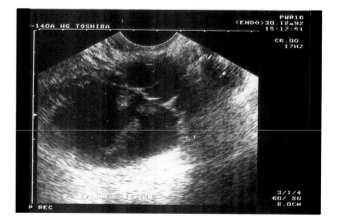

Figure 1 (b) *See legend above*

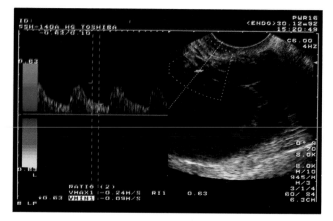

Figure 2 (b) Multilocular cyst: normal pulsatility index

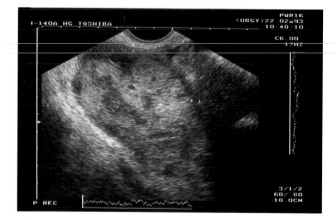

Figure 1 (c) *See legend above*

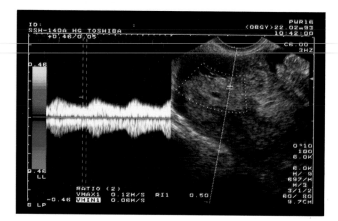

Figure 2 (c) Multilocular cyst with hyperechogenic areas. Low-resistant intratumoral blood vessels, suggesting malignancy

CA-125 in excess of 65 U/ml distinguished malignant from benign disease with a specificity of 92% and a sensitivity of 75% when both premenopausal and postmenopausal patients were studied together[11]. Greater specificity and sensitivity were observed in postmenopausal subjects, in whom the specificity of the assay was 97% and the sensitivity 78%[11].

CT and MRI

CT provides high quality images of the ovaries but does not give more information than ultrasound, except in cases of dermoid cysts (Figure 3). In our experience, CT is less sensitive and less specific than transvaginal echography in the detection of intracystic structures or septa (Figure 3).

MRI provides soft tissue contrast and clear pictures of pelvic organs (Figure 4). This modality is biologically safe and more sensitive than CT in the diagnosis of intracystic structures, and more sensitive and specific than either CT or ultrasound in the evaluation of an ovarian mass.

As a result of the accuracy, convenience, relatively low cost and availability of high-resolution ultrasound equipment, this technique has remained the principal imaging modality in assessing pelvic pathology. In our department, CT and MRI are indicated in cases of suspected malignant lesions.

INDICATIONS

Indications for laparoscopic cystectomy include serous, mucous, dermoid and endometriotic cysts. The internal wall of the endometriotic cyst, whose complete dissection from the ovarian cortex could be difficult, can also be vaporized with the CO_2 laser as previously described[12,13].

The indications for laparoscopic oophorectomy usually include large endometriotic cysts and benign ovarian cysts in patients aged over 40 years.

The laparoscopic aspiration of unilocular, smooth-walled, translucent ovarian cysts remains controversial. The main concern is spillage of malignancy. Thorough preoperative evaluation of the patient, combining ultrasonography of ovarian tumors with the measurement of tumor markers, may greatly improve the accuracy of diagnosis of ovarian malignancy. Moreover, laparoscopy is, in the first place, used as a diagnostic tool whereby the pelvis and the abdominal cavity are thoroughly evaluated.

The ovaries are inspected carefully to ensure that the cyst wall is smooth and that there is no vegetation (Figure 5). The interior wall of the cyst can also be carefully examined (Figure 6) and a biopsy with frozen histological evaluation can be carried out.

In a retrospective study of 226 patients, Mage and colleagues[14] reported that the diagnosis of malignant tumors by laparoscopy was 100% accurate.

The anatomopathological examination of specimens in benign conditions was never wrong. They concluded that laparoscopy is a reliable way of diagnosing the type of ovarian cyst.

According to these data, we have proposed the scheme outlined in Figure 7 for the laparoscopic management of ovarian cysts. In patients aged under 35 years, hormonal therapy is first attempted for 3 months if the echography reveals a unilocular, smooth-walled cyst without septa or intracystic structures. If the cyst persists, an ultrasound examination is carried out and the CA-125 level is measured, in order to exclude a malignant lesion. In patients under 40 years of age, a cystectomy is usually performed. In patients aged over 40 years, the preoperative evaluation (echography and CA-125) is made directly. If data suggest malignancy, a laparotomy is performed after computerized tomography and/or magnetic resonance imaging have been performed. Only when a malignant lesion can be excluded is a laparoscopy performed. If at all possible, the cyst is removed intact. Otherwise, the interior wall of the cyst is examined to exclude the presence of any suspect vegetation, which would require a biopsy and a frozen histological examination.

In patients over age 40 years, a cystectomy is rarely performed and a unilateral oophorectomy is the preferred procedure. If the frozen histological examination reveals the presence of malignant cells, a laparotomy and total abdominal hysterectomy is mandatory.

In patients aged over 50 years, after all the same precautions have been taken, a bilateral oophorectomy is carried out, even if the contralateral ovary is normal.

SURGICAL PROCEDURES

The procedure is performed under general anesthesia. After induction of a pneumoperitoneum, a 12-mm trocar is inserted subumbilically. The laparoscope is connected to a video camera. Three 5-mm trocars are systematically inserted suprapubically: one in the midline approximately 3 cm above the symphysis pubis, and the other two a few centimeters on either side, taking care to avoid the epigastric vessels.

The initial phase of the laparoscopy is purely diagnostic. First, the abdominal cavity is inspected thoroughly and a peritoneal sampling is sent for cytology. The ovaries are examined carefully in order to exclude the presence of excrescences or other evidence suggesting malignancy.

It is important to differentiate between organic and functional cysts during laparoscopy; 10–20% of functional cysts do not disappear after 3 months of treatment with combination oral contraceptive pills containing 50 μg of ethinylestradiol. According to Mage and associates[14], there are five laparoscopic criteria which allow us to distinguish between functional and organic cysts (Table 1).

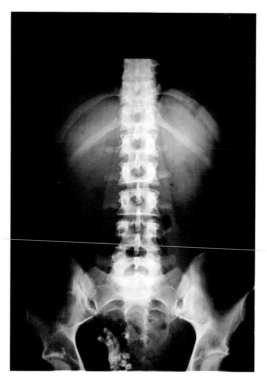

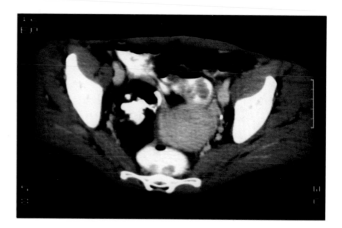

Figure 3(b)   *See legend opposite*

Figure 3(a) and (b)   Computerized tomography; in case of dermoid cyst, high quality images are obtained

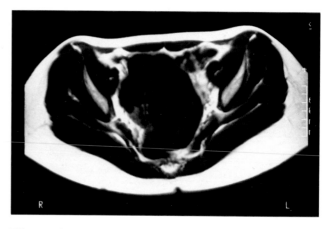

Figure 4(b)   *See legend opposite*

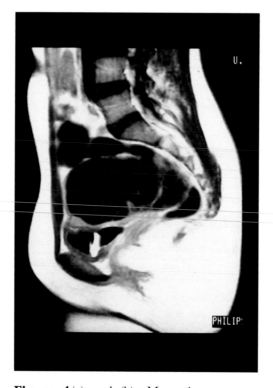

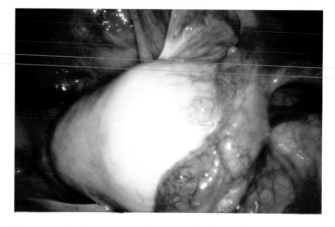

Figure 4(a) and (b)   Magnetic resonance imaging provides soft tissue contrast and clear pictures of pelvic organs. Multilocular cyst (histology: mucinous cyst)

Figure 5   Laparoscopic examination of the external cyst wall which must have a smooth appearance

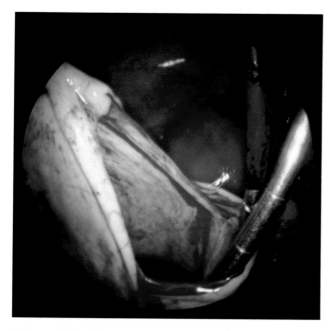 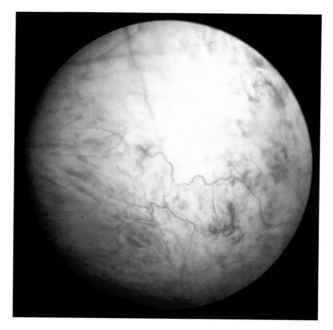

Figure 6(a)   Laparoscopic examination of the internal cyst wall; (b) internal view of the cyst. Note the absence of intracystic vegetations (no biopsy required)

Figure 6(b)   *See legend opposite*

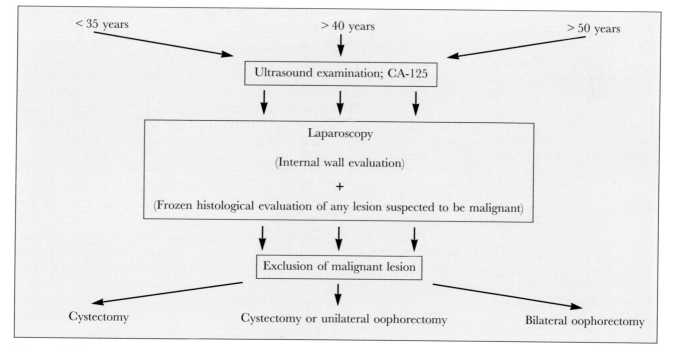

Figure 7   Laparoscopic management of ovarian cysts

Table 1 Laparoscopic criteria for differentiation between functional and organic ovarian cysts (from reference 14)

Criterion	Organic cysts	Functional cysts
Utero-ovarian ligament	lengthened	normal
Cyst wall	thick	thin
Ovarian vessels	numerous and regular starting from the mesovarium	more scanty, coral-like
Cyst fluid	clear, dark, brown, or demoid	saffron yellow
Internal cyst wall appearance	smooth or fibrotic with areas of hypervascularization	retina-like aspect

Intraperitoneal cystectomy

The utero-ovarian ligament is grasped with an atraumatic forceps introduced on the side of the tumor, in order to completely expose the ovary (Figure 8).

The first step consists of making an incision in the ovarian cortex with the scissors or with the CO_2 laser (Figure 9). The incision must be made in the ovarian cortex overlying the cyst and it must be long enough to permit a straightforward cystectomy. In some cases, the cyst is first aspirated and the liquid examined (Figure 10).

The interior wall of the cyst can be checked by introducing the laparoscope into the ovarian cyst (Figure 11). If there is any intracystic vegetation, a biopsy with frozen histological evaluation can be carried out before a decision is made whether to perform a cystectomy or oophorectomy. In fact, ideally, the cyst should be removed intact from the ovary, without aspirating any of the contents.

The second step is the separation of the ovarian cyst capsule from the surrounding ovarian cortex. The ovarian cyst is held using an atraumatic forceps and the ovarian cortex is grasped with another forceps placed close to the ovarian cyst (Figure 12). By traction and counter-traction, the dissection is easily carried out and the cyst is removed.

Nezhat and colleagues[5] inject 3–5 ml of dilute vasopressin between the capsule and ovarian cortex, to create a tissue plane (hydrodissection) and to reduce oozing from the ovarian bed. We do not consider this procedure to be useful and it is not used in our department.

The surgeon must constantly observe the tissue tension, and the grasping forceps must be moved often in order to apply the traction in just the right place to avoid tearing the ovary.

At the ovarian hilus, the dissection is often more difficult, but nevertheless, the dissection should continue until the cyst is completely removed from the ovary (Figure 13).

Thereafter, the interior ovarian surface is examined and rinsed. Hemostasis is usually achieved spontaneously but, if necessary, bipolar coagulation can be used. However, aggressive electrocoagulation can be the cause of ovarian destruction and premature ovarian failure.

Generally, there is no bleeding and the ovary is left to heal without suturing (Figure 14). Indeed, the ovarian edges approximate spontaneously. In cases of large cysts where approximation does not occur spontaneously, closure can be undertaken using the following techniques.

Suturing

The ability to suture during laparoscopy was initially developed by Semm[16]. Loop ligation using the endoloop or Roeder loop is most often used as an adjuvant to hemostasis, and as a classic ligature in the case of salpingo-oophorectomy or oophorectomy.

With the advent of endoligature and the intra- and extracorporeal operative knotting techniques, classic methods used at laparotomy were introduced in endoscopic surgery and have become a mainstay. The intracorporeal knotting technique has been recommended by Semm[16] for fine ovarian sutures. Two lower abdominal puncture sites are necessary, and through these, laparoscopic needle holders are introduced to manipulate the suture, needle and involved tissue. The suture material used is 4/0 or 6/0 polydioxanone.

Clips

Clips can also be used for closing the ovarian cortex after cystectomy. The clip is of medium to large size and is made of titanium, an inert, non-reactive metal (Autosuture (Eudohernia®); Ethicon). Three to four clips are applied using the 10-mm clip applicator; this is usually sufficient to achieve ovarian closure (Figure 15). For ovarian surgery, a titanium clip is preferred to one made of polydioxanone material.

Fibrin sealant

Fibrin sealant[13] is useful in controlling microvascular or capillary bleeding from ruptured or surgically dissected tissue. It is particularly beneficial during surgery on patients with increased bleeding tendencies. It might also

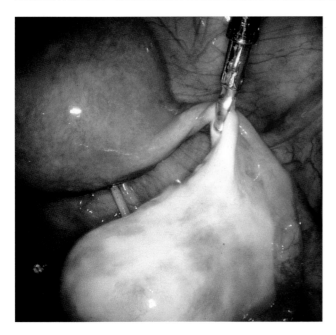

Figure 8 The ovarian cyst is exposed using a grasping forceps

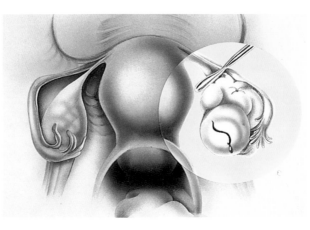

Figure 9(a)–(c)   Ovarian cortex incision with scissors

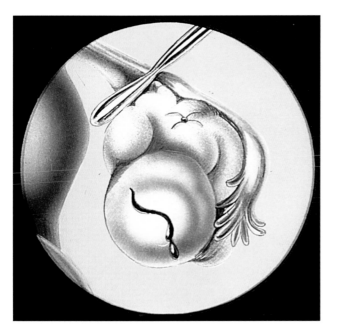

Figure 9(b)   *See legend above*

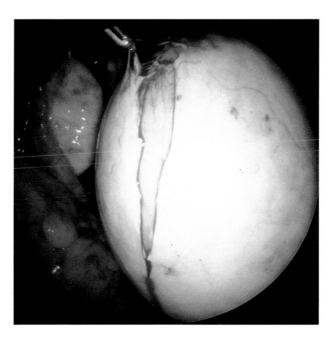

Figure 9(c)   *See legend above*

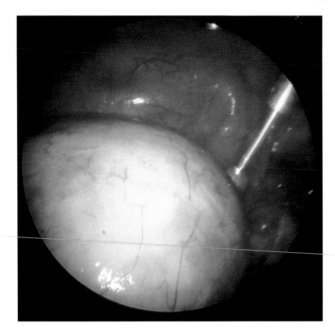

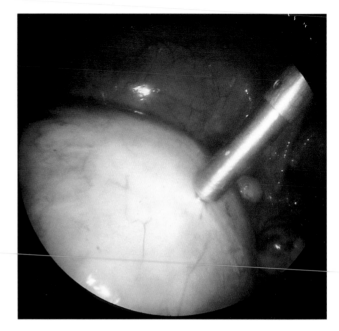

Figure 10(a) and (b)   In order to perform an ovarian cystoscopy, the aspiration of the intracystic contents can be carried out in some instances

Figure 10(b)   *See legend opposite*

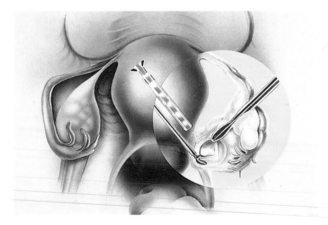

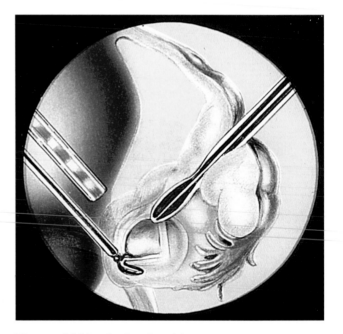

Figure 11(a) and (b) Ovarian cystoscopy by the introduction of the laparoscope into the cyst

Figure 11(b)   *See legend oppisite*

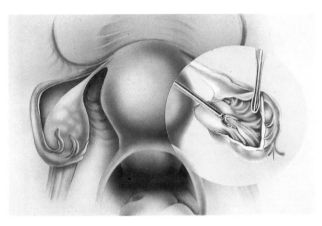

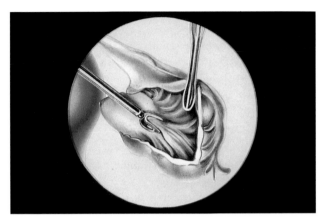

Figure 12(a)–(e) Separation of the ovarian cyst from the ovarian cortex using two atraumatic forceps

Figure 12(b) *See legend opposite*

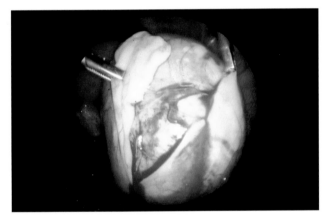

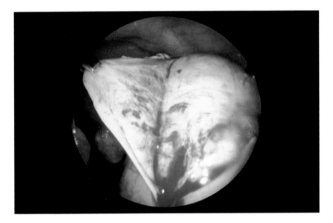

Figure 12(c) *See legend above*

Figure 12(d) *See legend above*

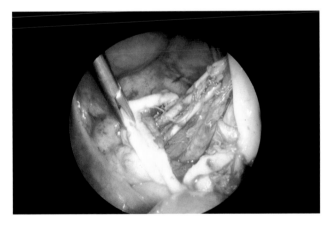

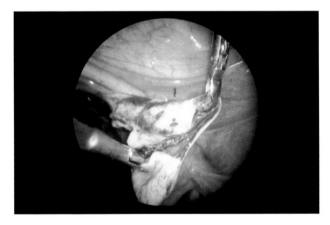

Figure 12(e) *See legend above*

Figure 13 Complete removal of the cyst. The remaining ovarian cortex is grasped with the help of two atraumatic forceps

be used to seal tissue with different kinds of biomaterials. Thus, fibrin sealant has a place in all surgical disciplines for the purposes of tissue sealing, hemostasis and support of wound healing. There seem to be a few drawbacks, such as the risk of viral transmission; however, the benefits of combining fibrin sealing with modern-day surgery far outweigh any known risks.

For the optimal use of fibrin sealant, the application technique should meet the following requirements:

(1) The sealant components should be fully dissolved and kept at a temperature of 37° C (which is easy with the Fibrinotherm system).

(2) The wound surfaces should be as dry as possible (though application to wet surfaces is feasible).

(3) The components should be mixed thoroughly on application.

(4) The thrombin and aprotinin concentrations may be adjusted to the purpose of application.

(5) The sealant should be applied as a thin film through a catheter introduced into one of the trocars.

(6) After clotting has occurred, further mechanical stresses should be avoided for about 3–5 min. The edges of the ovarian cortex are approximated with atraumatic forceps (Figure 16).

Laparoscopic oophorectomy

In most cases, the tube is removed with the ovary intact unless a previous salpingectomy has been performed. Different methods of laparoscopic oophorectomy have been described. The initial technique described the placement of pre-tied loop ligatures[16]; three chromic endoloop sutures were placed around the ovary and the tube and pulled tight. The ovary was then cut away from its pedicle, cut into strips, and removed laparoscopically.

The second method of laparoscopic oophorectomy was bipolar coagulation with excision (Figure 17(a) and (b)). This technique involved four punctures, with traction (Figure 17(c)) on the adnexum. A bipolar coagulation forceps was then used to coagulate the ovarian pedicle (Figure 17(d) and (e)). After total desiccation of the tissue, 5-mm scissors or the CO_2 laser were used to cut (Figure 17(f) and (g)). Successive portions of the meso-ovarium and mesosalpinx were treated in a similar fashion (Figure 17(h)), and the proximal tube and ovarian ligament were also coagulated (Figure 17(i)) and cut (Figure 17(j)). Once the tube and ovary had been separated, they were removed laparoscopically using a Lap sac (Figure 17(k)–(m)). Recent studies have shown equally good results using tissue desiccation with bipolar coagulation followed by excision without ligatures.

The most recent technique for laparoscopic oophorectomy is the automatic laparoscopic stapling device. Disposable stapling instruments for laparoscopic surgery are now available. The Multifire GIA surgical stapler (United States Surgical Corporation, Newark, NJ, USA) is readily available and is proving to be effective for appendicectomy, hysterectomy and adnexectomy (Figure 18).

A staple cartridge 3 cm in length is fired across the infundibulopelvic vessels. Two triple-staggered lines of titanium staples are automatically placed, with a knife cutting between them (Figure 18). In most cases, two firings of the automatic stapling device are necessary to accomplish removal of the tube and ovary. They are then extracted in a similar way to that used in other laparoscopic techniques. The automatic stapling device reduces operating time but is nevertheless more expensive than bipolar coagulation.

In certain cases, it is impossible to use pre-tied ligatures as the primary method because the ovary adheres too strongly to the sidewall to allow the placement of the ligature around the adnexa. In such cases, dissection and bipolar coagulation are necessary before beginning the oophorectomy. Similarly, the automatic stapling device, which is 12 mm in diameter, cannot be placed around the whole adnexa; it must be mobile and free before the automatic stapling device can be used[17]. Aquadissection, blunt probing, scissors and judicious use of bipolar coagulation are necessary in certain cases to mobilize the ovary for laparoscopic removal using any of the three techniques described. Aggressive ovariolysis increases the risk of ureteral or bowel injury, or severe bleeding.

The absence of ovarian adhesiolysis before oophorectomy can lead to the incomplete removal of all functional ovarian tissue. The endoloop sutures must be placed below the ovary, to avoid trapping ovarian tissue in the pedicle. Persistent ovarian remnant syndrome after laparoscopic oophorectomy has been described by several authors[15].

Cyst or adnexa removal

There are several techniques used for the removal of a cyst or of the adnexa:

(1) After enucleation from the ovaries or after oophorectomy, the tissue is grasped with the grasping forceps introduced through the operating channel of the laparoscope and removed from the abdominal cavity. Such removal can be performed only in cases of small ovarian cysts or after aspiration of the cyst.

However, in cases where spillage should be avoided at all costs (septate cysts or CA-125 > 35 U/ml), an impermeable bag can be used (Lap sac, Ethicon or Cook) (Figure 17(l) and (m)). The bag is introduced through a second puncture trocar. The cyst or the ovary with the intact cyst is

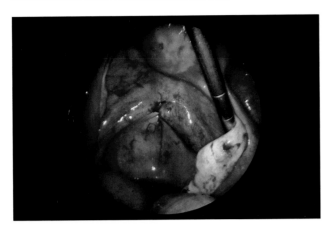

Figure 14 Final aspect of the ovarian cortex. The dermoid cyst was removed through a colpotomy incision whose closure is clearly visible between the utero-sacral ligaments

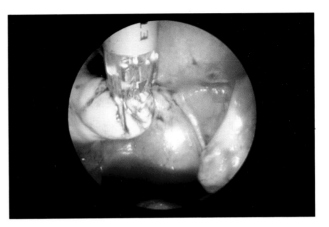

Figure 15 Ovarian closure using titanium clips

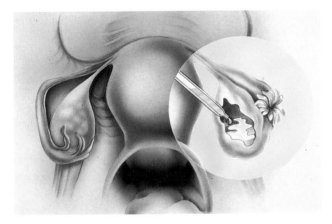

Figure 16(a) and (b) Ovarian closure by using fibrin sealant; (c) and (d) approximation of the ovarian cortex with two atraumatic forceps

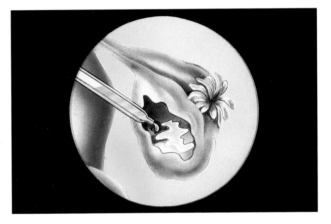

Figure 16(b) *See legend opposite*

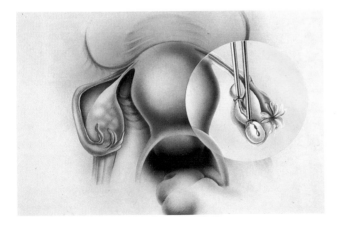

Figure 16(c) *See legend above*

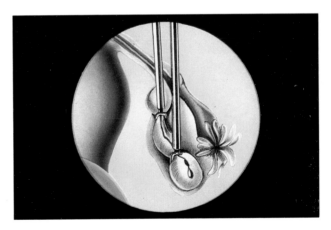

Figure 16(d) *See legend above*

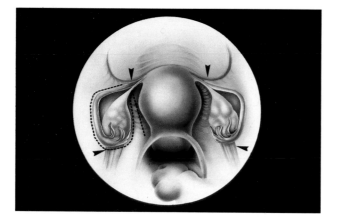

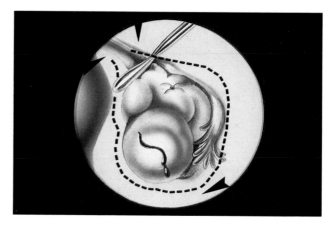

Figure 17 Laparoscopic annexectomy: (a) and (b) illustration of the technique – coagulation of the ovarian pedicle, the ligament, the Fallopian tube and the utero-ovarian ligament

Figure 17(b)   *See legend opposite*

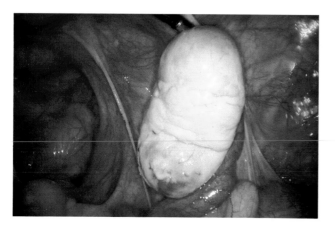

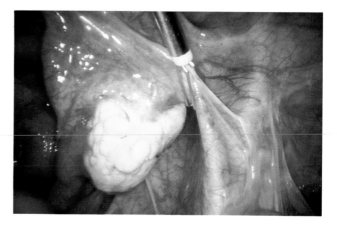

Figure 17(c) Laparoscopic view of a 3-cm multilocular cyst in a perimenopausal woman; the ovarian pedicle is grasped, elevated (d) and then coagulated (e)

Figure 17(d)   *See legend opposite*

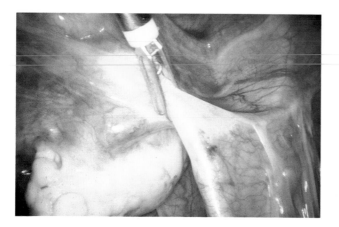

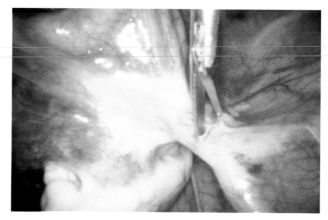

Figure 17(e)   *See legend above*

Figure 17(f) and (g)   Section of the ovarian pedicle with scissors

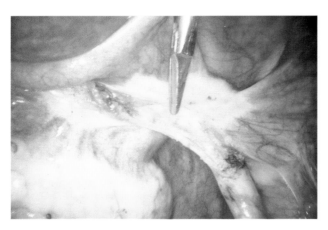

Figure 17(g)   *See legend on opposite page*

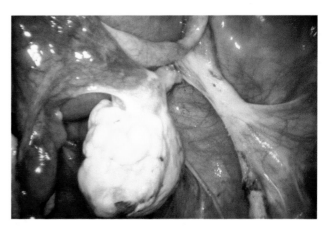

Figure 17(h)   The broad ligament is cut up to the round ligament

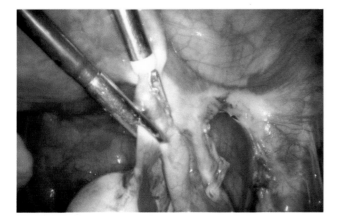

Figure 17(i)   Coagulation (i) and section (j) of the proximal part of the annexa; the annexa is dissected free (k). To avoid spillage, the ovary with intact cyst is placed in the bag (l) which is closed by pulling its drawstring (m)

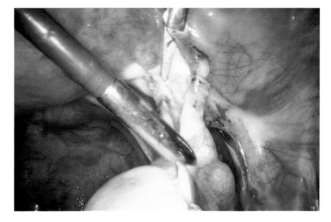

Figure 17(j)   *See legend opposite*

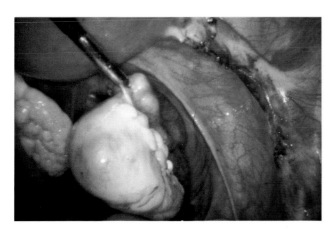

Figure 17(k)   *See legend above*

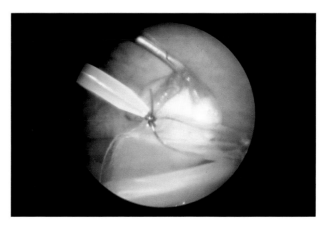

Figure 17(l)   *See legend above*

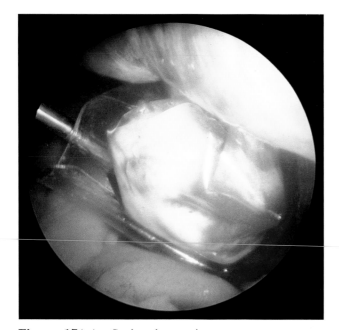

Figure 17(m)   *See legend on previous page*

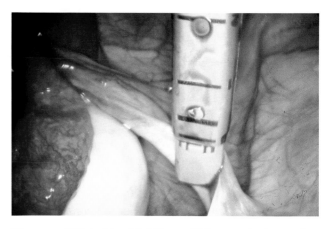

Figure 18(a)–(c)   Multifire GIA surgical stapler: application on the ovarian vessels

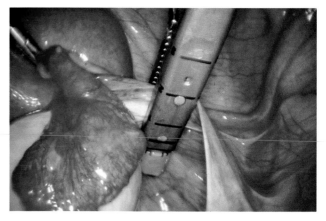

Figure 18(b)   *See legend above*

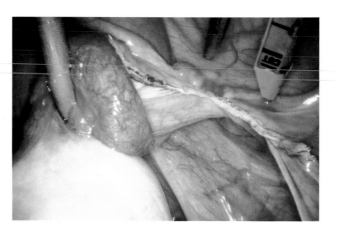

Figure 18(c)   *See legend above*

placed in the bag, which is closed by pulling its drawstring. The bag is raised to just beneath the abdominal wall and a needle is introduced into the bag in order to aspirate the cyst and decompress it. Then the bag is removed without spillage from the abdominal cavity through a 2-cm suprapubic incision. Reich[18] describes a different technique: the bag is inserted intraperitoneally through the colpotomy incision and it is removed by pulling the drawstring through the posterior vaginal incision. The bag is opened and the intact specimen visually identified, decompressed and removed.

(2) In some cases, the tissue is grasped directly with an instrument introduced through a suprapubic incision without using a bag. Theoretically, removing the cyst through a puncture site could lead to a surviving ovarian remnant in the abdominal wall. Nezhat and co-workers[15] have not observed this phenomenon in their 1–3-year follow-up in the patients who underwent this technique of cyst wall removal. However, Canis (personal communication) has recently reported induced endometriosis at the trocar site after removal of an endometriotic cyst through the abdominal wall. A metastatic tumor has been reported in three cases on the anterior abdominal wall at the trocar site, following biopsy of ovarian cancer[19]. It is suggested that any suspicious ovarian tissue must be removed from the abdomen while avoiding direct contact with the abdominal incision.

(3) In cases of large dermoid cysts, the cyst can be placed in the cul-de-sac of Douglas using a grasping forceps. A colpotomy incision is made and the cyst is then removed intact or aspirated through the vagina[20]: a needle is directed through the vagina for cyst decompression. The thick cyst contents can be evacuated by introducing the suction cannula into the cyst after making an incision of 5–6 mm. When the mass is small enough, it can be pulled through the vaginal incision. Copious vaginal and intraperitoneal irrigation with antiseptic solution is performed after cyst removal.

In our department, a colpotomy incision is made through the vagina and the overlying peritoneum using scissors. We have never encountered any complications – no bleeding, rectal injuries or infections – using this technique. However, Reich[18] suggests that a posterior colpotomy incision using the CO_2 laser or electrosurgery through the cul-de-sac of Douglas into the vagina is preferable to a vaginal incision because complete hemostasis is obtained while making the colpotomy incision. The anatomical relationship between the rectum and the posterior vagina must be confirmed before making the laparoscopic colpotomy incision to avoid cutting the rectum. Reich[18,21,22] uses an instrument placed in the uterus for elevation and anteversion. The posterior vaginal fornix is identified by placing a wet sponge in a ring forceps just behind the cervix. A rectal probe can also be used in order to ensure that the rectum is out of the way.

DISCUSSION

Risk of borderline tumor

The advantages of the laparoscopic treatment of ovarian cysts have been described for women under the age of 35 years with simple ovarian cysts, for whom the overall risk of malignancy is only 4.5 per 100 000 cases[14].

The risk is much higher in postmenopausal women. Indeed, a ten-year study[23] suggested that when a postmenopausal woman undergoes surgery for an ovarian neoplasm, the rate of malignancy may be as high as 45%. Very often, a malignant tumor is diagnosed or suspected by means of echography, CA-125, CT or MRI. We have tried to evaluate the 'true' risk of under-diagnosing an ovarian tumor preoperatively.

In a series of 114 postmenopausal women who underwent bilateral adnexectomy, 78 were found to have a serous or mucinous cystadenoma, ten an endometrial cyst, eight a paraovarian cyst, 14 a dermoid cyst and four (< 4%) a borderline tumor (Table 2). In this series, all patients had a preoperative check-up including the measurement of the CA-125 level and an ultrasound examination. Three of the four borderline tumor cases presented abnormalities at the preoperative check-up (Table 3). Indeed, in two cases, in spite of a normal CA-125 level, the echography showed a multilocular cyst. In one case, the cyst was unilocular but the CA-125 level was elevated. In the last case, however, there were no evident abnormalities (unilocular cyst, normal CA-125 level); therefore an accurate preoperative diagnosis was impossible (0.9%) (Figure 19). In these four borderline cases, the abnormal cells could not be detected on frozen pathology. These four patients underwent hysterectomy 2 weeks later. Peritoneal sampling for cytology did not reveal any abnormal cells, and the histology did not show any residual malignant tissue; to date, no sign of recurrence has been demonstrated.

The preoperative check-up of a mass diagnosed in postmenopausal women is, in most cases, accurate. Indeed, in our series only one case (< 1%) went undetected preoperatively. However, when an abnormality is observed (Figure 20), certain peroperative precautions must be taken to avoid spillage of the intracystic contents.

Risk of spillage

Spillage of benign material in cases of benign cystic teratomas or endometriomas can theoretically produce

Table 2 Bilateral adnexectomy ($n = 114$ postmenopausal women)

Pathology	Number
Serous or mucinous cystadenoma	78
Endometrial cyst	10
'Para-ovarian' cyst (Wolffian)	8
Dermoid	14
Borderline tumor	4

Table 3 Borderline tumors ($n = 4$); preoperative check-up

Case number	Echography	CA-125 (IU/ml)	Frozen pathology
1	multilocular	< 35	negative
2	multilocular	< 35	negative
3	unilocular	56	negative
4	unilocular	< 35	negative

chemical peritonitis. Intraoperative spillage of a mucinous cystadenoma may theoretically initiate pseudomyxoma peritonei. The risk appears to be very low, since pseudomyxoma peritonei, when reported, is usually present at the time of initial surgery[24]. According to several authors, pseudomyxoma peritonei is almost always associated with mucinous cystadenocarcinoma[25]. Furthermore, pseudomyxoma peritonei does not appear to be a frequent complication of mucinous carcinoma, even when ruptured at laparotomy. To date, Mage and co-workers[1,14] have observed no cases of pseudomyxoma peritonei after laparoscopic treatment of mucinous cystadenoma. Similar results have been reported after laparotomy with cyst rupture. The treatment of the cyst must include careful and copious peritoneal lavage performed immediately, using several liters of Ringer's lactate, with the patient in a reverse Trendelenburg position. Operative spillage should be avoided as much as possible by using 5-mm aspiration systems or a Lap sac. In cases of large cysts, the cyst can be punctured before it is placed in the Lap sac, which is positioned directly beneath the cyst in order to catch any possible spillage. Moreover, peritoneal lavage and the appropriate surgical treatment, carried out immediately after diagnosis, seem to make the risks of spillage negligible[1,26] (also Donnez and Nisolle, present study). A recent re-evaluation of intraoperative spillage at laparotomy has demonstrated no adverse effect on the prognosis of stage I ovarian cancer[27]. According to this study, the survival term depends primarily on three factors:

(1) The tumor grading;

(2) The density of adhesions; and

(3) Ascites > 250 ml.

However, the capsule penetration, the tumor size, the histological type, the age of the patient and the rupture of the tumor were found to have no influence on the prognosis.

It is generally agreed that ovarian cancer should not be managed laparoscopically. One of the drawbacks of operative laparoscopy may be that, in certain cases, malignant cysts cannot be detected.

Risk of postoperative adhesions

What is the risk of postoperative adhesion formation following closure vs. non-closure of ovarian defects? It is well known that the ovary is particularly sensitive to surgical trauma, as demonstrated by the high incidence of adhesions after ovarian wedge resection. Buttram and Vaquero[28] performed bilateral ovarian wedge resection for polycystic ovarian disease in 173 patients. Of these, 34% underwent endoscopy or laparotomy at some time after bilateral wedge resection. Although the degree of severity varied, all 59 women were found to have adhesions.

Of nine women of reproductive age who underwent removal of dermoid cysts via laparoscopy without an ovarian suture, Nezhat and associates[15] performed a repeat laparoscopy in four for the evaluation of possible pelvic adhesion formation. Only one had mild periovarian adhesions and she had experienced no previous spillage of cyst contents; in the other three women without adhesions at the time of their second laparoscopy, spillage had previously occurred during the cystectomy. Because there is little adhesion formation after intraperitoneal cystectomy, most authors consider that no suture is required and that the ovary can be left open. In our department, ovarian closure is performed only in cases of large endometriotic cysts. Indeed, such cysts are vaporized using the CO_2 laser instead of dissection. Following this type of procedure, the ovarian edges do not approximate spontaneously, and adhesion formation can occur between the vaporized area and the fimbria[12,13]. For this reason, Tissucol® or clips can be used for the ovarian closure[13].

CONCLUSION: THE RIGHT WAY IS THE SELECTION OF PATIENTS

Selection of patients for laparoscopic treatment can be accomplished successfully by excluding those with elevated CA-125 levels, suspect ultrasound appearances of cysts containing > 3-mm thick septations, solid components within a cyst, matted loops of bowel, or ascites. Large series have demonstrated a reassuringly low incidence of inadvertently encountered malignancy at laparoscopy (0.4%[29,30], 0.9% (Nisolle and Donnez, present study), 1.1%[24], 1.2%[1]), but intraoperative

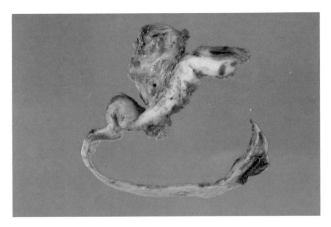

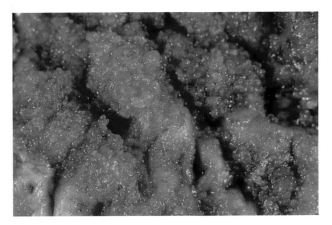

Figure 19 Borderline ovarian tumor: (a) unilocular cyst with a normal CA-125 level; (b) small (< 1 mm) papillary lesions were visible over an area of 1 cm²; (c)–(e) histology reveals the presence of an ovarian borderline tumor

Figure 19(b) *See legend opposite*

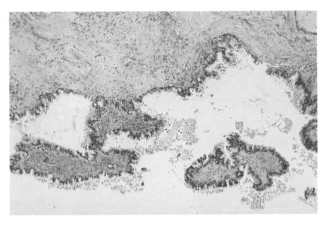

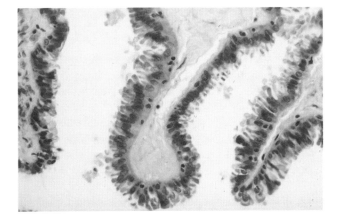

Figure 19(c) *See legend above*

Figure 19(d) *See legend above*

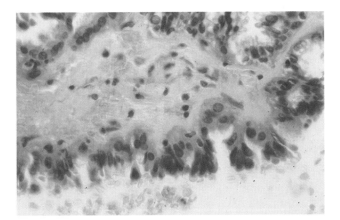

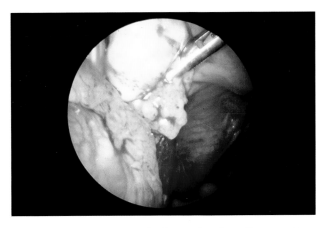

Figure 19(e) *See legend above*

Figure 20 Laparoscopic diagnosis of small vegetations on the surface of the ovary. These were not suspected by echography. Frozen histology revealed a 'borderline' tumor. Ovariectomy was carried out. The ovary was removed by using a Lap-Sac

surveillance and numerous biopsies are necessary if unsuspected cancer is to be correctly diagnosed.

We are of the opinion that careful preoperative and peroperative examination will eliminate the high rate of mistakes published in 1991 by Maiman and colleagues[31]. For us, this manuscript reveals a lack of experience or the absence of strict guidelines of the 29 respondents who took part in a survey concerning the 'laparoscopic management of ovarian neoplasms subsequently found to be malignant'.

REFERENCES

1. Mage, G., Canis, M., Manhes, H., Pouly, J.L., Wattiez, A. and Bruhat, M.A. (1990). Laparoscopic management of adnexal cystic masses. *J. Gynecol. Surg.*, **6**, 71–9
2. Bruhat, M.A., Mage, G., Chapron, C., Pouly, J.L., Canis, M. and Wattiez, A. (1991). Presentday endoscopic surgery in gynecology. *Eur. J. Obstet. Gynecol. Reprod. Biol.*, **41**, 4–13
3. Campbell, S., Bhan, V., Royston, P., Whitehead, M.T. and Collins, W.P. (1989). Transabdominal ultrasound screening for early ovarian cancer. *Br. Med. J.*, **299**, 1363–7
4. Hermann, U.J., Locher, G.W. and Goldhirsch, A. (1987). Sonographic patterns of ovarian tumors: prediction of malignancy. *Obstet. Gynecol.*, **69**, 777–81
5. Bourne, T., Campbell, S., Steer, C., Whitehead, M.I. and Collins, W.P. (1989). Transvaginal colour flow imaging: a possible new screening technique for ovarian cancer. *Br. Med. J.*, **299**, 1367–70
6. Kurjak, A., Schulman, H., Sosic, A., Zalud, I. and Shalan, H. (1992). Transvaginal ultrasound, color flow, and Doppler waveform of the postmenopausal adnexal mass. *Obstet. Gynecol.*, **80**, 917–21
7. Kawai, M., Kano, T., Kikkawa, F., Maeda O., Oguchi, H. and Tomoda, Y. (1992). Transvaginal Doppler ultrasound with color flow imaging in the diagnosis of ovarian cancer. *Obstet. Gynecol.*, **79**, 163–7
8. Weiner, Z., Thaler, I., Beck, D., Rottem, S., Deutsch, M. and Brandes, J.M. (1992). Differentiating malignant from benign ovarian tumors with transvaginal color flow imaging. *Obstet. Gynecol.*, **79**, 159–62
9. Fleischer, A.C., McKee M.S., Gordon, A.N. *et al.* (1990). Transvaginal sonography of postmenopausal ovaries with pathologic correlation. *J. Ultrasound Med.*, **9**, 637–44
10. Hata, K., Hata, T., Manabe, A., Sugimura, K. and Kitao, M. (1992). A critical evaluation of transvaginal Doppler studies, transvaginal sonography, magnetic resonance imaging, and CA-125 in detecting ovarian cancer. *Obstet. Gynecol.*, **80**, 922–6
11. Malkasian, G.D., Knapp, R.C., Lavin, P.T.,

Zurawski, V.R., Podratz, K.C., Stanhope, R., Mortel, R., Berek J.S., Bast, R.C. and Ritts, R.E. (1988). Preoperative evaluation of serum CA 125 levels in premenopausal and postmenopausal patients with pelvic masses: discrimination of benign from malignant disease. *Am. J. Obstet. Gynecol.*, **159**, 341–6
12. Donnez, J., Nisolle, M., Karaman, Y., Wayembergh, M., Clerckx, F. and Casanas-Roux, F. (1990). CO_2 laser laparoscopy in peritoneal endometriosis and in ovarian cyst. *J. Gynecol. Surg.*, **5**, 391
13. Donnez, J. and Nisolle, M. (1991). Laparoscopic management of large ovarian endometrial cysts: use of fibrin sealant. *J. Gynecol. Surg.*, **7**, 163–7
14. Mage, G., Canis, M., Manhes, G., Pouly, J.L. and Bruhat, M.A. (1987). Kystes ovariens et coelioscopie. A propos de 226 observations. *J. Gynecol. Obstet. Biol. Reprod.*, **16**, 1053–61
15. Nezhat, C., Winer, W.K. and Nezhat, F. (1989). Laparoscopic removal of dermoid cyst. *Obstet. Gynecol.*, **73**, 278–80
16. Semm, K. and Mettler, L. (1980). Technical progress in pelvic surgery via operative laparoscopy. *Am. J. Obstet. Gynecol.*, **138**, 121–7
17. Daniell, J.F., Kurts, B.R. and Lee J. (1992). Laparoscopic oophorectomy: comparative study of ligatures, bipolar coagulation, and automatic stapling devices. *Obstet. Gynecol.*, **80**, 325–8
18. Reich, H. (1993). Difficulties in removing large masses from the abdomen. In Corfman, R.S., Diamond, M.P. and De Cherney, A. (eds.) *Complications of laparoscopy and hysteroscopy*, pp.103–7. (New York: Blackwell Scientific Publications)
19. Hsiu, J.G., Given, F.T. and Kemp, G.M. (1986). Tumor implantation after diagnostic laparoscopic biopsy of serous ovarian tumors of low malignant potential. *Obstet. Gynecol.*, **68**, 91–3
20. Nisolle, M. and Donnez, J. (1992). Laparoscopic ovarian cystectomy. Presented at the *Seventh International Symposium on Laser Endoscopic Surgery*, Brussels
21. Reich, H. (1987). Laparoscopic oophorectomy and salpingo-oophorectomy in the treatment of benign tubo-ovarian disease. *Int. J. Fertil.*, **32**, 233–6
22. Reich, H. (1989). New techniques in advanced laparoscopic surgery. In Sutton, C.J.G. (ed.) *Baillière's Clinical Obstetrics and Gynaecology. Laparoscopic Surgery*, **3**, 655–82
23. Koonings, R.P., Campbell, K., Mishell, D.R. and Grimes, D.A. (1989). Relative frequency of primary ovarian neoplasms: a 10-year review. *Obstet. Gynecol.*, **74**, 921–6
24. Tasker, M. and Langley, F.A. (1985). The outlook for women with borderline epithelial tumours of the ovary. *Br. J. Obstet. Gynaecol.*, **92**, 969
25. Fernandez, R.N., and Daly, J.M. (1980).

Pseudomyxoma peritonei. *Arch. Surg.*, **115**, 409

26. Lueken, R.P. (1993). Laparoscopic-ovarian surgery. In Lueken, R.P. and Gallinat, A. (eds.) *Endoscopic Surgery in Gynecology*, pp.43–7. (Berlin: Demeter Verlag GMBH)

27. Dembo, A.J., Davy, M., Stenwig, A.E., Berle, E.J., Bush, R.S. and Kjorstad, K. (1990). Prognostic factors in patients with stage I epithelial ovarian cancer. *Obstet. Gynecol.*, **75**, 263–73

28. Buttram, V.C. and Vaquero, C. (1975). Post-ovarian wedge resection adhesive disease. *Fertil. Steril.*, **26**, 874

29. Nezhat, C. and Nezhat, F. (1993). Complications of laparoscopic ovarian cystectomy. In Corfman, R.S., Diamond, M.P. and De Cherney, A. (eds.) *Complications of laparoscopy and kysteroscopy*, pp.108–12. (New York: Blackwell Scientific Publications)

30. Nezhat, F., Nezhat, C., Welander, C.E. and Benigno, B. (1992). Four ovarian cancers diagnosed during laparoscopic management of 1011 women with adnexal masses. *Am. J. Obstet. Gynecol.*, **167**, 790–6

31. Maiman, M., Seltzer, V. and Boyce, J. (1991) Laparoscopic excision of ovarian neoplasms subsequently found to be malignant. *Obstet. Gynecol.*, **77**, 563–5

Fertility following laparoscopic treatment of benign adnexal cysts

S. Bassil, M. Canis, J.L. Pouly, A. Wattiez, G. Mage and M.A. Bruhat

INTRODUCTION

Postoperative adhesions are the most unfortunate sequelae of ovarian surgery and may result in mechanical infertility. In cases of persistent ovarian cysts in women of reproductive age, surgical removal is necessary. Laparoscopy is now being used with increasing frequency[1-3] for the management of adnexal cysts. Laparoscopy procedures seem to be associated with decreased postoperative adhesion formation compared to laparotomy[4,5], but some controversy persists concerning the closure or non-closure of the ovarian wound. In animal studies[4,6,7] ovarian non-closure seems to be less adhesiogenic than surgical ovarian closure. In women, evaluation of the postoperative fertility rates is an objective method of evaluating the effectiveness of laparoscopic techniques. Since 1980 we have been using laparoscopic surgery for the management of benign adnexal cysts with a follow-up for all patients. The postoperative fertility rates are reported in this study.

MATERIALS AND METHODS

The preoperative selection of patients was based on the suspicion of a benign organic cyst; patients were selected if they presented an echogenic or heterogeneous cyst on sonography without signs of malignancy, an anechogenic cyst more than 8 cm in diameter or a persistent anechogenic cyst after 3 months of hormonal therapy.

The operative techniques and the laparoscopic instruments used have been described previously[2,8,9]. Laparotomy was performed if any sign of malignancy was observed by laparoscopy. After peritoneal cytology and careful examination of the peritoneal cavity, benign adnexal cysts were treated conservatively using three laparoscopic procedures:

(1) Intraperitoneal cystectomy using two atraumatic grasping forceps to separate the cyst wall from the ovarian cortex;

(2) Extraperitoneal cystectomy after the extraction of the ovary through a transverse abdominal incision of 2–3 cm in diameter;

(3) Puncture and aspiration of cystic fluid with partial resection of the cystic wall, only in cases of functional cysts.

In all cases the ovarian cortex was left open and no suture was used. When necessary, additional hemostasis was achieved using bipolar coagulation.

Patients were either followed up in our department, or both the patient and her referring physician were contacted by letter with a standard questionnaire.

The cumulative pregnancy rate was calculated using life-table analysis and the monthly fecundity rate according to Cramer and colleagues[10]. As most of the patients at the time of the retrospective study had been using contraception for several months or years following the laparoscopic procedure, the delay before pregnancy occurred was established either from charts or from the patient's recollection when she received the questionnaire. Because data obtained from the patients (50% of the cases) were likely to be subjective, both the cumulative pregnancy rate and the monthly fecundity rate should be interpreted cautiously.

Out of 767 patients followed up for more than 12 months after laparoscopic diagnosis and treatment of

Table 1 Pathological diagnosis and operative procedures

Pathology	n	Intrauterine pregnancy	Fertile (%)	Puncture, aspiration, partial resection of cyst wall	Intraperitoneal cystectomy	Extra-abdominal cystectomy
Functional	12	12	100	10	1	1
Serous + mucinous	10	10	100	—	6*	5
Teratoma	14	13	92.9	—	9†	7
Paraovarian	7	5	71.4	—	5	2
Total	43	40	93	10	21	15

*, one patient had bilateral mucinous cysts;   †, two patients had bilateral dermoid cysts

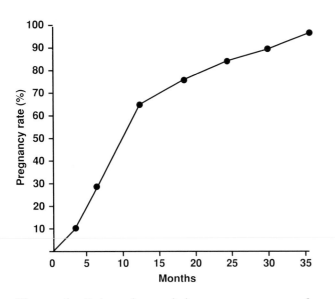

Figure 1 Estimated cumulative pregnancy rate after laparoscopic treatment of adnexal cysts

adnexal cysts of more than 3 cm in diameter, 43 women of reproductive age, treated conservatively, were finally included. Three patients presented a bilateral cyst. Their mean age was 27.7 ± 4.7 years (range 18–37 years); the mean duration of follow-up was 46 months (range 14–120 months).

Patients who had been using contraception since the procedure, who were previously infertile, or who had been treated by laparotomy were excluded from the analysis. Since both moderate and severe endometriosis are associated with decreased fertility[11], patients with endometriomas were also excluded.

The pathological diagnoses and the laparoscopic procedures are listed in Table 1.

A total of 46 cysts were removed in 43 patients (three patients had bilateral cysts); 12 patients had a functional cyst, seven a paraovarian cyst and 24 a benign organic cyst. The mean cyst diameter established from the pre-operative ultrasonographic examination was 5.9 ± 2 cm (range 3–11 cm). There were 16 patients with an adnexal cyst of 6 cm or more, including one functional cyst.

All patients had an uneventful postoperative recovery.

RESULTS

The overall rate of intrauterine pregnancy was 93% (40 patients). One patient (2.3%) had an ectopic pregnancy 37 months after an intraperitoneal cystectomy for the treatment of a paraovarian cyst of 12 cm in diameter. At the time of this study, two patients (4.3%) had failed to conceive more than two years after the treatment.

The cumulative pregnancy rate was 70.1% and 84.2% at 12 and 24 months, respectively (Figure 1). The monthly fecundity rate was 7.8% (95% confidence interval, 5.3–10.5%).

No differences in the intrauterine pregnancy rates were found according to the laparoscopic procedures. As shown in Table 2, the rate of intrauterine pregnancy was 100% after puncture and aspiration with partial resection of the cyst wall, 88.9% after intraperitoneal cystectomy and 93.3% after extraperitoneal cystectomy. Fertility was not associated with the diameter of the cysts (Table 3). There was no statistically significant difference between fertility rates associated with cysts less than 6 cm in diameter and with those of more than 6 cm in diameter.

DISCUSSION

Periadnexal adhesion formation is suggested as an important factor in infertility after ovarian surgery[12,13]. Microsurgery and laparoscopy have been advocated as non-traumatic techniques to avoid postoperative adhesion formation[8,14].

Microsurgical techniques have stressed the importance of reapproximation of the ovarian cortex with non-reactive suture, and endoscopic techniques have been described with the ovarian cortex left without suture[14,15]. In recent studies on animal models, the authors have shown that non-closure of the ovarian wound is less adhesiogenic than microsurgical closure[4,6,7]. Also, in a randomized trial concerning laparoscopy vs. laparotomy in the management of ectopic pregnancy, Lundorff[5] found significantly more postoperative adhesions in the group treated by laparotomy.

Table 2 Fertility according to the laparoscopic procedure

	Puncture, aspiration, partial resection of the cyst wall		Intraperitoneal cystectomy		Extra-abdominal cystectomy	
	n	%	n	%	n	%
Intrauterine pregnancy	10	100	16	88.9	14	93.3
Extrauterine pregnancy	0	0	1	5.5	0	0
No pregnancy	0	0	1	5.5	1	6.7
Total	10		18		15	

Table 3 Results according to ovarian cyst diameter

	Cyst diameter < 6 cm		Cyst diameter > 6 cm	
	n	%	n	%
Intrauterine pregnancy	24	100	11	91.7
Extrauterine pregnancy	0	0	—	—
No pregnancy	0	0	1	8.5
Total	24		12	

This study was not designed to compare laparoscopy to microsurgery directly, but the aim was to evaluate the effectiveness of laparoscopy in the management of benign adnexal cysts. From our results, laparoscopic procedures seem to improve fertility outcome. However, in this short series, only 33 patients were treated by laparoscopic cystectomy (10 patients were treated by puncture and aspiration of cystic fluid with partial resection of the cyst wall). Also, this study is an evaluation of a 10-year follow-up, and in the first 5 years difficult cases were treated by laparotomy. Therefore, this constituted a selection of cases. The present results will have to be confirmed by continuing the follow-up on larger series.

Only a few studies have evaluated fertility after treatment of adnexal cysts by laparotomy, and the majority of them include wedge resection of the ovaries; this procedure is known to be adhesiogenic and not valuable in the comparison with treatment of an isolated ovarian cyst[12,16,17]. Our results are similar to the 87% pregnancy rate reported by Leizerowitz and associates[18]. There was no difference in the intrauterine pregnancy rate according to the laparoscopic procedure or to the cyst diameter. One ectopic pregnancy occurred after the treatment of a paraovarian cyst. The intrauterine pregnancy rate after the treatment of organic ovarian cysts was 96.5% compared to a rate of 71.8% after treatment of paraovarian cysts. Laparoscopic cystectomy using the ovarian non-closure technique seems to be effective, with an overall intrauterine pregnancy rate of 93%.

From these results and our experience, some guidelines may be proposed to improve laparoscopic cystectomy:

(1) As in our study, the ovarian incision should be performed on the antimesenteric surface of the ovary, as far as possible from the fimbria, so that the edges of the incision will be approximated when the ovary falls back into the posterior cul-de-sac.

(2) The cystectomy should be performed using only one incision, which should be wide enough to avoid any additional tearing of the ovarian cortex.

(3) Careful hemostasis should be achieved.

(4) The shape of the ovary may be approximated using a minimal resection of the remaining ovarian tissue or a superficial coagulation or local vaporization of the internal wall of the ovarian cortex to induce an eversion of the ovary.

(5) Special care should be taken in the treatment of paraovarian cysts and the cystectomy must avoid deep dissection and tearing of the tubal serosa.

These procedures were applied to treat the patients included in this report and should be respected in the treatment of large ovarian or paraovarian cysts in future.

REFERENCES

1. Nezhat, C., Winer, W.K. and Nezhat, F. (1989). Laparoscopic removal of dermoid cysts. *Obstet. Gynecol.*, **73**, 278–81
2. Mage, G., Canis, M., Manhes, H., Pouly, J.L, Wattiez, A. and Bruhat, M.A. (1990). Laparoscopic management of adnexal cystic masses. *J. Gynecol. Surg.*, **6**, 71–9
3. Daniell, J.F., Kurtz, B.R. and Gurley, L.D. (1991). Laser laparoscopic management of large endometriomas. *Fertil. Steril.*, **55**, 692–5
4. Luciano, A.A., Maier, B.D., Koch, E.I., Nulsen, J.C. and Whitman, G.F. (1989). A comparative study of postoperative adhesions following laser surgery by laparoscopy versus laporotomy in the rabbit model. *Obstet. Gynecol.*, **74**, 220–4
5. Lundorff, P., Hahlin, M., Kallfelt, B., Thorburn, J. and Lindblom, B. (1991). Adhesion formation after laparoscopic surgery in tubal pregnancy: a randomized trial versus laparotomy. *Fertil. Steril.*, **55**, 911–15
6. Brumsted, J.R., Deaton, J., Lavigne, E. and Riddick, D.H. (1990). Postoperative adhesion formation after wedge resection with and without ovarian reconstruction in the rabbit. *Fertil. Steril.*, **53**, 723–6
7. Wiskind, A.K., Toledo, A.A., Dudley, A.G. and Zusmanis, K. (1990). Adhesion formation after ovarian wound repair in New Zealand white rabbits: a comparison of microsurgical closure with ovarian non-closure. *Am. J. Obstet. Gynecol.*, **163**, 1674–8
8. Bruhat, M.A., Mage, G., Pouly, J.L., Manhes, H., Canis, M. and Wattiez, A. (1991). *Operative Laparoscopy*, pp.187–202. (New York: MacGraw-Hill)
9. Canis, M., Mage, G., Wattiez, A., Bassil, S., Pouly, J.L., Manhes, H., Chapron, C. and Bruhat, M.A. (1992). Kystes de l'annexe. Place de la coelioscope en 1991. *Contracept. Fertil. Sex.*, **20**, 345–52
10. Cramer, D.W., Walker, A.M. and Schiff, I. (1979). Statistical methods in evaluating the outcome of infertility therapy. *Fertil. Steril.*, **32**, 80–6
11. Olive, D.L., Stohs, G.F., Metzger, D.A. and Franklin, R.R. (1985). Expectant management and hydrotubations in the treatment of endometriosis associated infertility. *Fertil. Steril.*, **44**, 35–41

12. Weinstein, D. and Polishuk, W.Z. (1975). The role of wedge resection of the ovary as a cause of mechanical sterility. *Surg. Gynecol. Obstet.*, **141**, 417–18

13. Donnez, J. and Thomas, K. (1983). Facteurs étiologiques de la stérilité tubaire. *J. Gynecol. Obstet. Biol. Reprod.*, **12**, 451–5

14. Levinson, C.J. and Swolin, K. (1980). Postoperative adhesions, etiology, prevention and therapy. *Clin. Obstet. Gynecol.*, **23**, 1213–20

15. Bruhat, M.A., Manhes, H., Mage, G. and Pouly, J.L. (1980). Treatment of ectopic pregnancy by means of laparoscopy. *Fertil. Steril.*, **33**, 411–14

16. Adashi, E.Y., Rock, J.A., Guzick, O., Wentz, A.C., Jones, C.S. and Jones, H.W. Jr (1981). Fertility following bilateral ovarian wedge resection: a critical analysis of 90 consecutive cases of the polycystic ovary syndrome. *Fertil. Steril.*, **36**, 320–5

17. Buttram, V.C., Jr and Vaquero, C. (1974). Post-ovarian wedge resection adhesive disease. *Fertil. Steril.*, **26**, 874–6

18. Leizerowitz, D.M., Ellenbogen, A., Jaschevatzky, O.E. and Grunstein, S. (1977). Fertility following adnexal surgery. *Acta Eur. Fertil.*, **8**, 239–43

The place of endoscopic surgery in the management of polycystic ovarian disease

16

J. Donnez and M. Nisolle

In 1935, Stein and Leventhal[1] described the clinical syndrome of polycystic ovarian disease (PCOD). Women with PCOD have a number of hormonal abnormalities: elevated levels of serum luteinizing hormone (LH) and plasma androgen concentrations leading to clinical signs of hirsutism, acne and anovulation.

During the same year, Stein and Leventhal[1] advocated ovarian wedge resection as a therapeutic measure; this became widely accepted as it was the only treatment available before the 1960s. Indeed, they reported an ovulation rate of 95% and a pregnancy rate as high as 85% after wedge resection. More than 10 years later, Adashi and colleagues[2] confirmed the ovulation rate but the pregnancy rate after wedge resection was lower than that published previously by Stein and Leventhal.

Much later, ovarian wedge resection by laparotomy was found to be the cause of periovarian adhesions (Figure 1). Thus, the endocrinological infertility of polycystic ovarian disease was transformed into a mechanical infertility[3]. Moreover, histological analysis of a biopsy taken from the site of an ovarian wedge resection (performed more than 1 year before) revealed fibrosis of the ovarian cortex (Figure 2).

To avoid such postoperative adhesions, endoscopic surgery was proposed for women with PCOD instead of laparotomy. Ovarian electrocautery was performed through the laparoscope and each ovary was cauterized in multiple places using a monopolar system. This procedure was described by Gjonnaess in 1984[4]. He reported that the ovulation rate was similar to that obtained after laparotomy.

This report was confirmed by Greenblatt and Casper in 1987[5]. Using the same technique, they showed that serum androstenedione, testosterone, estradiol and luteinizing hormone were significantly reduced postoperatively. In 1989, Daniell and Miller[6] published not only a very high ovulation rate but also a very high pregnancy rate with the laser. They vaporized and drained all the visible subcapsular follicles on each ovary to drill craters in the ovarian stroma. The CO_2, KTP and argon lasers were used (Figure 3).

At the same time, in our group, the CO_2 laser was used during operative laparoscopy for ovarian drilling in ten cases of polycystic ovarian disease. We also reported a high ovulation rate (70%), but the pregnancy rate was 20%. Moreover, the long-term efficacy (more than 6 months) in the reduction of testosterone secretion was less than 50%.

The aim of this report is to evaluate the efficacy of laparoscopic techniques and their place in the management of polycystic ovarian disease.

Table 1 Comparison of the ovulation and pregnancy rates found in the different types of management of polycystic ovarian disease

Author	Management	Number	Ovulation rate (%)	Pregnancy rate (%)
Gadir et al. (1990)[7]	electrocautery	29	71.4	52.1
	hMG	30	70.6	55.4
	FSH	29	66.7	38.3
Donnez (personal data)	CO_2 laser	10	70.0	20.0
	GnRHa + hMG	10	80.0	60.0
Kovacs et al. (1991)[8]	electrocautery	10	70.0	40.0*
Gurgan et al. (1991)[9]	electrocautery	7	71.0	57.0[†]
	Nd : YAG laser	10	70.0	40.0[†]
Gadir et al. (1992)[10]	electrocautery + hMG	16	85.3	43.8
	GnRH + hMG	17	77.3	47.1

hMG = human menopausal gonadotropin; GnRH = gonadotropin releasing hormone; GnRHa = GnRH agonist; FSH = follicle stimulating hormone; *, two cases after hMG therapy, one case after *in vitro* fertilization; [†], after a second-look laparoscopy and adhesiolysis

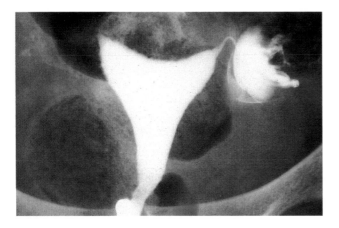

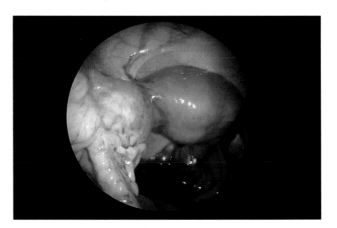

Figure 1 Hysterography (a) and laparoscopic aspect (b) after bilateral ovarian wedge resection: postoperative adhesion at the site of ovarian wedge resection

Figure 1(b)   *See legend opposite*

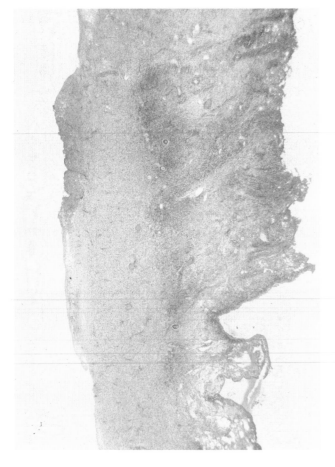

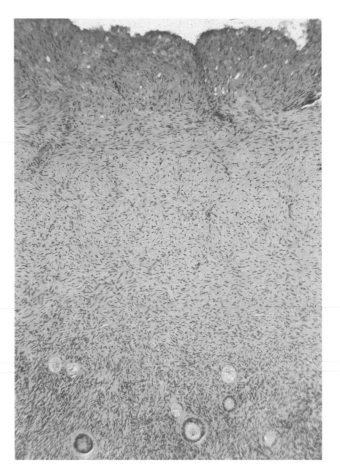

Figure 2 Postoperative ovarian fibrosis (Gomori's trichrome (a) × 56; (b) × 110). Note the presence of abundant connective tissue. Oocytes are found deep in the ovarian structure, far from the ovarian surface

Figure 2(b)   *See legend opposite*

REVIEW AND DISCUSSION OF THE LITERATURE

In a review of the literature of the past 2 years, some interesting articles have been found. Their conclusions are summarized in Table 1.

There are three laparoscopic techniques used in the management of polycystic ovarian disease: electrocautery; the CO_2 laser; and the Nd : YAG or KTP laser.

In 1990, Gadir and co-workers[7] compared ovarian electrocautery with human menopausal gonadotropin (hMG) therapy and with pure follicle stimulating hormone (FSH). All the patients were non-responders to clomifene citrate (150 mg/day for 5 days). The ovulation rate ($\pm 70\%$) was found to be similar in all groups and the pregnancy rate ($\pm 50\%$) was similar in the groups of patients treated by electrocautery and hMG. The authors concluded that electrocautery must be considered as the first line of therapy in polycystic ovarian disease.

However, these excellent results were not confirmed by Kovacs and associates in 1991[8]; they treated ten women, non-responders to medically induced ovulation (clomifene citrate), by laparoscopic ovarian cautery. A reduction in testosterone levels was observed after the procedure. The ovulation rate was 70% and the pregnancy rate 40%. Nevertheless, the efficacy of electrocautery is doubtful because out of the four patients who became pregnant, only one conceived without adjuvant therapy. Indeed, two patients conceived after gonadotropin therapy and one after an *in vitro* fertilization procedure.

In 1991, Rossmanith and colleagues[11] published the hormonal changes after Nd : YAG laser photocoagulation in women who failed to ovulate with 100 mg of clomifene citrate taken for 5 days. The serum androgen concentrations of ovarian origin were dramatically reduced following laparoscopic laser coagulation of ovarian surfaces and cysts. Mean LH concentrations declined because the LH pulse amplitudes were markedly reduced, while the LH pulse frequencies were unchanged.

In 1991, Gurgan and co-workers[9] published the incidence of adhesions after ovarian electrocautery vs. ovarian Nd : YAG laser photocoagulation. All patients were also non-responders to clomifene citrate. The ovulation rate was similar in both groups and the pregnancy rate was 57% in the electrocautery group and 40% in the Nd : YAG laser group. This pregnancy rate was achieved after a second-look laparoscopy performed after 4 weeks. During this second-look laparoscopy, adhesions were diagnosed and treated in 85% of cases in the electrocautery group and in 80% of cases in the Nd : YAG laser group. Keckstein and associates[12] also reported adhesion formation after CO_2 laser ovarian coagulation.

In 1992, Gadir and colleagues[10] compared ovarian electrocautery + hMG vs. gonadotropin releasing hormone agonist (GnRHa) + hMG. All patients failed to conceive during the first six treatment cycles with hMG. The ovulation rates (85% and 77%, respectively) and the pregnancy rates (43% and 47%, respectively) after 6 months of therapy were similar in both groups. The multiple pregnancy rate was lower in the group of patients treated by electrocautery + hMG (14%) than that observed in the group of women treated by GnRHa + hMG (25%). The only significant difference in this study was in the dose of hMG, which was higher in the group of patients treated by GnRH agonist + hMG. There was no significant difference in the duration of induction nor in the estradiol levels at midcycle. The authors concluded that electrocautery + hMG was better than GnRH agonist + hMG; however, this conclusion was not proved by their results.

PERSONAL EXPERIENCE

The aim of the treatment of PCOD is to produce a decrease in serum androgen levels without inducing pelvic adhesions which could reduce the pregnancy rate.

The efficacy of GnRH agonist + hMG was compared to CO_2 laser laparoscopy. All patients had free testosterone levels more than 3 nmol/l, LH more than 10 U/l and a LH:FSH ratio more than 2:1, and echography confirmed the presence of polycystic ovaries. Four weeks after CO_2 laser laparoscopy or after the GnRHa (Zoladex or Decapeptyl) injection, the testosterone levels were significantly decreased but in the same way in both groups (Figure 4). The ovulation rate was 70% after CO_2 laser therapy and 80% after GnRH agonist + hMG. The pregnancy rate was only 20% in the group of patients treated by CO_2 laser (follow-up: 9 months) and 60% after GnRH agonist + hMG (follow-up: 9 months; six cycles of GnRH agonist + hMG therapy). After 9 months, the eight non-pregnant women from the group of women treated by CO_2 laser received GnRH agonist and hMG. Pregnancy was achieved in six out of the eight women.

CONCLUSION

Bilateral wedge resection, ovarian electrocoagulation or photovaporization result in the restoration of cyclic ovulation, but the pregnancy rate is low[2,8,13]. This may be due to the short-lived hormonal changes; indeed, the marked decrease in testosterone and androstenedione production after surgery is transitory[11] (also Donnez and Nisolle, unpublished results). The low pregnancy rate may also be explained by postoperative pelvic adhesions. The high incidence of formation of periovarian adhesions after wedge resection has been known for a long time[3]. Laparoscopic procedures do not seem to

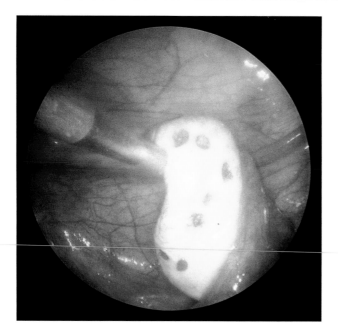

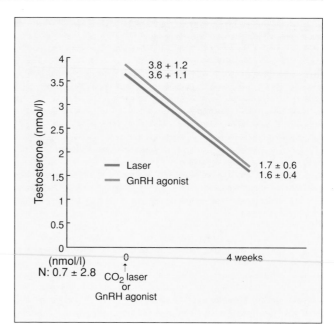

Figure 3 Ovarian drilling: the visible subcapsular follicles on each ovary are drained; the CO_2 laser is used to drill craters in the ovarian stroma

Figure 4 Testosterone levels (nmol/l) before and 4 weeks after CO_2 laser laparoscopy or after injection of gonadotropin releasing hormone agonist

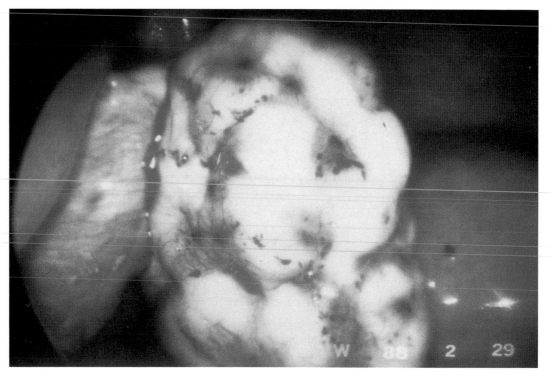

Figure 5 Second-look laparoscopy after CO_2 laser vaporization of the ovaries. The ovarian surface shows dot-like sears (a result of carbonized debris) and small vascularized area; periovarian adhesions are noted. (From ref. 13)

prevent postoperative adhesion formation after ovarian electrocautery. Indeed, Lyles and colleagues[14] reported the rate of adhesion formation as 100% after either mode of therapy. Keckstein and co-workers[12] and Gurgan and associates[9] also reported periovarian adhesion formation (Figure 5).

Ovarian electrocautery, CO_2 laser vaporization or YAG laser coagulation are effective in reducing serum testosterone and LH levels. A further advantage could be the increase in the serum FSH level after laparoscopic therapy[12]. However, there is no evidence in randomized studies that electrocautery is better than medical therapy.

A decrease in serum androgen levels may also be produced in PCOD with a long-acting GnRH agonist[15]. The correction of the endocrine abnormalities is probably explained by the suppression of the abnormal gonadotropin secretion of PCOD and, as a result, a reduction in ovarian androgen secretion.

There is no difference in the ovulation rate and the pregnancy rate between electrocautery + hMG and GnRH agonist + hMG. Some possible advantages can nevertheless be noted:

(1) Electrocautery is less expensive.

(2) The number of cycles with multiple dominant follicles tends to be reduced.

(3) There is an increase in the FSH level which could be beneficial for follicular maturation.

Laparoscopic ovarian drilling must *not* be considered as a first line of therapy because it can provoke adhesions and because there is no evidence of a better efficacy when compared with medical therapy as a first line of treatment. PCOD is a *medical* problem which should be treated *hormonally* on all but rare occasions.

In our department, the scheme of therapy for polycystic ovarian disease is as follows:

(1) Clomifene citrate 100 mg/day for 5 days.

(2) If no response, the dose is increased up to 250 mg/day.

(3) If no response, hMG is given.

(4) If failure to conceive, GnRH agonist + hMG.

(5) Finally, laparoscopic electrocautery, CO_2 or YAG therapy is indicated only if multiple follicular recruitment or hyperstimulation is present after GnRH agonist + hMG, or if there is failure to conceive.

REFERENCES

1. Stein, I.F. and Leventhal, M.L. (1935). Amenorrhea associated with bilateral polycystic ovaries. *Am. J. Obstet. Gynecol.*, **29**, 181

2. Adashi E.Y., Rock, J.A., Guzick, D., Colston Wentz, A., Seegar Jones, G. and Jones, H.W. (1981). Fertility following bilateral ovarian wedge resection: a critical analysis of 90 consecutive cases of the polycystic ovary syndrome. *Fertil. Steril.*, **36**, 320–5

3. Buttram, V.C. and Vaquero, C. (1975). Post-ovarian wedge resection adhesive disease. *Fertil. Steril.*, **26**, 874–6

4. Gjonnaess, H. (1984). Polycystic ovarian syndrome treated by ovarian electrocautery through the laparoscope. *Fertil. Steril.*, **41**, 20

5. Greenblatt, E. and Casper, R.F. (1987). Endocrine changes after laparoscopic ovarian cautery in polycystic ovarian syndrome. *Am. J. Obstet. Gynecol.*, **156**, 279

6. Daniell, J.F. and Miller, W. (1989). Polycystic ovaries treated by laparoscopic laser vaporisation. *Fertil. Steril.*, **51**, 232

7. Gadir, A.A., Mowafi, R.S., Alnaser, H.M., Arrashid, A.H., Alonezi, A.M. and Shax, R.W. (1990). Ovarian electrocautery versus human menopausal gonadotrophins and pure follicle stimulating hormone therapy in the treatment of patients with polycystic ovarian disease. *Clin. Endocrinol.*, **33**, 585–92

8. Kovacs, G., Buckler, H., Bangah, M., Outch, K., Burger, H., Healy, D., Baker, G. and Phillips, S. (1991). Treatment of anovulation due to PCO syndrome by laparoscopic ovarian electrocautery. *Br. J. Obstet. Gynaecol.*, **98**, 30–5

9. Gurgan, T., Kisnisci, H., Yarali, H., Develioglu, O., Zeyneloglu, H. and Tarik, A. (1991). Evaluation of adhesion formation after laparoscopic treatment of polycystic ovarian disease. *Fertil. Steril.*, **56**, 1176–8

10. Gadir, A.A., Alnaser, H.M.I., Mowafi, R.S. and Shaw, R.W. (1992). The response of patients with polycystic ovarian disease to human menopausal gonadotropin therapy after ovarian electrocautery of a luteinizing hormone-releasing hormone agonist. *Fertil. Steril.*, **57**, 309–13

11. Rossmanith, W.G., Keckstein, J., Spatzier, K. and Lauritzen, C. (1991). The impact of ovarian laser surgery on the gonadotrophin secretion in women with polycystic ovarian disease. *Clin. Endocrinol.*, **34**, 223–30

12. Keckstein, G., Rossmanith, W., Spatzier, K., Schneider V., Börchers, K. and Steiner, R. (1990). The effect of laparoscopic treatment of polycystic ovarian disease by CO_2 laser or Nd:YAG laser. *Surg. Endosc.*, **4**, 103–7

13. Goldzieher, J.W. (1981). Polycystic ovarian disease. *Fertil. Steril.*, **35**, 371–94

14. Lyles, R., Goldzieher, J.W., Betts, J.W., Franklin, R.R., Buttram, V.C., Feste, J.R. and Malinack, L.R. (1989). Early second-look laparoscopy after the treatment of polycystic ovarian disease with laparoscopic ovarian electrocautery and/or Nd : YAG laser photocoagulation. Presented at the *45th Annual Meeting of The American Fertility Society*, San Francisco, California, November 13–16, 1989.

In the *Program Supplement*, p.S26 (Abstr. 0-061). (Birmingham, Alabama: American Fertility Society)

15. Calogero, A.E., Macchi, M., Montanini, V., Mongioi, A., Maugeri, G., Vicari, E., Coniglione, F., Sipione, C. and D'Agata, R. (1987). Dynamics of plasma gonadotropin and sex steroid release in polycystic ovarian disease after pituitary–ovarian inhibition with an analog of gonadotropin-releasing hormone. *J. Clin. Endocrinol. Metab.*, **64**, 980–5

Laparoscopic management of adnexal torsion: a review of 41 cases

17

M. Canis, G. Mage, A. Wattiez, H. Manhes, J.L. Pouly and M.A. Bruhat

Laparoscopy is useful for the accurate diagnosis of adnexal torsion. Early diagnosis prevents adnexal necrosis[1,2] and allows conservative treatment of this rare condition[3,4]. We assumed it would be possible to perform complete conservative treatment by laparoscopy in most cases. Here we present our experience of 33 cases treated by laparoscopy from a series of 41 cases.

MATERIAL AND METHODS

Patients

A total of 41 cases of adnexal torsion were diagnosed between June 1978 and June 1988. Only cases with at least a 360° rotation of the ovarian pedicle or the tube were included in this study. Malignant tumors, always treated by laparotomy, were excluded. According to their clinical data, patients were divided into two groups.

Group 1

This group consisted of 30 patients (73.2% of the total) with acute pelvic pain; the interval between the onset of pain and laparoscopy ranged from 6 h to 4 days. The preoperative diagnosis was correct in about 70% of cases.

Group 2

In this group of 11 cases (26.8%), laparoscopy was performed for the surgical evaluation of adnexal cystic tumors. The time lapse between the first visit to our department and laparoscopy ranged from 1 to 3 months. Torsion was never suspected before laparoscopy.

Method

Laparoscopy was performed under general anesthesia with endotracheal intubation. The technique and the instrumentation used have been described previously[5,6,7]. After diagnosis, the laparoscopic management included two stages: management of ischemic lesions and treatment of the etiology (Figures 1 and 2).

Management of ischemic lesions

As recommended by Way[4], the organs involved were always untwisted to assess ischemic lesions. This procedure was performed slowly with an atraumatic forceps to avoid additional adnexal damage. Treatment was chosen according to the initial lesions and the speed of recovery. The women were assigned to one of the following groups:

(1) Group A: no evidence of ischemia, or mild lesions with immediate and complete recovery;

(2) Group B: severe ischemia (tube and ovary were dark red or black at the time of diagnosis) with partial recovery 10 min after the pedicle was untwisted;

(3) Group C: gangrenous adnexa without recovery.

In group A and B, conservative management was chosen whenever it was possible to treat the etiology in this way. In group B a second-look laparoscopy was performed 6–8 weeks after the initial procedure to assess definitive recovery. In group C gangrenous adnexa were removed either by laparotomy or by laparoscopy.

Table 1 Adnexal torsions

Pathological findings	Tube (n = 9)	Ovary (n = 1)	Adnexa (n = 31)	Total (n = 41)
Paroophoritic cysts	6	—	7	13
Functional ovarian cysts	—	—	5*	5
Organic ovarian cysts	—	—	12	12
Ectopic pregnancy	2	—	—	2
Adhesions	1	—	1*	2
Congenital malformation	—	1	1	2
Normal adnexa	—	—	6	6

*, One case with adhesions associated with a functional cyst

Table 2   Management of adnexal torsions according to laparoscopic findings

Laparoscopic findings	Radical treatment		Conservative treatment	
	Laparoscopy	Laparotomy	Laparoscopy	Laparotomy
Mild ($n = 25$)	1	1	19	4
Severe ($n = 9$)	0	0	8	1
Gangrenous ($n = 7$)	5	2	0	0

Treatment of the etiology

Various laparoscopic procedures such as the treatment of ectopic pregnancy[6], adhesiolysis[8] or ovarian cystectomy[5], were used for the treatment of the etiology. All patients were closely followed clinically, looking for any recurrence of torsion after conservative management.

RESULTS

Laparoscopy permitted a diagnosis in all cases. The whole adnexa was involved in 31 cases, the tube in nine cases and the ovary in one case.

Detorsion

The laparoscopic unwinding of torsion was possible in 38 cases. In the three remaining cases, the manipulation of gangrenous tubes resulted in a salpingectomy without any bleeding. Ischemic lesions were mild in 25 cases (group A), severe in nine cases (group B), and beyond recovery in seven cases. All patients with chronic pelvic pain were included in group A.

Etiology

Pathological findings are listed in Table 1. Paroophoritic and ovarian cysts were the most common etiologies. In two cases the etiology was thought to be congenital; we found a rather short mesovarium (4 mm in length) in one case and a utero-ovarian ligament which was too long in the other case. Normal-size adnexa underwent spontaneous torsion; in such cases several ovarian punctures were performed to rule out the presence of a small ovarian cyst.

Management

Management is shown in Table 2. Laparoscopic treatment was achieved in 33 cases (80.5%). Indications for laparotomy are listed in Table 3. Conservative management was possible in 32 cases and was performed by laparoscopy in 27 cases (Table 4) and by laparotomy in five cases.

There were no significant postoperative problems. Although heparin therapy was never used, we observed no thromboembolic complications. Patients were discharged 2–3 days after a laparoscopic procedure and 6 days after laparotomy.

In group B, six patients had a second-look laparoscopy which showed a complete and even surprising recovery of ischemic lesions (Figure 3). Ovarian biopsy was performed in only one case and histological examination showed a thickened ovarian capsule with a normal follicular population.

Follow-up

The duration of follow-up ranged from 9 months to 6 years. Ten patients were lost to follow-up 1 month after the treatment. Two recurrences were observed:

(1) One recurrence involved the same adnexa: 12 months after a laparoscopic ovariopexis using a Fallopian ring to treat an over-long utero-ovarian ligament, a second laparoscopy was performed to evaluate an ovary which was 6 cm in diameter; a recurrence of torsion was found with four twists without any evidence of ischemia. A bilateral surgical ovariopexis was then performed by laparotomy;

(2) The second recurrence involved the contralateral adnexa and was diagnosed 12 months after the initial procedure (which included a right ovariopexis and a right ovarian cystectomy); the recurrence was explained only by an over-long utero-ovarian ligament. This recurrence was treated conservatively; a laparoscopic ovariopexis was performed using non-absorbable suture and fibrin glue.

DISCUSSION

In our experience laparoscopy always permits an accurate diagnosis of adnexal torsion, an infrequent condition[9,10]. As the clinical symptoms can be associated with more common diseases such as ectopic pregnancy, salpingitis or corpus luteum hemorrhage which can be managed by laparoscopy, we and others[9,10] believe that surgical exploration should be carried out in this way.

In group C (gangrenous adnexa), laparoscopy was performed more than 72 h after the onset of pain in five

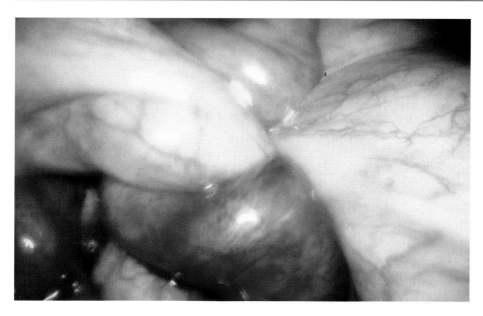

Figure 1 Torsion of the right adnexa

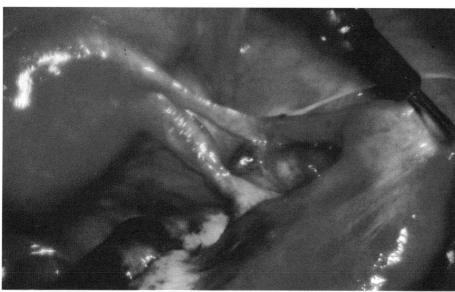

Figure 2 Partial ovarian recovery at the end of the laparoscopy

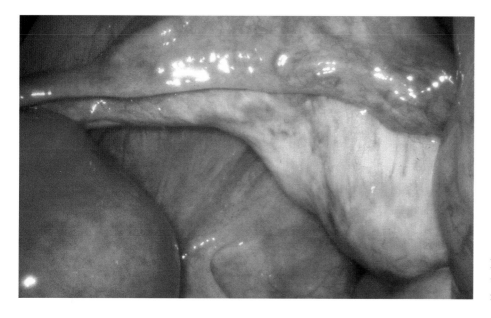

Figure 3 The same ovary at the second-look laparoscopy 3 months later

Table 3 Treatment of adnexal torsions; indications are given for cases in which laparotomy was performed

Treatment	Number of cases (%)
Laparoscopic	33 (80.5)
Laparotomy	8 (19.5)
gangrenous organs	2
ovarian cystectomy	4
ovariopexis	1
oophorectomy for large dermoid cyst	1

cases, emphasizing the need for an early diagnosis of torsion. Indeed a delayed exploration will find a gangrenous adnexa which must be removed; and spontaneous evolution probably results in spontaneous tubo-ovarian auto-amputation[11,12].

Conservative management was possible in 78% of our patients and appeared necessary as many patients were under 30 years of age. Conservative management requires first the unwinding of the torsion, a procedure which was previously condemned for fear of freeing a potentially fatal embolus[13,14]. In a recent report, fear of this complication appeared to be one of the main indications for radical management of adnexal torsion[10]. We and other authors[3,4] have never observed any embolic complications; prompt diagnosis and treatment probably account for this. Embolic complications could have been encountered when adnexal torsion was managed in a phlegmatic manner and twisted organs were found to be obviously gangrenous at laparotomy. Furthermore, in many cases of gangrenous adnexa, an unwinding of the torsion appears to be impossible; indeed, in three of our patients, gentle exploration of the adnexa with a probe resulted in spontaneous salpingectomy. As we observed no bleeding in these cases, we feel that no embolus is likely to be freed during this procedure. Conservative management remains questionable in cases of mild ischemia (group A). Indeed, Azoury[2] reported that histological examination of a tube removed in spite of a complete recovery from mild ischemia showed definite mucosal damage. He concluded that conservative management should be attempted only in young women with bilateral adnexal torsion. Our experience differs from this since one of our patients had an intrauterine pregnancy following conservative treatment of a solitary twisted adnexa with severe ischemic damage. Furthermore, tubal patency was previously confirmed by hysterosalpingography[4]. Therefore, conservative management of mild and severe ischemic lesions appears to be safe and effective even if further studies are required to assess fertility after this procedure.

A complete laparoscopic treatment was achieved in 33 cases (80.5%). Physical stress, postoperative recovery and economic cost are reduced with such treatment, making it more acceptable and more desirable than conventional surgical management. This method should, however, be restricted to physicians trained in operative laparoscopy with a complete set of instruments available.

Many etiological factors have been discussed previously in the literature. The main problem is the correct and safe management of ovarian cysts. When an organic cyst is diagnosed or even suspected, a complete cystectomy must be performed for histological examination, either by laparoscopy or by laparotomy[5]. Infarction makes accurate pathological diagnosis quite difficult and Lomano[15] reported 26 non-specific ovarian cysts among 44 cases of twisted ovarian cysts. We encountered this problem in only one case.

When ischemic lesions are severe, laparoscopic differentiation between torsion of a normal tube and torsion of a tubal pregnancy is quite difficult. We believe that, if a hematosalpinx is diagnosed in women of reproductive age, a salpingotomy with tubal aspiration must be performed in every case[6]. In our series, two cases of adnexal torsion were attributed to congenitally unusual ovarian attachment. In one of these patients, a laparoscopic ovaropexis, using a Fallopian ring, resulted 12 months later in a recurrence of torsion with the disappearance of the utero-ovarian ligament. Although we observed no complication when the utero-ovarian ligament was shortened after the treatment of a paroophoritic cyst, we believe that this procedure should not be used to prevent recurrence of torsion. Laparoscopic ovariopexis should use non-absorbable sutures. Several authors report that a routine ovariopexis is required during every conservative treatment of adnexal torsion[9,14]. In our study and in other reports[1,3,4], a recurrence of torsion seems to be quite rare, so we believe that, once an etiology has been found and correctly treated, the risk of recurrence is quite low. In our opinion, ovariopexis should be performed in cases of unusual ovarian attachment and/or immediate recurrence of torsion but it is questionable in cases of normal adnexa.

Table 4 Adnexal torsions: secondary laparoscopic procedures

Procedure	Number
Adhesiolysis	2
Puncture biopsy of functional cysts	5
Conservative treatment of ectopic pregnancy	1
Paroophoritic cystectomy	10
Ovarian cystectomy	4
Oophorectomy	2
Salpingectomy	4
Ovariopexis with Fallopian ring	3

REFERENCES

1. Lee, R.A. and Welch, J.S. (1967). Torsion of the uterine adnexa. *Am. J. Obstet. Gynecol.*, **97**, 974
2. Azoury, R.S. Chemab, R.M. and Muffarrij, I.K. (1980). The twisted adnexa: a clinical pathological review. *Diagn. Gynecol. Obstet.*, **2**, 185
3. MacGowan, L. (1964). Torsion of cystic or diseased tissue. *Am. J. Obstet. Gynecol.*, **88**, 135
4. Way, S. (1946). Ovarian cystectomy of twisted cysts. *Lancet*, **2**, 47
5. Mage, G., Canis, M., Manhes, H., Pouly, J.L. and Bruhat, M.A. (1987). Kystes ovariens et coelioscopie. *J. Gynecol. Obstet. Biol. Reprod.*, **16**, 1053–61
6. Pouly, J.L., Manhes, H., Mage, G., Canis, M. and Bruhat, M.A., (1986). Conservative laparoscopic treatment of 321 ectopic pregnancies. *Fertil. Steril.*, **46**, 1093
7. Bruhat, M.A., Mage, G., Pouly, J.L., Manhes, H. and Wattiez, A. (1989). Coelioscopie Opératoire. *Editions Medsi*, Juin (Paris: McGraw Hill)

8. Bruhat, M.A., Mage, G., Manhes, H., Soualhat, C., Ropert, J.F. and Pouly, J.L. (1983). Laparoscopic procedures to promote fertility: result of 93 selected cases. *Acta Eur. Fertil.*, **14**, 113
9. Nicols, D.H. and Julian, P.J. (1985). Torsion of the adnexa. *Clin. Obstet. Gynecol.*, **28**, 375–80
10. Hibbart, L.T. (1985). Adnexal torsion. *Am. J. Ostet. Gynecol.*, **152**, 456
11. Sebastian, J.A., Baker, R.L. and Cordray, F., (1973). Asymptomatic infarction and separation of ovary and distal uterine tube. *Obstet. Gynecol.*, **41**, 531–5
12. Beyth, Y. and Barin, E. (1984). Tubo-ovarian autoamputation and infertility. *Fertil. Steril.*, **42**, 932
13. James, D.F., Barber, H.R.K. and Graber, E.A. (1970). Torsion of uterine adnexa in children. Report of 3 cases. *Obstet. Gynecol.*, **365**, 226
14. Powell, J.L., Foley, F.P. and Llorens, A.S. (1972). Torsion of the Fallopian tube in post menopausal women. *Am. J. Obstet. Gynecol.*, **111**, 113–15
15. Lomano, J.M., Trelford, J.D. and Ullery, J.C. (1970). Torsion of the uterine adnexa causing an acute abdomen. *Obstet. Gynecol.*, **35**, 221

Laparoscopic myomectomy

18

J.B. Dubuisson, C. Chapron, M. Mouly, H. Foulot,
F.X. Aubriot and J. Bouquet de Jolinière

The indications for operative laparoscopy have expanded greatly over the past decades as its many advantages over laparotomy have been recognized[1-3]. Myomectomy may be performed by laparoscopy in selected cases, particularly in subserous and interstitial myomas[4,5].

PREOPERATIVE EVALUATION

Preoperative evaluation is important in determining the operative strategy, which depends on the number, size and localization of myomas. In addition, a preoperative ultrasound with measurement of all myomas is necessary in all cases before instituting medical treatment[6]. Hysteroscopy must be performed in patients with menometrorrhagia, in cases of multiple myomas, in cases of suspected intrauterine abnormalities at hysterosalpingography or ultrasound and in infertile patients. Hysteroscopy allows the surgeon to differentiate between a deep interstitial myoma and a submucous myoma or polyp. Comparison of the results of the ultrasound and the hysteroscopy is important to determine the operative strategy.

Hysterosalpingography is also performed in some patients. In cases of infertility, it permits an evaluation of the distortion of the uterine cavity and the tubal status (diverticula, tuba erecta). If adenomyosis is suspected by hysteroscopy or ultrasound, hysterosalpingography is also indicated.

The blood count is always checked before operative laparoscopy, particularly in patients with menometrorrhagia.

PREOPERATIVE TREATMENT WITH GONADOTROPIN RELEASING HORMONE

In patients undergoing laparoscopic myomectomy, preoperative treatment with gonadotropin releasing hormone agonists (GnRHa) may be beneficial. These agents cause myoma shrinkage by reducing circulating estrogen levels[7]. Maximal reduction of myoma size is achieved by 12 weeks of therapy, with no further change observed after 24 weeks of treatment[8]. Matta and colleagues[9] observed that GnRHa reduce uterine blood flow. A marked reduction in blood loss during myomectomy has been demonstrated[10]. However, Friedman

and co-workers[10] observed a significant reduction in total intraoperative blood loss only in patients with uterine volumes of $> 600 \, cm^3$ treated with leuprolide acetate. In our experience, GnRHa has the advantage of reducing bleeding during operative laparoscopy[4]. Thus, preoperative treatment is indicated in patients with myomas larger than 5 cm in diameter, and in patients with anemia due to menometrorrhagia.

INDICATIONS FOR OPERATIVE LAPAROSCOPY

The indications depend on the number, size and localization of myomas[4]. The number of myomas may be a problem during operative laparoscopy. If myomas are numerous, the risk of bleeding and the problems of extraction of all the myomas are increased. In our experience, the procedure should not be attempted when more than four myomas are present.

The size may also be a problem during operative laparoscopy. Large myomas should not be removed by laparoscopic surgery because of the increased risk of bleeding and the prolonged operating time needed to fragment and remove the myoma. In our experience, a myoma of more than 10 cm in diameter should not be treated in this way.

The localization of the myomas is important to consider. Subserous and interstitial myomas are an indication for elective operative laparoscopy. Myomas situated in the broad ligament or at the uterine isthmus can also be treated by operative laparoscopy, taking care not to damage the ureter and the uterine vessels. The ablation of a submucous myoma is generally performed by operative hysteroscopy when its diameter is less than 5 cm. However, a submucous myoma of more than 5 cm may be treated laparoscopically in our experience: the hysterotomy is performed with the opening of the cavity on the side where the myometrium is thinnest. In such cases, the uterus is closed using interrupted sutures in one or two layers, depending on the depth of the incision. In cases of multiple myomas, the association of a submucous myoma less than 5 cm in diameter with subserous and interstitial myomas has to be considered. In our experience, the submucous myoma is treated first by operative hysteroscopy. The laparoscopic treatment of the other myomas will be discussed later. We rarely associate operative hysteroscopy with operative laparoscopy (only one case since 1990); we consider that

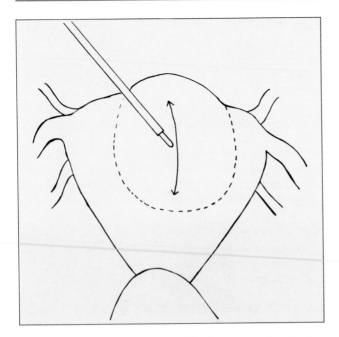

Figure 1 Uterine incision with the monopolar hook

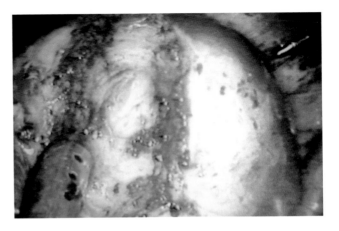

Figure 2 Cleavage of the myoma using a pelvicleaner

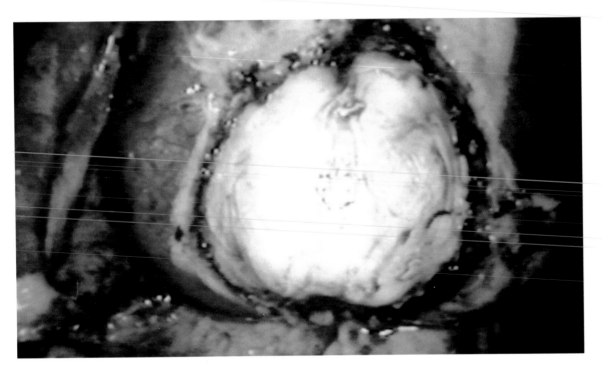

Figure 3 Myoma appearance during enucleation

the association usually increases the duration of the operation and consequently the risk of complications.

TECHNIQUE

Under general anesthesia, before the laparoscopy, a rigid cannula is introduced into the uterus to facilitate its mobilization. Laparoscopy is performed transumbilically using a 10-mm endoscope adapted to a video camera. The instruments are introduced through three suprapubic puncture sites. We use 5-mm trocars laterally and a 10-mm trocar at the median site. The following instruments are used: 5-mm atraumatic forceps, 5-mm monopolar hook, 5-mm bipolar forceps, 5-mm needle holder, Semm claw forceps and pelvicleaner (Storz-France). High-frequency electrosurgical generators are employed.

Myomectomy is performed according to the principles of atraumatic infertility surgery in all cases: magnification, meticulous hemostasis and precise closure of the myometrium in cases of deep myomas. A microsurgical technique prevents bleeding, adhesion formation and postoperative complications.

For pediculated myomas, the technique consists of coagulation and section of the implantation surface. A monopolar hook is used to coagulate and cut, but complementary hemostasis with a bipolar forceps is often necessary. When the implantation surface is small (< 1 cm^2), no sutures are required.

For subserous myomas with a large implantation surface, and for interstitial myomas, a hysterotomy is perfomed at the site of the myoma. The direct incision limits the bleeding. A vertical incision is usually made, although in some cases we prefer a horizontal incision. For the incision, we use the monopolar hook (Figure 1). Complementary coagulation of the vessels of the myometrium is often performed using the bipolar forceps. Vasoconstrictive agents are not employed. The enucleation is performed using atraumatic forceps and a Semm claw forceps is introduced through the suprapubic puncture (Figures 2–4). The uterine cavity is not opened except in cases of submucous myomas. After the myomectomy, it is important to ensure complete hemostasis. Uterine incisions are closed by laparoscopy with sutures, to prevent rupture of the myometrium in case of pregnancy and to reduce the risk of adhesion formation on a large raw surface (> 1 cm^2). We close the uterus in one layer or two with interrupted (Figures 5, 6 and 7) (or running) 3-0 Vicryl (Polyglactine 910, 20-mm needle, Ethicon). Extra-abdominal sutures may also be used (2-0 polysorb, 20-mm needle and 122 cm-long thread with delivery system, Auto Suture France). Usually, sutures are placed every 5 mm along the hysterotomy.

The myoma may be removed through the suprapubic puncture site after enlargement of the incision (20 mm) with one or two single-tooth tenaculums. The myoma is brought up to the suprapubic incision and held against the peritoneum to prevent loss of CO_2. The myoma is then fragmented under laparoscopic control, using a small blade passed through the incision.

The myoma may also be removed through a posterior colpotomy. The colpotomy may be performed by laparoscopy using the monopolar hook or the CO_2 laser. The incision is facilitated by the introduction of a compress into the vagina. The colpotomy may also be performed conventionally through the vagina. The colpotomy is alway closed vaginaly.

We generally use the suprapubic route when the myoma measures less than 5 cm because the fragmentation takes a short time. When the myoma is bigger, we prefer to perform a colpotomy. After the removal of the myoma, the peritoneal cavity is irrigated with saline solution. Hemostasis is checked again. More sutures may be needed if bleeding persists.

Laparoscopic myomectomy is a safe technique which has several advantages. The risk of complications is low in selected cases.

RECOMMENDATIONS FOR OPERATIVE MYOMECTOMY

With regard to operative myomectomy, the following are recommended:

(1) Ultrasound and hysteroscopic evaluation, especially in cases of menometrorrhagia or multiple myomas;

(2) Preoperative blood count control;

(3) Administration of gonadotropin releasing hormone agonists for 2-3 months before laparoscopy in cases of voluminous myomas or anemia;

(4) The use of high-frequency electrosurgical generators and monopolar hook;

(5) Uterine closure with intraperitoneal sutures to prevent bleeding, weakening of the myometrium and adhesions if deep hysterotomy is performed; and

(6) Colpotomy for the extraction of the myoma.

REFERENCES

1. Bruhat, M.A., Manhes, H., Choukroun, J. and Suzanne, F. (1977). Essai de traitement per coelioscopique de la grossesse extra-uterine. A propos de 26 observations. *Rev. Française Gynécol. Obstét.*, **72**, 667

2. Donnez, J. (1987). CO_2 laser laparoscopy in infertile women with endometriosis and women with adnexal adhesions. *Fertil. Steril.*, **48**, 39

3. Murphy, A.A. (1987). Operative laparoscopy. *Fertil. Steril.*, **47**, 1

4. Dubuisson, J.B., Lecuru, F., Foulot, H. *et al.* (1992).

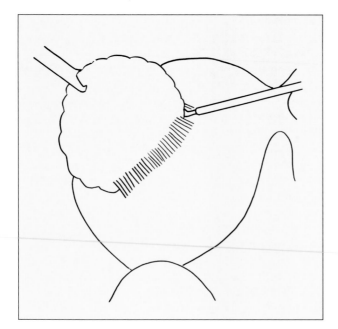

Figure 4 Myoma enucleation using traction with the 10-mm Semm forceps and coagulation section

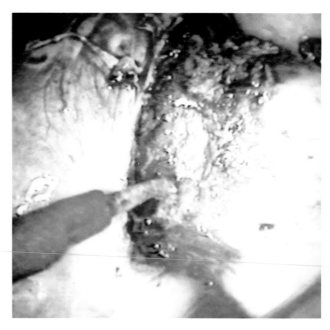

Figure 5 Coagulation and section with the hook at the end of the procedure

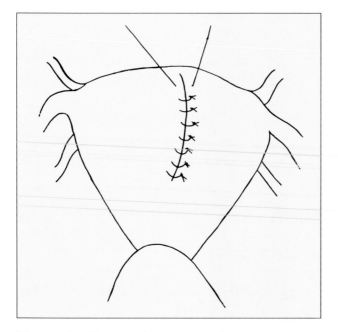

Figure 6 Closure of the uterus in one layer with interrupted sutures

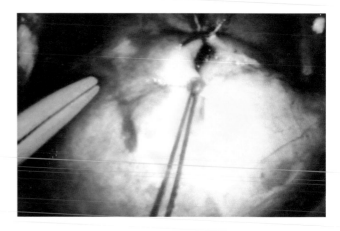

Figure 7 Closure of the uterus with interrupted sutures

Myomectomy by laparoscopy: a preliminary report of 43 cases. *Fertil. Steril.*, **56**, 827

5. Semm, K. and Mettler, L. (1980). New techniques in advanced laparoscopic surgery. In Sutton, C.J.C. (ed.) *Baillière's Clinical Obstetrics and Gynecology*, **138**, 121

6. Fedele, L., Vercellin, P., Bianchi, S., Brioschi, D. and Dorta, M. (1990). Treatment with GnRH agonists before myomectomy and the risk of short-term myoma recurrence. *Br. J. Obstet. Gynaecol.*, **97**, 393

7. Friedman, A.J., Harrison-Atlas, D., Barbieri, R.L. *et al.* (1989). A randomized, placebo-controlled, double-blind study evaluating the efficacy of leuprolide acetate depot in the treatment of uterine leiomyomata. *Fertil. Steril.*, **51**, 251

8. Lumsden, M.A., West, C.P. and Baird, D.T. (1987). Goserelin therapy before surgery for uterine fibroids. *Lancet*, **1**, 36

9. Matta, W.H.M., Stabile, I., Shaw, R.W. and Campbell, S. (1988). Doppler assessment of uterine blood flow changes in patients with fibroids receiving the gonadotropin-releasing hormone agonist buserelin. *Fertil. Steril.*, **49**, 1083

10. Shaw, R.W. (1989). Mechanism of LHRH analogue action in uterine fibroids. *Horm. Res.*, **32**, 150

11. Friedman, A.J., Rein, M.S., Harrison-Atlas, D., Garfield, J.M. and Doubilet, P.M. (1989). A randomized placebo-controlled, double-blind study evaluating leuprolide acetate depot treatment before myomectomy. *Fertil. Steril.*, **52**, 728

Laparoscopic myolysis with the Nd : YAG laser

19

M. Nisolle, M. Smets, S. Gillerot, V. Anaf and J. Donnez

INTRODUCTION

Uterine fibroids are common, benign, solid tumors of the genital tract and, depending on their size and location, can lead to hysterectomy. Advanced operative laparoscopy techniques have been developed and large uterine fibroids can now be removed laparoscopically in patients wishing to avoid hysterectomy[1-3].

In our department, laparoscopic myolysis has been proposed in cases of subserous or intramural myomas as an alternative to myomectomy or hysterectomy.

The purpose of this chapter is to describe the technique and the results of the use of the Nd : YAG laser for laparoscopic myolysis, according to a research protocol. The aim is to evaluate the long-term effects of the technique on myoma growth.

MATERIALS AND METHODS

Between 1989 and 1991, 243 patients suffering from uterine leiomyomas were treated in our department. Out of the 243 women, 142 underwent a complete investigation for infertility (including hysterosalpingography and hysteroscopy), which proved the presence of large, partially submucosal intramural myomas. All underwent laparotomy and classical myomectomy. The 101 remaining women with fibroids were treated endoscopically: 53 by laparoscopic myomectomy and 48 by laparoscopic myolysis. The technique of laparoscopic myolysis, described here, was proposed only to women who did not wish to bear any more children.

The mean age was 42 years (ranging from 35 to 48 years). Myomas were diagnosed by pelvic examination. Their size and location were confirmed by ultrasonography (Figure 1). The vascularization was evaluated by means of Doppler ultrasound with color flow imaging (Figure 2). No previous laparoscopy had been performed in these women.

Hysterosalpingography was carried out in all cases of abnormal uterine bleeding.

Patients with symptomatic submucosal uterine fibroids were treated hysteroscopically as previously described[4,5]. They were thus excluded from the study. Myolysis was proposed to women of more than 35 years of age with intramural myomas up to 8 cm in diameter. Indications for myolysis were:

(1) Pelvic pain;

(2) Compression symptoms; and

(3) Global uterine volume between 9 and 12 weeks (in order to avoid hysterectomy).

In only five cases, asymptomatic intramural myomas were treated by myolysis at the time of laparoscopic sterilization.

Myolysis was also considered as an alternative to laparoscopic myomectomy if myomectomy was judged to be too difficult or not mandatory, or in cases of multiple intramural myomas to avoid a time-consuming laparoscopic myomectomy. A total of 28 patients with more than two myomas were treated by myolysis.

TECHNIQUE

Laparoscopy was performed transumbilically using a 10-mm endoscope adapted to a video camera. The instruments were introduced through three suprapubic puncture sites (5 mm in diameter).

The bare laser fiber was introduced as perpendicularly as possible into the fibroid through a second puncture trocar to a depth depending on the myoma diameter (Figure 3(a) and (b)). During the application of laser energy, the fiber was introduced, reaching the central part of the fibroid, and was then removed slowly in order to provoke a 'strong coagulation'. The power used was 80 W. The procedure was repeated on the entire surface of the myoma in order to coagulate most of the myoma volume. The surface of the myoma was rinsed with 0.9% saline solution during the laser application to reduce thermal conduction through the uterine wall. The distance between holes was about 5–7 mm (Figure 4).

Vasopressin was never used to infiltrate the myometrium adjacent to the fibroid to induce temporary myometrial ischemia, reducing blood loss. However, in one case, diluted vasopressin was required to obtain complete uterine hemostasis: 5 U of vasopressin in 20 ml of saline solution was injected just around the hemorrhagic site at the end of the procedure.

Immediately following myolysis, many laser scars can be seen on the myoma, which appears paler than normal (Figure 5). In the last ten cases, an Interceed graft (Johnson and Johnson, New Brunswick, NJ) was used to cover the coagulated area after hemostatic control was

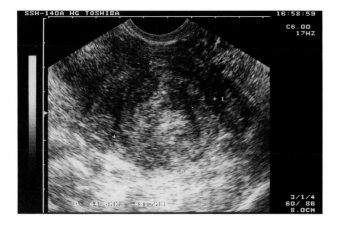

Figure 1 Preoperative echography: size is determined

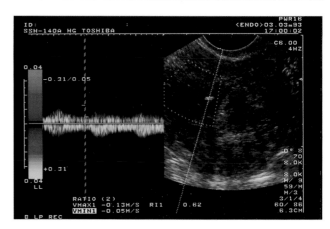

Figure 2 Myoma: the vascularization is evaluated by means of Doppler ultrasound with color flow imaging

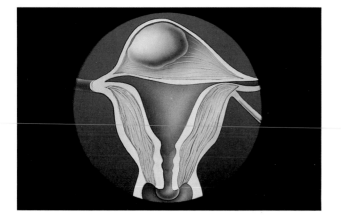

Figure 3(a)–(c) Intramural myoma: illustration and laparoscopic view; (d)–(g) myolysis technique: the laser fiber is introduced at an angle perpendicular to the fibroid and removed during the application of laser energy

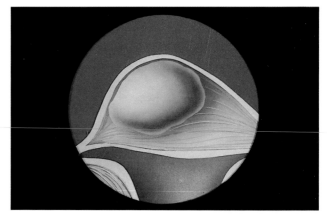

Figure 3(b) *See legend opposite*

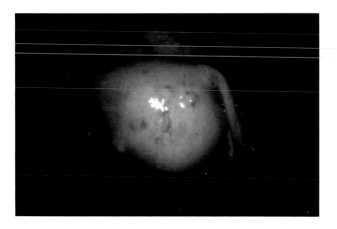

Figure 3(c) *See legend above*

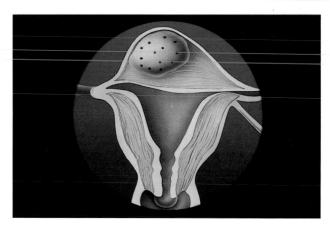

Figure 3(d) *See legend above*

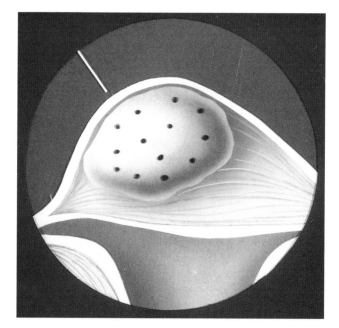

Figure 3(e)   *See legend on opposite page*

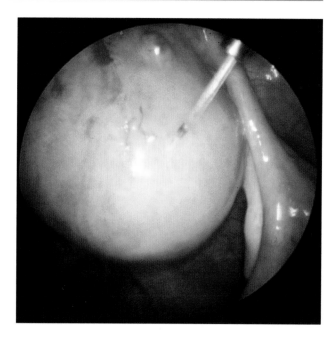

Figure 3(f)   *See legend on opposite page*

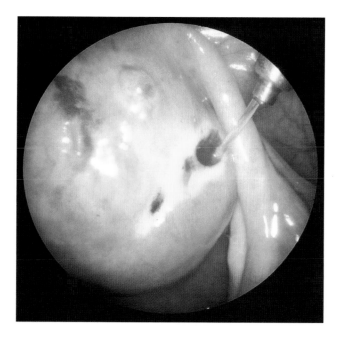

Figure 3(g)   *See legend on opposite page*

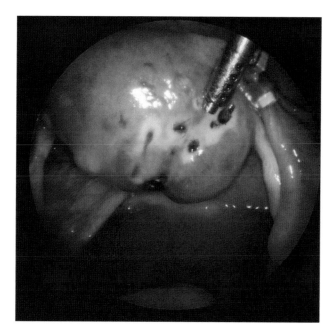

Figure 4   Laparoscopic view: the distance between holes was about 5-7 mm

obtained, in order to decrease the risk of adhesions. Careful aspiration of peritoneal fluid was then carried out and a suction catheter was left in the pouch of Douglas.

EVALUATION OF MYOMA SIZE

The number, size and location of the myomas were evaluated by vaginal echography before laparoscopic myolysis. The size of the myomas, measured by ultrasound, ranged from 3 to 8 cm in diameter.

Postoperatively, myoma evaluation was echographically performed at weeks 6 and 12, after 6 months and after 1 year; 15 patients were evaluated after 3 years.

RESULTS

Fibroids treated by myolysis ranged from 3 to 8 cm in diameter. The mean decrease in the myoma diameter after myolysis was 4% (range 0–6%) at week 6, 12% (range 2–18%) at week 12 and 41% (range 18–62%) after 6 months. The results observed after 1 year were similar to those seen after 6 months; there was neither any further decrease in size nor a regrowth of the myoma (Figure 6).

After 3 years, 15 patients were evaluated by echography. In ten of them who had two to three myomas (between 3 and 5 cm in diameter), echography revealed only small areas (< 1 cm in diameter) whose echographic structure was slightly different from the normal myometrium. Among the five remaining patients, three were stable and two showed a reappearance of myomas in other sites.

Failure of the treatment, indicated by an absence of any significant decrease in the myoma diameter, was never observed.

In our series of 48 patients, none required laparotomy for bleeding, and no bladder or bowel injury was reported. During surgery, some problems arose because of difficult accessibility to posterior myomas by the laser fiber, introduced through a second puncture. In such cases, the laser fiber can be introduced directly through the laparoscope to achieve better accessibility.

The estimated blood loss was minimal (< 50 ml) in all cases but one. The operating time varied from 20 to 45 min, depending on the myoma diameter and number.

All patients were released in good physical condition the following day; none experienced any postoperative infection or hemorrhage.

FOLLOW-UP

Changes in the myoma structure and size were analyzed by echography. In the first 3 weeks, areas of necrosis were suspected by the presence of numerous anechogenic areas (Figure 7) in the myoma. Subsequently, a more echogenic structure appeared. Finally, after 6 months, the echostructure of the coagulated myoma was such that only experienced echographists could really distinguish the limits of the myoma.

Second-look laparoscopy

In seven patients (out of the first 20 treated), a second-look laparoscopy was proposed 6 months after myolysis in order to evaluate the appearance of the myoma. In all cases but one, dense and fibrous adhesions were observed between the myoma and, most frequently, the small bowel and/or epiploon. After adhesiolysis, the myoma appeared white without any apparent vessels. Dissection of the myoma from the normal myometrium was surprisingly easy and the myomas were removed in order to evaluate histologically the efficacy of myolysis (Figure 8). There was necrosis in most myoma areas, characterized by edema and an absence of viable cells. In other areas, giant cells and macrophages containing carbonized particles very close to the necrotic sites suggested that necrosis was really induced by the laser coagulation (Figure 9).

DISCUSSION

Myomas are very common in women of reproductive age and may be responsible for menorrhagia, anemia, pelvic pain, compression, infertility or miscarriage. However, myomas are often asymptomatic and may not require treatment. In such asymptomatic patients, indications for myomectomy are debatable; therapy may be considered in some cases to prevent complications related to the growth of the myoma. Uterine fibroids can now be treated endoscopically[1-3,6]. As previously described, in cases of submucosal uterine fibroids, hysteroscopic myomectomy[4,5] is carried out if the greater diameter of the leiomyoma is inside the uterine cavity.

In cases of very large fibroids whose largest diameter is not inside the uterine cavity, the protruding portion is removed and the intramural portion is devascularized by introducing the laser fiber into the myoma, at a length depending on the depth of the remaining intramural portion[5,7].

This technique proved to be effective in provoking myoma shrinkage, with a dramatic decrease in size and a marked devascularization of the myoma. The technique was then applied to the laparoscopic approach in the treatment of intramural myomas in women who do not desire further pregnancy.

In cases of subserosal and intramural fibroids, myomectomy can also be carried out laparoscopically by an incision through the uterine serosa with a needle tip

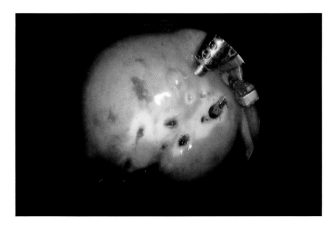

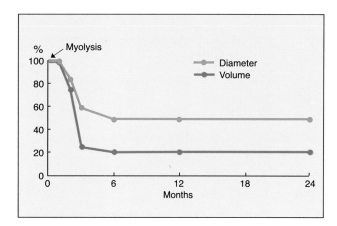

Figure 5(a) At the end of the procedure, numerous laser scars are seen; the paler color of the myoma is due to the coagulation; (b) and (c) to avoid adhesions, Interceed® is used to cover the laser scars

Figure 6 Decrease in the myoma diameter, area and volume after myolysis

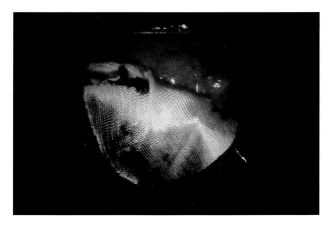

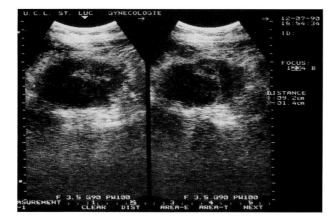

Figure 5(b) *See legend above*

Figure 7 Ultrasound evaluation of the myoma 3 weeks after myolysis: areas of necrosis, characterized by anechogenic structures, are observed

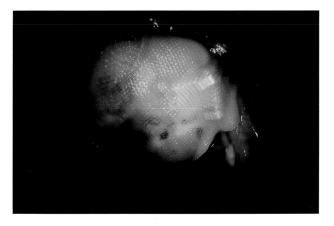

Figure 5(c) *See legend above*

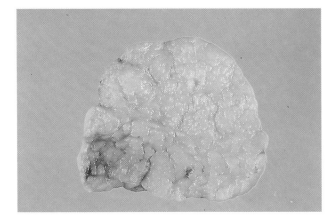

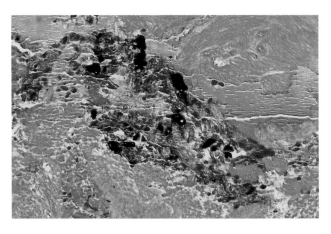

Figure 8 Specimen of myoma, 6 months after myolysis: (a) histological evaluation of the myoma; in some areas carbonized particles are visible (b); (c) there is necrosis characterized by edema and the absence of viable cells

Figure 9 Histological evaluation of the myoma after myolysis: in some areas, giant cells and macrophages containing carbonized particles very close to the necrotic sites suggest that necrosis was really induced by the laser coagulation

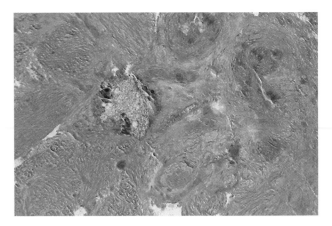

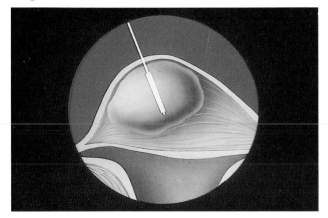

Figure 8(b)   *See legend above*

Figure 10(a) and (b)   ITT fiber can also be used to induce myoma shrinkage

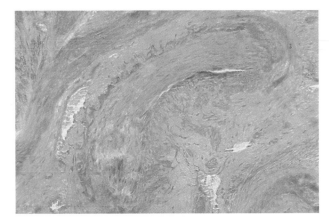

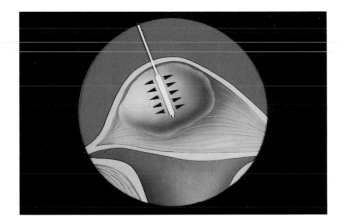

Figure 8(c)   *See legend above*

Figure 10(b)   *See legend above*

or knife electrode unipolar cautery, a KTP/YAG laser in KTP mode, or hook scissors. The exposed fibroid is separated from the myometrium and removed by the combination of traction, twisting and cutting[2]. Serosal reapproximation can be accomplished with a bipolar coagulator in cases of small fibroids (< 3 cm), sutures or fibrin glue (Tissucol®). The excised fibroids are removed from the abdominal cavity via a posterior colpotomy, through suprapubic anterior wall incisions or through the operating channel of the laparoscope after fragmentation, depending on the size of the tumor.

Sometimes, in cases of large intramural fibroids or multiple myomas, laparoscopic myomectomy can be difficult or time-consuming[3]. Laparoscopic myolysis can be proposed as an alternative to myomectomy, performed by laparoscopy or laparotomy in cases of large or multiple intramural fibroids[8]. The fibroids are not removed but coagulated with the help of the YAG laser. The myoma coagulation is followed by necrosis and the size of the myoma decreases dramatically. Myoma coagulation can also be achieved with bipolar probes[6].

The patients must be *selected*: only those aged over 40 years or those not desiring to bear any more children but wishing to avoid a future hysterectomy can undergo a myolysis. Indeed, the possibility of coagulation and devascularization of the myometrium exists, as does, at least theoretically, the possibility of uterine rupture in cases of pregnancy.

Long-term follow-up has shown that there is no regrowth of the myoma. Histology proved the complete devascularization of the myoma with subsequent necrosis. However, when performed, the second-look laparoscopy demonstrated the presence of very dense adhesions. In order to reduce the risk of adhesions, Interceed was placed on the coagulated area. Randomized studies must be carried out in the future in order to prove the efficacy of Interceed in this indication.

In order to reduce adhesions, new laser fibers (ITT fibers) are now being evaluated (Figure 10). In this type of fiber, diffusion of the heat inducing the necrosis occurs along the terminal part of the fiber. Only one hole is required and this reduces the lesion of the myoma serosa.

In conclusion, myolysis is effective in the reduction of myoma size and can be proposed as an alternative to myomectomy, but only in selected patients. Because of the risk of bowel adhesions and of coagulation of the myometrium, this type of surgery must be reserved for large, intramural, symptomatic myomas if endoscopic myomectomy is considered to be too difficult or time-consuming.

REFERENCES

1. Daniell, J.F. and Gurley, L.D. (1991). Laparoscopic treatment of clinically significant symptomatic uterine fibroids. *J. Gynecol. Surg.*, **7**, 37–9

2. Dubuisson, J.B., Lecuru, F., Foulot, H., Mandelbrot, L., Aubriot, F.X. and Mouly, M. (1991). Myomectomy by laparoscopy: a preliminary report of 43 cases. *Fertil. Steril.*, **56**, 827–30

3. Nezhat, C., Nezhat, F, Silfen, S.L., Shaffer, N. and Evand, D. (1991). Laparoscopic myomectomy. *Int. J. Fertil.*, **36**, 275–80

4. Donnez, J., Schrurs, B., Gillerot, S., Sandow, J. and Clerckx, F. (1989). Treatment of uterine fibroids with implants of gonadotropin releasing-hormone agonist: assessment by hysterography. *Fertil. Steril.*, **51**, 947–50

5. Donnez, J., Gillerot., S, Bourgonjon, D., Clerckx, F. and Nisolle, M. (1990). Neodymium : YAG laser hysteroscopy in large submucous fibroids. *Fertil. Steril.*, **54**, 999–1003

6. Gallinat, A. and Leuken, R.P. (1993). Current trends in the therapy of myomata. In Leuken, R.P. and Gallinat, A. (eds.) *Endoscopic Surgery in Gynecology*, pp. 69–71. (Berlin: Demeter Verlag GmBH)

7. Donnez, J. (1993). Nd : YAG laser hysteroscopic myomectomy. In Sutton, C. and Diamond, M. (eds.) *Endoscopic Surgery for Gynaecologists*, pp.331–7. (London: W.B. Saunders Company Ltd)

8. Nisolle, M., Smets, M., Gillerot, S., Anaf, V. and Donnez, J. (1993). Laparoscopic myolysis with the Nd-YAG laser. *J. Gynecol. Surg.*, **9**, 95–9

LASH: laparoscopic supracervical (subtotal) hysterectomy

20

J. Donnez and M. Nisolle

The development of new accessories and improved technology has enabled gynecologists to perform laparoscopic hysterectomy. Reich and colleagues[1] described the technique of laparoscopic hysterectomy for the first time in 1989. Laparoscopy-assisted vaginal hysterectomies (LAVH) and bilateral salpingo-oophorectomies have been performed routinely since 1990 in cases of endometrial cancer and benign gynecological disease in our department as well as in others[2-4].

In 1990, we performed the first laparoscopic subtotal (supracervical) hysterectomy (LASH) in our department[5]. The technique, the results and the indications are discussed.

INDICATIONS AND TECHNIQUE

In 1990, 214 hysterectomies were performed in our department. Out of this series (Table 1), 98 women underwent vaginal hysterectomy for genital prolapse or myomas; 51 underwent laparoscopic adnexectomy and vaginal hysterectomy for ovarian disease with or without associated uterine pathology, or for endometrial carcinomas; 17 women underwent laparoscopic adhesiolysis followed immediately by vaginal hysterectomy; and the first four cases of laparoscopic subtotal hysterectomy were also performed during the same period. In 1990, a total of 44 women underwent abdominal hysterectomy.

The incidence of LASH in a series of 251 hysterectomies performed in 1992 was 18% (Table 1). Thus, it increased from an incidence of 2% to 18%. The wider use of LASH has been proposed in cases of:

Table 1 Comparison of methods of hysterectomy in the authors' series between 1990 and 1992

	1990 (n = 214)		1992 (n = 251)	
Vaginal hysterectomy	98		64	
LAVH	51	(77%)	87	(74%)
Laparoscopic adhesiolysis and vaginal hysterectomy	17		11	
LASH	4	(2%)	44	(18%)
Abdominal hysterectomy	44	(21%)	45	(18%)

(1) Enlarged uterus with multiple fibroids (up to a 13-week gestational volume) and normal cervix (even in nulligravida);

(2) Failures of endometrial ablation and/or myomectomy (failure demonstrated by the recurrence of menometrorrhagia);

(3) Myomatous uterus in women who have a medical history of Cesarean section;

(4) Multiple submucosal myomas even if the uterine volume is < 7 gestational weeks.

All patients had a normal Pap smear, colposcopy and hysteroscopic cervical canal evaluation. All patients received general anesthesia. Following induction of general endotracheal anesthesia, the patient was placed in the dorsal lithotomy position. The abdomen and the vagina were prepared with a diluted iodine solution. A Foley catheter was inserted. Two Pozzi forceps were placed on the cervix and a non-metallic intrauterine cannula was inserted into the uterine cavity in order to manipulate the uterus easily.

A four-puncture technique was used for LASH: three 5-mm second-puncture trocars were inserted on the suprapubic line (± 3 cm above the pubis): one was inserted midline and the others 4–5 cm laterally, in each lower quadrant within the safety triangles (between the midline and the epigastric artery area). A 10-mm laparoscope connected to a video camera was placed intraumbilically. After careful inspection of the entire peritoneal cavity, the patient was moved into the Trendelenburg position (Figure 1(a)–(c)). Two surgical methods were used to transect pelvic ligaments and achieve hemostasis: either bipolar coagulation and transection or an Endo GIA automatic stapling device (Auto Suture). Because endoscopic staplers are very expensive, bipolar coagulation (Bipolar grasping forceps, Storz n°26176FB, 3 mm wide) and transection were more frequently used. Bipolar coagulation was used to desiccate the utero-ovarian ligaments and vessels and the isthmic portion of both Fallopian tubes. Scissors or CO_2 laser were then used to transect the structures within the coagulated areas (Figure 1(d)–(f)). Meticulous hemostasis was achieved by the repeated bipolar coagulation of transected vessels. The round ligaments were treated similarly (Figure 2).

When the automatic stapler device was used, the multifire Endo GIA surgical stapler delivered two staggered triple rows of staples onto the Fallopian tubes, the utero-ovarian ligaments and the round ligaments.

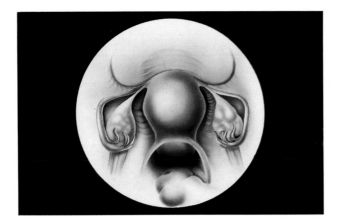

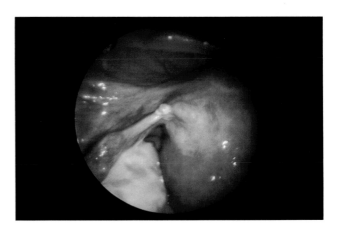

Figure 1(a) and (b) Laparoscopic view before LASH; (c) and (d) desiccation of the isthmic portion of the Fallopian tubes, utero-ovarian ligaments and vessels with bipolar coagulation; (e) transection of the structures within the coagulation area

Figure 1(b) *See legend opposite*

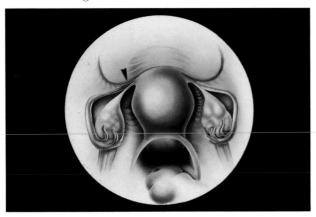

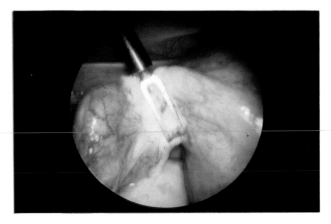

Figure 1(c) *See legend above*

Figure 1(d) *See legend above*

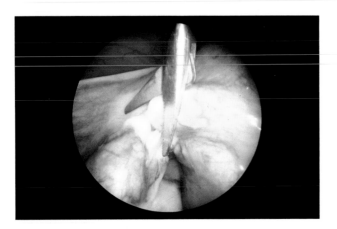

Figure 1(e) *See legend above*

The anterior and posterior leaves of the broad ligament were then opened with scissors. Hydrodissection made the procedure easier and allowed the surgeon to expose the uterine vessels (Figure 3). Thereafter, the vesicouterine peritoneum was opened with scissors. The vesicocervical space was dissected no more than 2 cm below the limit between the cervix and the corpus uteri (Figure 4).

After careful identification of the uterine vessels and ureters, the uterine vessels were electrocoagulated with the bipolar coagulation forceps and transected (Figure 5).

The unipolar knife (Coagulating electrode, Storz n°26178S) or the CO_2 laser were then used to cut and separate the cervix from the corpus (Figure 6). Hemostasis was achieved by meticulous coagulation. Longitudinal (vertical or horizontal) posterior colpotomy can be performed either by laparoscopy or through the vagina. A Pozzi forceps, introduced through the colpotomy incision, grasped the uterus, which was previously pushed into the pouch of Douglas (Figure 7). The uterus was then removed (Figure 8) and the longitudinal colpotomy incision was sutured in one layer. Whenever possible, the uterosacral ligaments were caught in the stitches and sutured together. This technique had the advantage of preventing cervical prolapse and enterocele.

The patient was then repositioned for a second-look laparoscopic examination. After reinsufflation, irrigation fluid was instilled into the pelvis and the operative sites were inspected. A titanium clip (Figure 9) was then applied to the uterine artery to insure complete hemostasis. After each point of bleeding had been coagulated, the instruments were removed from the abdomen and the four incisions were reapproximated with 3-0 nylon suture.

If necessary, loop resection of the cervical transformation zone can be performed. Prophylactic antibiotics (cephalosporin (Zinacef®) 2 g/day and tinidazole (Fasygyn®) 2 g/day) were administered during the procedure and for the first 3 postoperative days.

EVALUATION OF LASH

All of our LASH procedures were successful. The patients' ages ranged from 38 to 45 years. In all cases (except the first, which required more time), the average duration of surgery did not exceed 90 min. In experienced hands, the average duration in 1992 was 60 min.

The estimated blood loss was consistently less than 100 ml. There were no intraoperative complications such as bowel or ureteral injuries. No patient experienced fever. All patients were able to leave the hospital the day following surgery.

In our department, the length of hospital stay after surgery ranged from 4 to 5 days for vaginal hysterectomy, 3 to 4 days for LAVH and 5–8 days for abdominal hysterectomy (mostly dependent on the age of the patient).

Patients who underwent LASH reported much less discomfort than patients who underwent other types of hysterectomy. No patients required major analgesic drugs. Patients were able to ambulate very soon after LASH (the same day), just as patients who underwent laparoscopic adhesiolysis, ovarian cystectomy or salpingoneostomy. Sexual intercourse was permitted 3 weeks after surgery.

There were no signs of cervical prolapse or enterocele in patients reviewed in a 1-year follow-up. There were no complaints of urinary incontinence. Only 10% of patients required analgesic drugs a few hours after surgery, but no patients required drugs the day after surgery.

Patients were requested to undergo a Pap-smear and a colposcopy every year.

DISCUSSION

The indications for laparoscopic surgery have increased greatly over the past decades. Some expansion has also been seen in hysteroscopic surgery[6–9]. Endometrial ablation performed endoscopically has been proposed as an alternative to hormonal therapy or hysterectomy in dysfunctional bleeding without intrauterine lesions[10]. Hysteroscopic myomectomy has also been proposed for large submucosal myomas[6–8]. In a recent study, the long-term results of Nd : YAG laser hysteroscopic myomectomy were found to be excellent in cases of less than three large submucosal fibroids[7,8]. Indeed, the recurrence of menorrhagia did not exceed 5% after a 2-year follow-up. But in cases of multiple (four or more) submucosal fibroids, the recurrence of bleeding due to recurrent myomas was found to be as high as 25%, even when endometrial ablation was performed concomitantly[7,8].

In 1990, we performed the first laparoscopic subtotal hysterectomy (LASH)[5]. This technique was not used frequently in our department in that year. Indeed, out of 214 hysterectomies carried out in the department, only four LASH procedures (2%) were performed. At that time the disadvantage of the technique – the remaining cervix – was considered as a potential risk for the development of cervical cancer. However, loop resection of the cervical transformation zone can be carried out, if necessary, at the time of posterior colpotomy, so that the risk of cervical cancer is greatly reduced.

Subsequently, the number of LASH procedures performed increased from 2 to 18% of the total number of hysterectomies by 1992 (Table 2). Colpotomy incisions were made either vertically or horizontally. There was no difference in the surgical procedure or in the postoperative healing between the two types of incision. No patients required major analgesics the day after surgery.

Numerous advantages were noted, although our data were not generated from a randomized study. The advantages were:

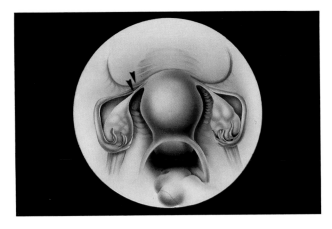

Figure 2(a)–(c)   Coagulation and section of the round ligaments

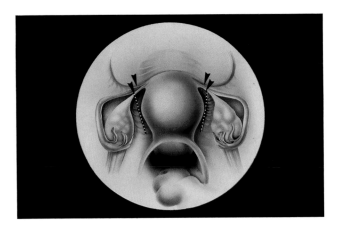

Figure 3(a) and (b)   The anterior leaf of the broad ligament is opened in order to visualize the uterine vessels

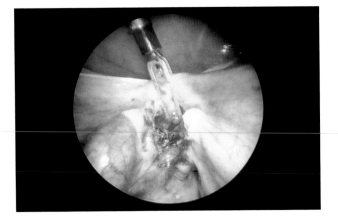

Figure 2(b)   *See legend above*

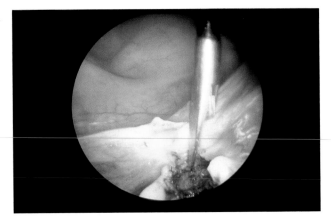

Figure 3(b)   *See legend above*

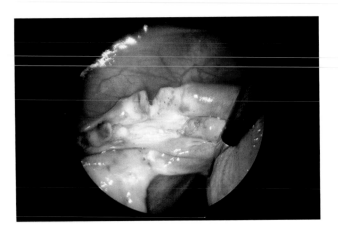

Figure 2(c)   *See legend above*

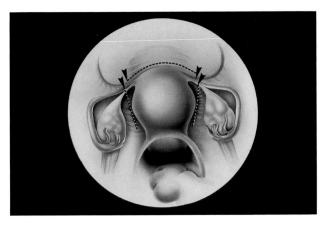

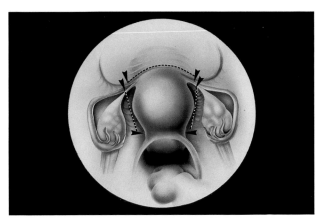

Figure 4(a)–(c) The vesico-uterine peritoneum is opened with scissors or with CO_2 laser

Figure 5 The uterine vessels are electrocoagulated (a) and (b) and transected (c)

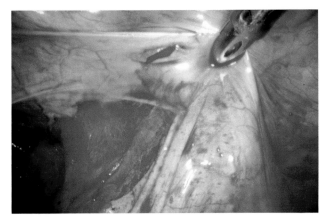

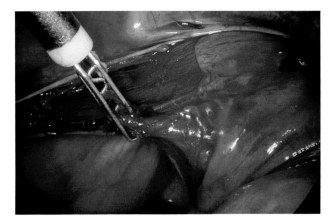

Figure 4(b)   *See legend above*

Figure 5(b)   *See legend above*

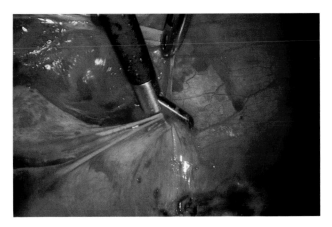

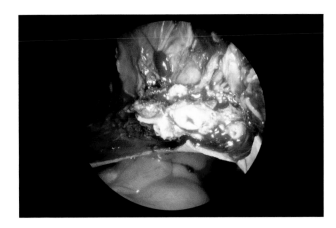

Figure 4(c)   *See legend above*

Figure 5(c)   *See legend above*

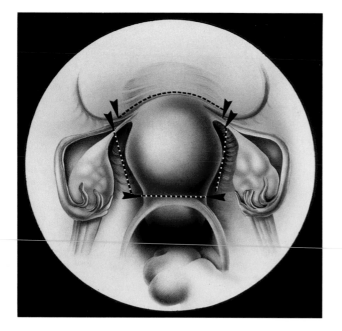

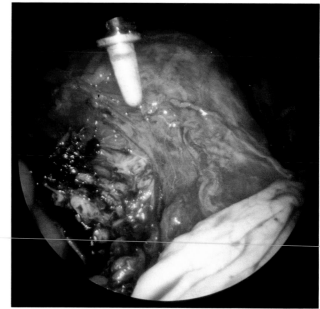

Figure 6(a)–(c)   The unipolar knife or the CO_2 laser is used to cut and separate the cervix from the corpus; (d) a plastic cannula is inserted into the cervix to avoid electrical conduction

Figure 6(b)   *See legend opposite*

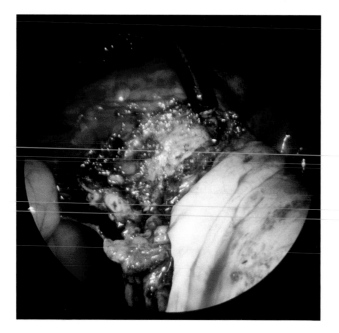

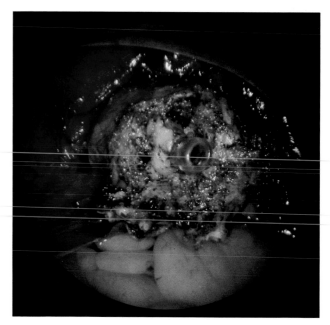

Figure 6(c)   *See legend above*

Figure 6(d)   *See legend above*

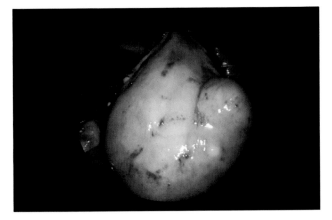

Figure 7 A posterior colpotomy is then carried out (either by laparoscopy or through the vagina) and a Pozzi forceps grasps the body of the uterus, which is removed through the colpotomy incision

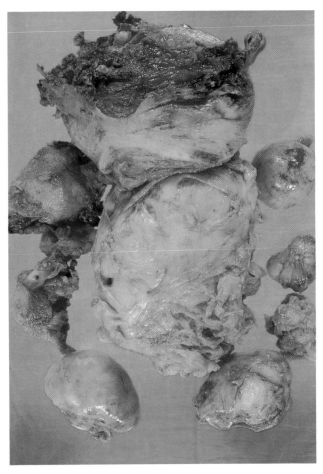

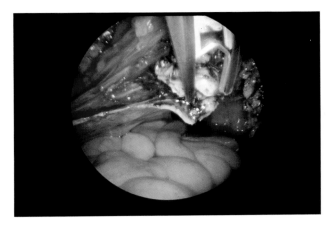

Figure 9(a) and (b)   A titanium clip is then applied

Figure 8 Supracervical hysterectomy (LASH): the volume of the uterus was > 14 weeks

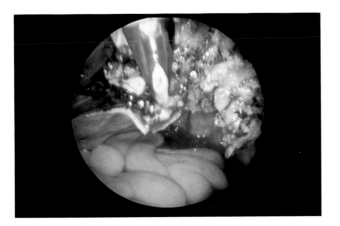

Figure 9(b)   *See legend above*

Table 2 'Laparoscopy-assisted' hysterectomy in 1992

Vaginal hysterectomy	64 (25%)
Abdominal hysterectomy	45 (18%)
Laparoscopic assisted hysterectomy (LAVH, LH, LASH)	142 (57%)
Total	251

(1) The reduced operative time when compared to LAVH;

(2) The rapid recovery, similar to that observed after laparoscopic surgery for infertility; and

(3) The reduced postoperative discomfort and shorter hospital stay.

A serious complication rate of 3% was recently reported after laparoscopy-assisted vaginal hysterectomy (LAVH) and laparoscopic hysterectomy (LH) in a multicentric study conducted in the UK (Garry, personal communication) as well as in Belgium[10]. Ureteral and/or bladder damage occurred at a rate of 2% after laparoscopic hysterectomy. In our series, no major complications were noted. The technique of LASH reduces the risk of ureteral and bladder injury.

One other advantage of LASH is the preservation of the cardinal and uterosacral ligaments which probably play a role in pelvic organ suspension and in the control of bladder continence.

When performing LASH, we have not found endoscopic automatic staplers, CO_2 or Nd : YAG lasers beneficial. Bipolar coagulation and scissors allow the surgeon to perform this procedure very safely.

Because the technique is easy to perform, has a very low morbidity rate and a quick recovery, LASH could be suggested as a strictly laparoscopic approach for some indications and especially in cases of a uterus with multiple submucosal myomas. Indeed, we know that in such cases, the rate of recurrence of bleeding after hysteroscopic myoma resection and endometrial ablation is more than 25% after a 2-year follow-up[7,8]; LASH could be proposed instead of hysteroscopic surgery to women with this type of pathology.

Failures of endometrial ablation (endometrial laser ablation and partial endometrial laser ablation) for dysfunctional bleeding in a normal-sized uterus occur in about 3 to 5% of cases[9]. Failed endometrial ablation must also be considered as an indication for LASH.

Because of the good results and the absence of complications, the technique of LASH is proposed in our department in cases of:

(1) Enlarged uterus with multiple fibroids (up to a 13-week gestational volume) and normal cervix (even in nulligravida);

(2) Failures of endometrial ablation and/or myomectomy (failure demonstrated by the recurrence of menometrorrhagia);

(3) Myomatous uterus in women who have a medical history of Cesarean section;

(4) Multiple submucosal myomas even if the uterine volume is < 7 gestational weeks.

As for other new laparoscopic techniques, further studies, possibly controlled trials, are needed before the efficacy compared to other procedures can be established. After this preliminary report, we suggest that a greater number of surgeons perform LASH in order to gain broader experience and to permit a comparative study with vaginal hysterectomy.

REFERENCES

1. Reich, H., De Caprio, J. and MacGlynn, F. (1989). Laparoscopic hysterectomy. *J. Gynecol. Coll. Surg.*, **5**, 213

2. Nezhat, C., Nezhat, F. and Silfen, S.L. (1990). Laparoscopic hysterectomy and bilateral salpingo-oophorectomy using multifire GIA surgical stapler. *J. Gynecol. Coll. Surg.*, **6**, 287

3. Mage, G., Canis, M., Wattiez, A., Pouly, J.L. and Bruhat, M.A. (1990). Hystérectomie et coelioscopie. *J. Gynecol. Obstet. Biol. Reprod.*, **19**, 573–6

4. Padial, J.G., Sotolongo, J., Casey, M.J., Johnson, C. and Osborne, N.G. (1992). Laparoscopy-assisted vaginal hysterectomy: report of seventy-five consecutive cases. *J. Gynecol. Surg.*, **8**, 81

5. Donnez, J. and Nisolle, M. (1993). LASH: laparoscopic supracervical (subtotal) hysterectomy. *J. Gynecol. Surg.*, **9**, 91–4

6. Donnez, J., Gillerot, S., Bourgonjon, D., Clerckx, F. and Nisolle, M. (1990). Neodymium : YAG laser hysteroscopy in large submucous fibroids. *Fertil. Steril.*, **54**, 999

7. Donnez, J. and Nisolle, M. (1992). Hysteroscopic surgery. *Curr. Opin. Obstet. Gynecol.*, **4**, 439

8. Donnez, J. (1993). Nd - YAG laser hysteroscopic myomectomy. In Sutton, C. and Diamond, M. (eds.) *Endoscopic Surgery for Gynecologists*, pp.331–7. (London: W.B. Saunders Company Ltd)

9. Nisolle, M., Grandjean, P., Gillerot, S. and Donnez, J. (1991). Endometrial ablation with the Nd-YAG laser in dysfunctional bleeding. *Min. Invas. Ther.*, **1**, 35

10. Cusumano, P.G., Deprest, J., Hardy, A., Van Herendael, B. and Verly, M. (1992). Multicentric registration on laparoscopic hysterectomy: a one year experience. *Proceedings of the First European Congress of Gynecologic Endoscopy*, Clermont-Ferrand, France, September, p.46

Laparoscopy-assisted vaginal hysterectomy and laparoscopic hysterectomy in benign diseases

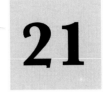

J. Donnez, M. Nisolle and V. Anaf

INTRODUCTION

In the United States, hysterectomy is one of the most commonly performed surgical procedures (656 000 hysterectomies in 1987 alone[1]). Approximately 70% are performed using the abdominal approach and 30% are performed vaginally[2]. Contraindications to vaginal hysterectomy depend essentially on the skill of the surgeon[2-5]. The most frequent contraindications are:

(1) Endometriosis (moderate or severe);

(2) Previous Cesarean section;

(3) Significant uterine enlargement or limited uterine mobility in a nulligravida;

(4) Previous pelvic surgery; and

(5) Previous uterine suspension.

In many cases, however, careful examination of the pelvis by diagnostic laparoscopy reveals the absence of contraindications to vaginal hysterectomy. In addition, a large proportion of patients are candidates for vaginal hysterectomy after adhesiolysis.

Most of the endoscopic procedures can be applied to treat adhesions, extensive pelvic endometriosis, adnexal disease and myomas, and hysterectomies that require an abdominal approach may be performed with laparoscopic dissection (partial or total) followed by vaginal removal. A major benefit of both laparoscopic and vaginal hysterectomy is the avoidance of an abdominal incision, which typically requires a longer hospitalization (5 days) and recuperation time (4–6 weeks) than does the combination of laparoscopy and vaginal removal.

Laparoscopic hysterectomy[6] is a substitute for abdominal hysterectomy and not for vaginal hysterectomy.

DEFINITIONS

Laparoscopic hysterectomy was first performed by Reich in January 1988[6]. According to Reich[6] and Mage and colleagues[7], there are at least four types:

(1) Type 1: laparoscopy performed for diagnostic purposes, where indications for a vaginal approach are equivocal, in order to determine whether vaginal hysterectomy is possible.

(2) Type 2: laparoscopy-assisted vaginal hysterectomy (LAVH), an initial laparoscopic surgical procedure after which vaginal hysterectomy is carried out.

(3) Type 3: laparoscopic hysterectomy, denoting the laparoscopic ligation of the uterine arteries[6].

(4) Type 4: complete laparoscopic hysterectomy (LH); laparoscopic dissection continues until the uterus is free of all attachments in the peritoneal cavity.

Laparoscopic supracervical hysterectomy has recently regained advocates after Kilkku and co-workers[8] reported a reduction in orgasms after hysterectomy as compared with supravaginal amputation. Laparoscopic subtotal hysterectomy (LASH) was recently described by Donnez and Nisolle[9].

A staging system was devised in order to standardize terminology (Table 1)[5].

Table 1 Laparoscopy-assisted vaginal hysterectomy staging (according to Johns, 1993[5])

Stage	
0	diagnostic laparoscopy without laparoscopic procedure prior to vaginal hysterectomy
1	procedure including laparoscopic adhesiolysis and/or excision of endometriosis
2	one or both adnexa freed laparoscopically
3	bladder dissected from uterus
4	uterine artery transected laparoscopically
5	anterior and/or posterior colpotomy or entire uterus freed

INDICATIONS

The indications for LH include benign pathologies such as endometriosis, fibroids, adnexal masses, adhesions from a previous Cesarean section, inflammatory disease or previous surgery, which usually require an abdominal approach to hysterectomy. Laparoscopic hysterectomy may also be considered for Stage I endometrial, ovarian and cervical cancer[7,10-12] (see Chapter 22).

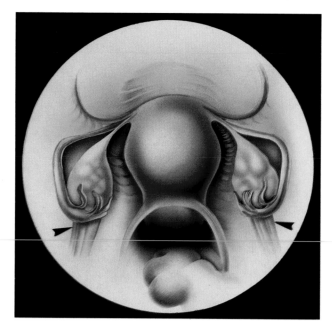

Figure 1(a)–(c) Coagulation of the infundibulopelvic ligament

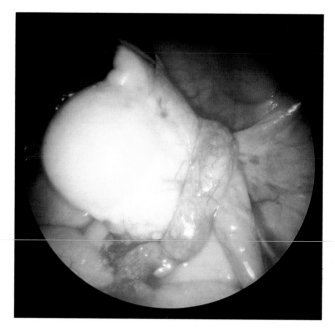

Figure 1(b) *See legend opposite*

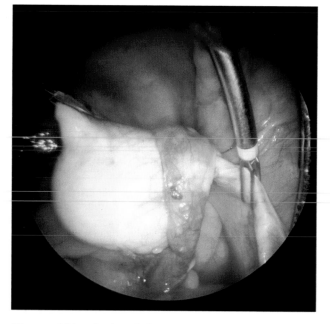

Figure 1(c) *See legend above*

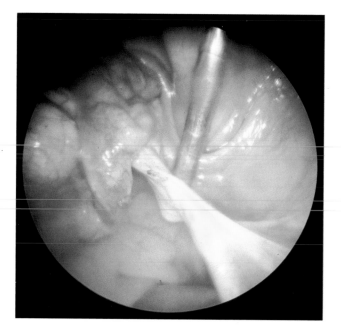

Figure 2 Section of the infundibulopelvic ligament using the CO_2 laser. Scissors can also be used

TECHNIQUES

All surgical procedures after uterine vessel ligation, including anterior and posterior vaginal incision, cardinal and intersacral ligament division, intact uterine removal and vaginal closure, can be performed vaginally or laparoscopically.

A Foley catheter is inserted during surgery to empty the bladder. Four laparoscopic puncture sites, including the umbilicus, are used: 10 mm umbilical, 5 mm right, 5 mm medial and 5 mm left lower quadrant. These are placed just above the pubic hairline; lateral incisions are made next to the deep epigastric vessels. A cannula is placed in the cervix for appropriate uterine mobilization. Abdominal and adnexal adhesions, if present, are lysed to mobilize the uterus, and the ureters are identified.

The adnexa are removed first. The infundibulopelvic ligament is identified and exposed by applying traction to the adnexa with an opposite forceps. The bipolar forceps is used to compress and desiccate the vessels (Figure 1), which are then cut with scissors (Figure 2). Bipolar coagulation is used to coagulate the pedicle, or staples or sutures may be applied. Scissor division is carried out close to the line of desiccation to ensure that the pedicle remains compressed.

The peritoneum between the infundibulopelvic ligament and the round ligament is then cut (Figure 3). The round ligaments are desiccated (Figure 4) and cut with scissors (Figure 5). The leaves of the broad ligament are separated and cut (Figure 6).

The peritoneum of the vesico-uterine space is then grasped and elevated with a forceps while scissors are used to dissect the vesico-uterine space (Figure 7). Aquadissection may be used to separate the leaves of the broad ligament, distending the vesico-uterine space and defining the tendinous attachments of the bladder in this area; these are coagulated and cut. Sharp dissection can also be used to divide the peritoneum down to the uterosacral ligaments.

The uterine vessels are identified (Figure 8) and skeletonized using aquadissection. When these are well identified, and after confirming the position of the ureters, the uterine vessels are desiccated with bipolar coagulation (Figure 9) and cut (Figure 10). In some departments, staples are used, but this is very expensive. Some authors[13] prefer suture ligation of the vascular bundle. Ligation of the uterine vessels can also be performed by the vaginal approach.

The rest of the operation is performed vaginally, as is suturing of the vaginal vault. At the end of the vaginal procedure, a laparoscopic check-up is performed and a Silastic catheter is left in the Douglas pouch for drainage for a period of 24 h.

The total procedure (type 4 according to Reich; Stage 5 according to Johns) may also be performed laparoscopically. Vaginal incision is achieved over a sponge placed between the vaginal anterior wall and the cervix (Figure 11). Tenting this area from below allows precise laparoscopic dissection of the bladder away from the vagina.

The vagina is entered over a sponge using a unipolar cutting current or a CO_2 laser (Figure 12). The same procedure is performed posteriorly over a sponge, exposing the area in the cul-de-sac where an incision can be made. The vaginal incision is completed and the uterosacral and cardinal ligaments are clamped and divided.

The completely freed uterus is then pulled into the vagina. The vagina may be sutured from below (Figure 13) or laparoscopically with three sutures. The first joins the uterosacral ligament across the midline. The second brings the cardinal ligament and underlying vagina across the midline. The third suture closes the anterior vagina and its fascia[5,6].

During laparoscopy, hemostasis is achieved by bipolar coagulation. Blood clots are removed. The pelvis is rinsed with an antiseptic solution which is left in the abdominal cavity for 2–3 h. The drain catheter is then opened without suction. Antibiotics (Zinacef® 2g/day, Fasygin® 2g/day) are given peroperatively and for 3–5 days postoperatively.

SPECIFIC EQUIPMENT AND COMMENTS

Bipolar coagulation

Reich[13] suggests monitoring electrical current flow with a flow meter to ensure total coagulation of the tissue between the tips of the bipolar forceps. Current flow between the tips of the bipolar electrodes ceases only when complete desiccation (dehydration) has occurred. Kleppinger bipolar forceps are excellent for large-vessel hemostasis. Specially insulated bipolar forceps allow the current to pass only through their tips, so that precise hemostasis can be obtained. For Reich[13], the Kleppinger bipolar forceps with a matched power source is an indispensable tool for all operative laparoscopies. The visual current flow meter ensures that desiccation of the tissue held by the forceps is complete.

Uterine mobilizer

The uterine mobilizer is inserted to antevert the uterus and delineate the posterior vagina. Reich[13] uses the Valtchev uterine mobilizer. We prefer to use an intra-uterine cannula similar to that used for methylene blue injection and a sponge held in a forceps to delineate the 'anterior' and 'posterior' vaginal cul-de-sac.

Ureter dissection

Reich[6,13] begins surgery with identification of the ureters, usually at the pelvic brim, and their mobilization.

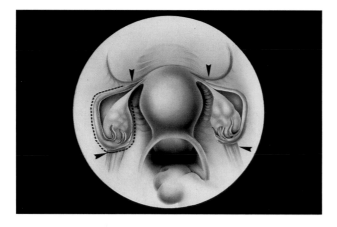

Figure 3(a)–(c) Section of the peritoneum between the infundibulopelvic ligament and the round ligament

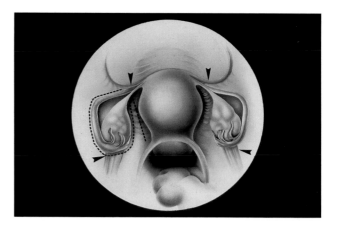

Figure 4(a) and (b) Coagulation of the round ligament

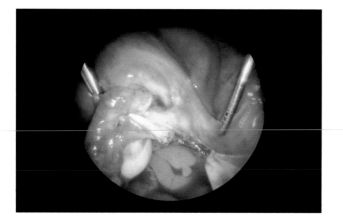

Figure 3(b) *See legend above*

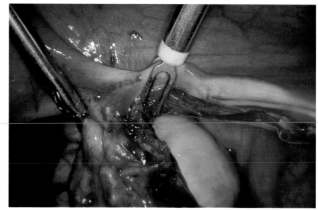

Figure 4(b) *See legend above*

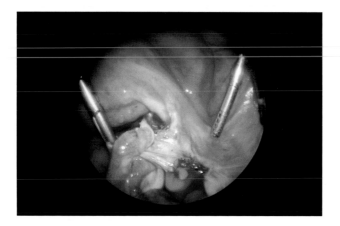

Figure 3(c) *See legend above*

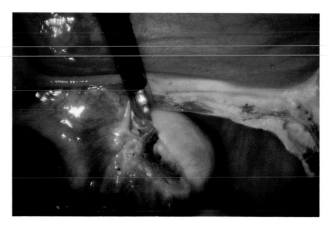

Figure 5 Section of the round ligament

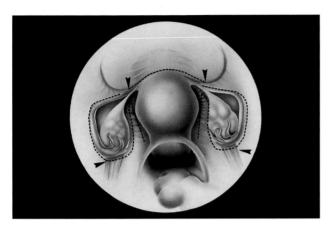

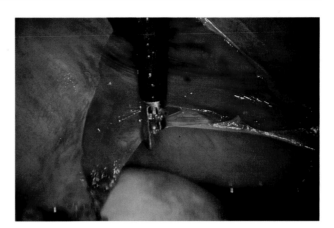

Figure 6(a) and (b) Dissection of the leaves of the broad ligament

Figure 6(b) *See legend opposite*

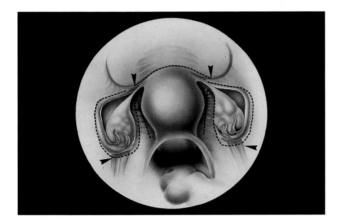

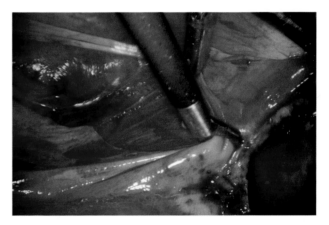

Figure 7(a) and (b) Dissection of the vesico-uterine space

Figure 7(b) *See legend opposite*

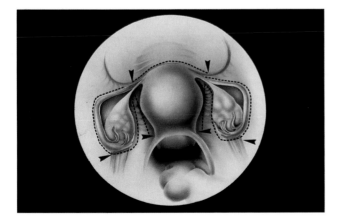

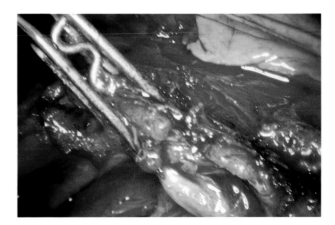

Figure 8(a) and (b) Identification of the uterine vessels and coagulation with bipolar forceps

Figure 8(b) *See legend opposite*

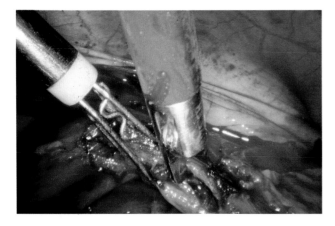

Figure 9(a) and (b)   Section of the uterine vessels

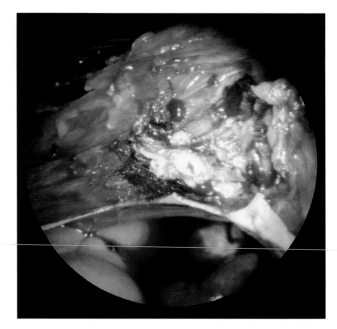

Figure 9(b)   *See legend opposite*

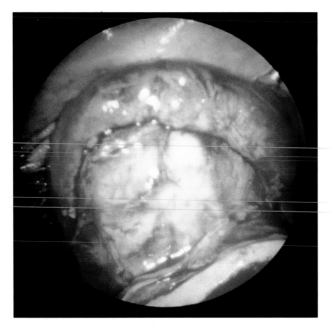

Figure 10   A sponge is placed in the anterior vaginal fornix

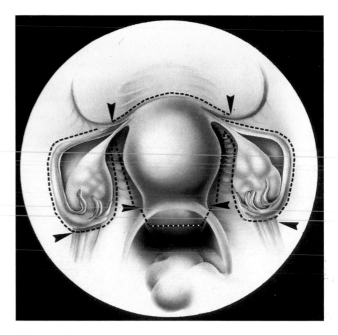

Figure 10   A sponge is placed in the anterior vaginal fornix

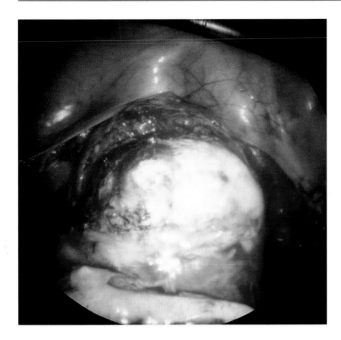

Figure 11(b)   *See legend opposite*

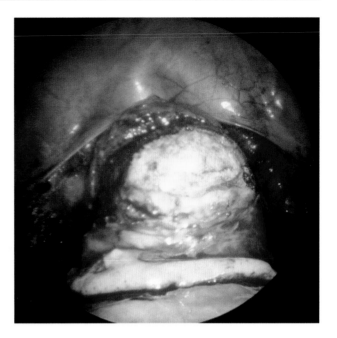

Figure 11(c)   *See legend opposite*

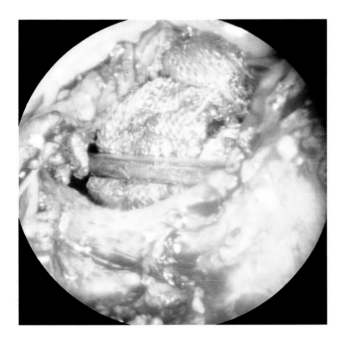

Figure 11(d)   *See legend opposite*

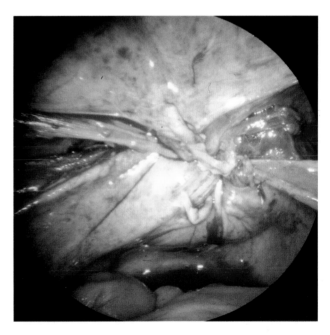

Figure 12   Final view after peritoneal and vaginal closure

Their dissection requires medial reflection of the recto-sigmoid, to expose the ovarian vessels and the ureters as they cross over the iliac artery to enter the true pelvis.

The positions of the previously dissected ureters in the broad ligament are again checked before desiccation, stapling, or suturing of the uterine vessels. When the ureter is far from the uterine vessels, bipolar desiccation or stapling is carried out. Inspection of the ureter after positioning the stapler has been known to reveal entrapment of the ureter. Suture ligation of the vascular bundle is preferred by Reich[13]: this technique avoids such injury, as the ureter is visualized directly throughout the ligation process. Mage et al.[7] and Donnez et al.[12] prefer bipolar coagulation. In our department, the ureter is identified but only dissected in cases of endometriosis.

Vaginal closure

Reich[13] proposes laparoscopic vaginal closure in which the ligaments and vaginal epithelium are brought together. In our department, the closure is performed through the vagina: the peritoneum and uterosacral ligaments are brought together, then the vaginal mucosa is closed. Laparoscopy is then used to inspect the operative sites.

Drainage

One of the intraoperative advantages of a laparoscopic approach to hysterectomy is the ability to achieve complete hemostasis and evacuate all blood clots at the end of the procedure. This removal of all remaining clots and pelvic lavage may reduce postoperative infection associated with vaginal hysterectomy. At the end of surgery, we prefer to leave 300 ml iodine or Rifocine® solution in the abdominal cavity for 2–3 h. The drain is left in the Douglas pouch, closed for 2–3 h and then opened. In our series, no cases of infection were reported.

Is preoperative administration of a gonadotropin releasing hormone agonist useful?

Gonadotropin releasing hormone (GnRH) analogs may reduce the total uterine volume in patients with uterine leiomyomata by between 35% and 50%[14,15]. When hysterectomy is planned for the treatment of large myomas, women should be pretreated with a GnRH analog for at least 3 months, since shrinkage of the myoma should facilitate laparoscopic or vaginal hyster-ectomy. This preoperative therapy may also be used in women with an enlarged uterus of more than 13 weeks, but less than 17 weeks, in order to decrease the volume of the uterus.

COMPLICATIONS (Table 2)

In a series of 191 LAVH performed in our department from January 1990 to December 1992, the complication rate was very low at 1%. Most of the LAVH were type 2 according to the classification of Reich, or Stage 3 according to the classification of Johns. Adhesiolysis and/or bilateral adnexectomy were performed laparo-scopically and the bladder was laparoscopically dissected from the uterus. Most frequently (> 90%), ligation of the uterine artery was achieved vaginally, as was anterior and posterior colpotomy.

In one case, bladder injury (Table 2) occurred during the vaginal extraction of a large uterus (> 15 weeks). Morcellation of the uterus was carried out in order to extract it and bladder injury was found subsequently. The bladder was vaginally repaired without compli-cation. In another case, a secondary hemorrhage occurred on the second postoperative day. Vaginal closure stitches and the peritoneal closure stitches were cut, and the bleeding site was identified as the right uterine artery, which had been coagulated laparo-scopically 2 days before by bipolar coagulation. Ligation was performed easily through the vagina.

As a result of this occurrence, we now systematically apply one titanium clip to the uterine artery after the removal of the uterus and the rinsing of the pelvic cavity. It is important to apply the clip at the end of the procedure to avoid manipulation of the tissue, causing the clip to slip.

Table 2 Severe complications of laparoscopy-assisted vaginal hysterectomy (n = 191)

Bladder injury*	1	(0.5%)
Ureteral injury	0	
Bowel injury	0	
Secondary hemorrage†	1	(0.5%)
Fever > 38°C (after second postoperative day)	0	

*, Bladder laceration during extraction of a > 15-week uterus; †, In one case, where ligation was laparoscopically performed, a hemoperitoneum occurred. Bleeding was found coming from the uterine artery. Ligation was performed vaginally

CONCLUSION

Opponents of the concept of laparoscopic hysterectomy argue that vaginal hysterectomy is faster, less expensive, and results in a similar short hospital stay and convalescence. In the United States and in Europe, however, 75% of hysterectomies are performed by an abdominal approach. If laparoscopic hysterectomy is added to our surgical armamentarium, almost all hysterectomies (90%) will be carried out without an abdominal incision. In our department (Table 3), the rate of abdominal hysterectomy is 18%. The remaining indications for abdominal hysterectomy are myomas > 14–15 weeks (unless a GnRH agonist can be administered in order to reduce the volume), malignant (or suspected to be malignant) ovarian masses and cervical cancer stage IB (Wertheim-Meigs), and frozen pelvis, when a hysterectomy is mandatory.

Table 3 Methods of hysterectomy used in our department

	1990 (n = 214)		1992 (n = 251)	
Abdominal hysterectomy	44	(21%)	45	(18%)
Vaginal hysterectomy	98	(46%)	64	(25%)
Laparoscopic hysterectomy	72	(33%)	142	(57%)
LASH	4		44	
LAVH*	68		98	

*, Laparoscopic adnexectomy and/or adhesiolysis followed by vaginal hysterectomy. The bladder is dissected laparoscopically from the uterus. Most of the time, the uterine arteries are ligated and transected vaginally

REFERENCES

1. Findlay, S. (1990). The health-insurance factor. *US News World Rep.* **30**, 57
2. Kovak, S.R., Cruikshank, S.H. and Retto, H.F. (1990). Laparoscopic assisted vaginal hysterectomy. *J. Gynecol. Surg.*, **6**, 185–90
3. Isaacs, J.H. (1990). *Gynecology and Obstetrics. Clinical Gynecology*, vol.1, pp.1–11. (Philadelphia: J.B. Lippincott)
4. Smith, H.O. and Thompson, J.D. (1986). Indications and technique for sapinol hysterectomy. *Contemp. Obstet. Gynecol.*, 125
5. Johns, A. (1993). Laparoscopic assisted vaginal hysterectomy (LAVH). In Sutton, C. and Diamond, D. (eds.) *Gynecologic Endoscopy for Gynecologists*, pp.179–86. (London: Saunders)
6. Reich, H. (1989). New techniques in advanced laparoscopic surgery. *Clin. Obstet. Gynecol.*, **3**, 655–81
7. Mage, G., Wattiez, A., Chapron, C., Canis, M., Pouly, J.L., Pingeon, J.M. and Bruhat, M.A. (1992). Hystérectomie per-coelioscopique: résultats d'une série de 44 cas. *J. Gynecol. Obstet. Biol. Reprod.*, **21**, 436–44
8. Kilkku, P. (1983). Supravaginal uterine amputation vs hysterectomy: effects on libido and orgasm. *Acta Obstet. Gynecol. Scand.*, **62**, 141–5
9. Donnez, J. and Nisolle, M. (1993). LASH: laparoscopic supracervical hysterectomy. *J. Gynecol. Surg.*, **9**, 91–4
10. Querleu, D., Leblanc, E. and Castelain, G. (1991). Laparoscopic pelvic lymphadenectomy in the staging of early carcinoma of the cervix. *Am. J. Obstet. Gynecol.*, **164**, 579–81
11. Reich, H., McGlynn, F. and Wickie, W. (1990). Laparoscopic management of stage 1 ovarian cancer: a case report. *J. Reprod. Med.*, **35**, 601
12. Donnez, J., Nisolle, M. and Anaf, V. (1993). Place de l'endoscopie dans le cancer de l'endomètre. In DuBuisson, J.B., Chapron, C.H. and Bouquet de Jolinière, J. (eds.) *Coelioscopie et Cancerologie en Gynecologie*, pp.77–82. (Paris: Arnette)
13. Reich, H. (1993). New laparoscopic techniques. In Sutton, C. and Diamond, M. (eds.) *Endoscopic Surgery for Gynaecologists*, pp.28–39. (London: W.B. Saunders)
14. Donnez, J., Schrurs, B., Gillerot, S., Sandow, J. and Clerckx, F. (1989). Treatment of uterine fibroids with implants of gonadotropin-releasing hormone agonist: assessment by hysterography. *Fertil. Steril.*, **51**, 947–50
15. Donnez, J., Gillerot, S., Bourgonjon, D., Clerckx, F. and Nisolle, M. (1990). Neodymium : YAG laser hysteroscopy in large submucous fibroids. *Fertil. Steril.*, **54**, 999–1003
16. Canis, M., Mage, G., Wattiez, A., Pouly, J.L., Manhes, H. and Bruhat, M.A. (1990). La chirurgie endoscopique a-t-elle une place dans la chirurgie radicale du cancer du col utérin? *J. Gynecol. Obstet. Biol. Reprod.*, **19**, 921
17. Canis, M., Mage, G., Wattiez, A., Pouly, J.L., Chapron, C. and Bruhat, M.A. (1992). Vaginally assisted laparoscopic radical hysterectomy. *J. Gynecol. Surg.*, **8**, 103–5

The role of the laser in laparoscopic hysterectomy

22

H. Reich

INTRODUCTION

Laparoscopic hysterectomy and laser surgery have become popular procedures due to media attention and consumer interest. Most hysterectomies (75%) are performed using an abdominal incision[1].

Laparoscopic hysterectomy, defined as the ligation of the uterine vessels, is a substitute for abdominal hysterectomy, with more attention to ureteral identification[2–4]. It was first performed in January 1988[5]. Laparoscopic hysterectomy stimulated a laparoscopic approach to hysterectomy exemplified by laparoscopic assisted vaginal hysterectomy (LAVH) as gynecologists not trained in vaginal or laparoscopic techniques struggled to maintain a market share of the large and lucrative hysterectomy market. LAVH has become an expensive procedure, performed for indications for which skilled vaginal surgeons rarely find laparoscopy necessary. Laparoscopic hysterectomy remains a substitute for abdominal hysterectomy.

Most hysterectomies currently requiring an abdominal approach may be performed by laparoscopic dissection of part or all of the abdominal portion followed by vaginal removal. There are many surgical advantages, particularly magnification of anatomy and pathology, easy access to the vagina and rectum, and the ability to achieve complete hemostasis and clot evacuation during underwater examination. Patient advantages are multiple and are related to the avoidance of a painful abdominal incision. They include reduced duration of hospitalization and recuperation and an extremely low rate of cuff infection and ileus.

The goal to be realized with vaginal hysterectomy, laparoscopic assisted vaginal hysterectomy, or laporoscopic hysterectomy is the safe avoidance of an abdominal wall incision. Vaginal hysterectomy should be performed if it is possible after ligation of the utero-ovarian ligaments. Laparoscopic inspection at the end of the procedure will still allow the surgeon to control any bleeding and evacuate clot. Unnecessary operations should not be performed because of the surgeon's preoccupation with the development of new surgical skills. Laparoscopic hysterectomy is not indicated when vaginal hysterectomy is possible.

DEFINITIONS

There is a variety of operations in which the laparoscope is used as an aid to hysterectomy (Table 1).

Table 1 Laparoscopic hysterectomy classification

(1) Diagnostic laparoscopy with vaginal hysterectomy

(2) Laparoscopic assisted vaginal hysterectomy (LAVH)
   ? morcellation
   ? laparoscopic vault suspension

(3) Laparoscopic hysterectomy (LH)
   ? morcellation
   ? laparoscopic vault suspension

(4) Total laparoscopic hysterectomy (TLH)
   ? morcellation
   ? laparoscopic vault suspension

(5) Laparoscopic supracervical hysterectomy (LSH) including CISH (classical intrafascial Semm hysterectomy)

(6) Vaginal hysterectomy with laparoscopic vault suspension or reconstruction

(7) Laparoscopic hysterectomy with lymphadenectomy

(8) Laparoscopic hysterectomy with lymphadenectomy and omentectomy

(9) Laparoscopic radical hysterectomy with lymphadenectomy

It is important that these different procedures are clearly delineated:

(1) Diagnostic laparoscopy with vaginal hysterectomy indicates that the laparoscope is used for diagnostic purposes, when indications for a vaginal approach are equivocal, to determine whether *vaginal hysterectomy* is possible[6]. It also assures that vaginal cuff and pedicle hemostasis are complete and allows clot evacuation.

(2) Laparoscopic assisted vaginal hysterectomy (LAVH) is a vaginal hysterectomy performed after laparoscopic adhesiolysis, endometriosis excision, or oophorectomy[7–9]. Unfortunately, this term is also used when the upper uterine blood supply of a relatively normal uterus is staple-ligated. It must be emphasized that the easy part of both abdominal and vaginal hysterectomy is usually upper pedicle ligation.

(3) Laparoscopic hysterectomy (LH) denotes laparoscopic ligation of the uterine arteries, using electrosurgery desiccation, suture ligature or staples. All maneuvers after uterine vessel ligation can be performed vaginally or laparoscopically, including anterior and posterior vaginal entry, cardinal and uterosacral ligament division, uterine removal (intact

or by morcellation), and vaginal closure (vertically or transversely). Laparoscopic ligation of the uterine vessels is the *sine qua non* for laparoscopic hysterectomy. Ureteral isolation has always been advised.

(4) Total laparoscopic hysterectomy (TLH) is a laparoscopic assisted abdominal hysterectomy. Laparoscopic dissection continues until the uterus lies free of all attachments in the peritoneal cavity. The uterus is removed through the vagina, with morcellation if necessary. The vagina is closed with laparoscopically placed sutures.

(5) Laparoscopic supracervical hysterectomy (LSH) has recently regained advocates after suggestions that total hysterectomy results in a decrease in libido[10]. The uterus is removed by morcellation from above or below.

Semm's version of supracervical hysterectomy is called the CISH procedure (classical intrafascial Semm hysterectomy). It leaves the cardinal ligaments intact while eliminating the columnar cells of the endocervical canal. After perforating the uterine fundus with a long sound-dilator, a calibrated uterine resection tool (COURT) that fits around this instrument is used to core out the endocervical canal. Thereafter, at laparoscopy, suture techniques are used to ligate the utero-ovarian ligaments. An Endoloop is placed around the uterine fundus to the level of the internal os of the cervix and tied. The uterus is divided at its junction with the cervix and removed by laparoscopic morcellation.

LASER DISSECTION

Most laparoscopic hysterectomy procedures can be performed with the CO_2 laser, whose main effect on tissue is vaporization. This can be used for direct vaporization of lesions, but is more often used for division or separation of adhesions and for excision of tissue in a manner similar to using scissors. As with electrosurgery, blood vessels less than 1 mm in diameter are often coagulated in the process, but application of the beam to an actively bleeding vessel usually results in burnt, black blood.

The major advantages of the CO_2 laser are its 0.1-mm depth of penetration and poor conduction through water, allowing a greater margin of safety when working around the bowel, ureter, and major vessels, and its ability to work at a distance from tissue without contact while other instruments are used for traction. Backstops are rarely necessary because of this superficial penetration and the wet surgical field, especially, however, when the operator develops the skill of using the tissue to be treated as the backstop. It must be emphasized that laser surgery is still associated with a zone of thermal necrosis surrounding treated tissue, and in susceptible patients, adhesions will form. Laser surgery does not result in a reduced rate of adhesion formation when compared to other thermal energy sources.

Use of the CO_2 laser through the operating channel of a laser laparoscope converts the umbilical incision into a portal for performing surgery, reducing the need for an additional incision. This delivery system allows the surgeon a panoramic field of vision to cut or ablate tissue in otherwise inaccessible locations in the deep pelvis perpendicular to and in the middle of this field. The invisible CO_2 laser beam, composed of photons of electromagnetic radiation of 10.6 μm wavelength, is delivered to the laparoscope through mirrors fixed in an articulating arm. This beam then travels down the 5–8 mm diameter operating channel of an operating laparoscope. The focal point is approximately 2 cm from the end of the laparoscope, and the beam remains in focus for several centimeters beyond this point. This beam is adjusted into a 1-mm helium–neon (HeNe) spot with a standard coupler or one with a micromanipulator joystick; the depth of tissue affected will be slightly greater than 1 mm. A useful technique is to align the beam and its surrounding symmetrical halo emanating from the laparoscope into the center of the operating channel by using transparent tape or the cuff of the surgeon's glove over the scope tip to identify where the beam exits.

Major problems encountered when using CO_2 lasers through the operating channel of an operating laparoscope are jumping, blooming, and loss of the beam. Tension on the laser laparoscope as it traverses the trocar sleeve will modify the beam spot, as will the extent of hydration of tissue being vaporized, irrigant on the scope tip, and smoke in the peritoneal cavity. The alignment of the articulating arm mirrors may require frequent adjustment to ensure a reproducible tissue effect. An ice pack between the laserscope coupler and the surgeon's hand may be necessary to prevent skin burns when using lasers with large raw beams and beam–coupler mismatches.

Failure of the laser laparoscope coupler to connect with the laparoscope at precisely 90° causes asymmetric beam passage through the operating channel. The beam energy heats the CO_2 purge gas unevenly, causing it to act as an asymmetric lens and refracting the CO_2 laser energy to a spot other than where the HeNe aiming beam was located. Most new laser couplers correct this problem.

An effect similar to a blended current is accomplished with the CO_2 laser through the operating channel of an operating laparoscope when used at power settings > 50 W as a large spot size with diameter from 2 to 4 mm is obtained. This is extremely coagulative and provides very good hemostatic cutting[11]. A similar tissue effect is obtained with a defocusing coupler. Heraeus LaserSonics (Milpitas, CA) and Sharplan Laser (Tel Aviv, Israel) have recently introduced defocusing couplers for laparoscopy. With the Sharplan CVD (continuously variable defocus) system, spot size can be controlled to obtain a 1-mm spot size for cutting and a much larger defocused spot for coagulation (0.6–4.0 mm).

The passage of CO_2 gas through the laparoscope lumen, presently a necessity to purge this channel of debris, decreases both the power delivered to tissue and the power density at tissue because the 10.6 μm wavelength of the laser beam is absorbed and thus heats the CO_2 purge gas, which has the same wavelength. Power delivered to the tissue is reduced by 30–50% with a 7.2-mm laparoscopic operating channel (12-mm scope) and by 60% with a 5-mm operating channel (10-mm scope)[11]. While it is desirable to operate at high power density for a short time to minimize damage to surrounding tissue, heating of CO_2 gas in the laparoscope lumen increases spot size and thus reduces power density (the concentration of laser energy on the tissue) at higher power settings.

Considering these limitations, using a Sharplan 1100 laser through a 10-mm laparoscope with a 5-mm operating channel, a setting of 20–35 W in the superpulse mode is used for most procedures (<1000 W/cm^2 at the tissue). Between 80 and 100 W in the continuous mode is used to obtain a diffuse hemostatic effect for myomectomy and culdotomy.

Heraeus LaserSonics maintains a small spot size by performing rapid exchanges of gas through the operating channel of the laparoscope. The gas is exchanged faster than it can be heated up, a technique which also minimizes smoke in the peritoneal cavity during use of the laser.

Some new terms need defining. Superpulse mode implies very high power (500 W) released for brief surges (< 50 mJ), theoretically allowing tissue to cool between spikes to reduce surrounding thermal effect. Much higher energy pulses (> 200 mJ) are generated with Ultrapulse (Coherent, Palo Alto, CA) or Pulsar (Sharplan), allowing longer cooling intervals between pulses and resulting in char-free vaporization.

Coherent has recently advanced CO_2 laser technology by introducing the ^{13}C isotope of CO_2 to modify the 10.6 μm wavelength to 11.1 μm. This circumvents absorption of laser energy by the CO_2 purge gas in the operating channel of the laparoscope; the result is little interference in power transmission from the purge gas (Ultrapulse 5000L). A 6-mm raw beam enters the coupler from the end of the laser arm and emerges as a 1.5-mm spot 350–400 mm away. The 1.5-mm spot size is maintained at all settings. At high power settings the power density at impact is 10 times more than at similar settings with a 10.6-μm wavelength beam that results in a 4-mm spot from heating of the CO_2 purge gas. With the isotope laser, cutting with minimal coagulation is obtained at 200 mJ/pulse. If more coagulation with cutting is required, < 100 mJ should be used. Power settings of 10–20 W ultrapulse are used for

precise cutting and 50–80 W are used for extirpative procedures.

Using 200 mJ/pulse at 50 W with a conventional or ultrapulsed CO_2 laser, a beam spot size of 2–3 mm is obtained, resulting in excellent coagulation with cutting. With the Coherent 5000L, a 1.5-mm beam spot size is maintained at all settings, and 200 mJ at 50 W results in cutting with little coagulation.

When a laser is used in the continuous wave mode of operation (non-pulsed), the most important predictor of thermal damage is power density at the tissue. It is generally accepted that for continuous wave CO_2 lasers, the nature of the tissue interaction undergoes a gradual change as the power density crosses through a threshold at about 5000 W/cm^2. At or above this 'ablation threshold', cutting and ablation are achieved with minimal thermal damage. Below this threshold, more thermal damage is produced. With conventional CO_2 lasers and CO_2 purge gas, it is not possible to produce power densities > 1500 W/cm^2. Using isotopic $^{13}CO_2$, a power density of 3000 W/cm^2 can be reached.

For pulsed laser operation the single pulse ablation threshold that also produces minimal thermal damage is 2.8 J/cm^2. Ultrapulse lasers produce higher energy pulses than superpulse lasers. At a pulse energy > 125 mJ, an energy density above the single pulse ablation threshold is reached. At 200 mJ/pulse, very little thermal effect occurs.

The 12-mm operating laparoscope with a 7.5-mm operating channel gives a smaller spot size and higher power transmission than a 10-mm operating laparoscope with 5-mm channel. This difference is due to the diffraction limit, a result of physical optics that describes the limiting focus spot diameter that can be achieved at the end of an opaque tube of given length and diameter, and which has little dependence on the laser itself.

Fiber lasers (KTP, Argon, and YAG) are not used as they lack the versatility of electrosurgical electrodes for cutting, coagulation or fulguration. The energy from these lasers is converted in tissue to heat due to absorption by the tissue protein matrix. A much larger volume of tissue is involved in the laser thermal effect, with coagulation initially and vaporization only after protein is heated to > 100°C. In contrast, energy from the CO_2 laser is totally absorbed by water and converted rapidly to thermal energy, with a much smaller volume of tissue involved in the laser thermal effect as cutting proceeds.

INDICATIONS FOR LAPAROSCOPIC HYSTERECTOMY

Indications for laparoscopic hysterectomy presently include benign pathology such as endometriosis, fibroids, adhesions and adnexal masses, lesions which usually require an abdominal approach to hysterectomy. It is also appropriate when vaginal hysterectomy is contraindicated because of a narrow pubic arch, a narrow vagina with no prolapse, or severe arthritis that prohibits placement of the patient in a lithotomy position sufficient for vaginal exposure. Laparoscopic procedures in obese women allow the surgeon to make an incision above the panniculus and operate below it. Laparoscopic hysterectomy may also be considered for Stage I endometrial, ovarian, and cervical cancer[12–14].

The most common indication for laparoscopic hysterectomy is a symptomatic fibroid uterus. Morcellation is often necessary. Fibroids fixed in the pelvis or abdomen without descent are easier to mobilize laparoscopically. Rectocele repair may be accomplished from above, but cystocele repair usually requires a perineal approach.

Uterine size and weight are important indicators of the appropriateness of laparoscopic hysterectomies: most small uteri can be removed vaginally. The normal uterus weighs 70–125 g. At the twelfth week of pregnancy the uterus weighs 280–320 g, and at 24 weeks the weight is 580–620 g.

Hysterectomy should not be undertaken for Stage IV endometriosis with extensive cul-de-sac involvement unless the surgeon has the capability and time to resect all deep fibrotic endometriosis from the posterior vagina, uterosacral ligaments, and anterior rectum. Excision of the uterus using an intrafascial technique leaves the deep fibrotic endometriosis behind to cause future problems. It is much more difficult to remove deep fibrotic endometriosis when there is no uterus between the anterior rectum and the bladder; after hysterectomy, the endometriosis left in the anterior rectum and vaginal cuff frequently becomes densely adherent or invades the bladder and one or both ureters. In most cases, Stage IV endometriosis with extensive cul-de-sac obliteration is a reason to preserve the uterus to prevent future vaginal cuff, bladder and ureteral problems[15]. Obviously, this approach will not be effective when uterine adenomyosis is present. In these cases, after excision of cul-de-sac endometriosis, persistent pain will lead ultimately to hysterectomy. Oophorectomy is not necessary at hysterectomy; if the endometriosis is removed, it should not recur. Bilateral oophorectomy is rarely indicated in women under the age of 40 years undergoing hysterectomy for endometriosis.

Hysterectomy is performed in women of reproductive age for abnormal uterine bleeding, defined as excessive uterine bleeding or irregular uterine bleeding for > 8 days during more than a single cycle or as profuse bleeding requiring additional protection (large clots, gushes, or limitations on activity). There should be no history of a bleeding diathesis or use of medication that may cause bleeding. A negative effect on quality of life should be documented. The results of physical examination, laboratory data, ultrasound, and, if necessary, hysteroscopy and/or dilatation and curettage are frequently normal. Prior to hysterectomy, hormone treatment should be attempted and its failure, contraindication, or refusal documented. Any anemia should be corrected. If hysterectomy is chosen, a vaginal approach may be appropriate. Laparoscopic hysterectomy is performed when vaginal hysterectomy is not possible due to history of previous surgery, lack of prolapse (nulliparous or multiparous), or inexperience of the operator with the vaginal approach.

EQUIPMENT

High-flow CO_2 insufflation up to 10–15 l/min is necessary to compensate for the rapid loss of CO_2 during suctioning. The ability to maintain a relatively constant intra-abdominal pressure between 10 and 15 mmHg during laparoscopic hysterectomy is essential.

Operating-room tables capable of achieving a 30° Trendelenburg position are extremely valuable for laparoscopic hysterectomy. Unfortunately these tables are rare, and great difficulty can be encountered with the limited degree of body tilt produced by ordinary tables. The steep Trendelenburg position (20–40°), with shoulder braces and the arms at the patient's sides, has been used without adverse effects.

A Valtchev uterine mobilizer (Conkin Surgical Instruments, Toronto, Ont.) is the best available single instrument to antevert the uterus and delineate the posterior vagina. The uterus can be anteverted to about 120° and moved in an arc about 45° to the left or right by turning the mobilizer around its longitudinal axis. The 100-mm long, 10-mm thick or the 80-mm long, 8-mm thick obturator is used for uterine manipulation during hysterectomy. When this device is in the anteverted position, the cervix sits on a wide pedestal, making the cervicovaginal junction readily visible between the uterosacral ligaments when the cul-de-sac is inspected laparoscopically[16].

If a Valtchev uterine mobilizer is not available, a sponge on a ring forceps is inserted into the posterior vaginal fornix and a No.81 French rectal probe (Reznik Instruments, Skokie, IL) is placed in the rectum to define the rectum and posterior vagina for excision of endometriosis, or to open the posterior vagina (culdotomy). In addition, a No.3 or 4 Sims curette or Hulka uterine elevator is placed in the endometrial cavity to antevert the uterus markedly and stretch out the cul-de-sac. The rectal probe and intraoperative rectovaginal examinations remain important techniques even when the Valtchev mobilizer is available. Whenever rectal location is in doubt, it is identified by placing a probe.

Trocar sleeves are available in many sizes and shapes. For most cases, 5.5-mm cannulae are adequate. Newer electrosurgical electrodes which eliminate capacitance and insulation failures (Electroshield from Electroscope, Boulder, CO), require 7/8-mm sleeves. Laparoscopic stapling is performed through 12/13-mm Surgiports (US Surgical Corporation, Norwalk, CT).

A short trapless 5-mm trocar sleeve with a retention screw grid around its external surface (Richard Wolf Medical Instruments, Vernon Hills, IL; Apple Medical, Bolton, MA) is used on the left to facilitate efficient instrument exchanges and evacuation of tissue while allowing unlimited freedom during extracorporeal suture tying[17]. An experienced laparoscopic surgical team exchanges instruments so fast that little pneumo-peritoneum is lost.

Bipolar forceps use high-frequency low-voltage cutting current (20–50 W) to coagulate vessels as large as the ovarian and uterine arteries. The Kleppinger bipolar forceps (Richard Wolf) are excellent for large vessel hemostasis. Specially insulated bipolar forceps (Apple Medical) are available that allow current to pass only through their tips, so that precise hemostasis can be obtained. Microbipolar forceps contain a channel for irrigation and a fixed distance between the electrodes. They are used to irrigate bleeding sites, to identify vessels before coagulation and to prevent sticking of the electrode to the eschar. Irrigation is used during underwater examination to remove blood products and clots from the bleeding vessel, making its identification before coagulation more precise.

Disposable stapling instruments (US Surgical) are rarely used during laparoscopic hysterectomy because of their expense. A laparoscopic stapler (Multi-fire Endo GIA 30) places six rows of titanium staples, 3 cm in length, and simultaneously divides the clamped tissue. The standard staple compresses on firing to 1.5 mm, while the vascular cartridge compresses to 1 mm. The disposable handle is designed to fire up to six staple cartridges through a 12-mm cannula before being discarded.

PREOPERATIVE PREPARATION

The preoperative administration of gonadotropin releasing hormone (GnRH) analogs for at least 2 months before hysterectomy for large myomas is encouraged as it may reduce both the total uterine volume and the volume of the leiomyoma itself, making laparoscopic or vaginal hysterectomy easier[18,19]. During treatment with depot leuprolide (Lupron Depot) at a dose of 3.75 mg intramuscularly monthly for 3–6 months, anemia secondary to hypermenorrhea resolves, and autologous blood donation can be considered prior to laparoscopic hysterectomy. Packed red blood cells have a shelf life of 35 days if stored at 1–6°C. In addition, Lupron Depot is often administered after ovulation in the cycle preceding surgery to avoid operating on ovaries containing a corpus luteum.

Patients are encouraged to hydrate and eat lightly for 24 h before admission on the day of surgery. When extensive cul-de-sac involvement with endometriosis is suspected, a mechanical bowel preparation is ordered (polyethylene glycol-based isosmotic solution: Golytely or Colyte)[15]. Lower abdominal, pubic and perineal hair is not shaved. A Foley catheter is inserted during surgery and is removed the next morning. Antibiotics (usually cefoxitin) are administered in all cases.

POSITIONING OF PATIENT

All laparoscopic surgical procedures are performed under general anesthesia with endotracheal intubation. The routine use of an orogastric tube is recommended to diminish the possibility of a trocar injury to the stomach and to reduce small bowel distension. The patient is flat (0°) until after the umbilical trocar sleeve has been inserted and is then placed in steep Trendelenburg position (20–30°). Lithotomy position with the hip extended (thigh parallel to abdomen) is obtained with Allan stirrups (Edgewater Medical Systems, Mayfield Heights, OH) or knee braces, which are adjusted to each individual patient before she is anesthetized. A pelvic examination after the patient is anaesthetised is always performed prior to preparing the patient.

Laparoscopy was never thought to be a sterile procedure before the incorporation of video, as the surgeon operated with his head in the surgical field, attached to the laparoscopic optic. Since 1983, this author has maintained a policy of not sterilizing or draping the camera or laser arm. Infection has been rare: less than 1/200 cases. The umbilical incision is closed with a single 4-0 Vicryl suture opposing deep fascia and skin dermis, the knot being buried beneath the fascia to prevent the suture from acting as a wick and transmitting bacteria into the soft tissue or peritoneal cavity.

HYSTERECTOMY TECHNIQUE (Figures 1–17)

The technique described is for total laparoscopic hysterectomy.

Incisions

Three laparoscopic puncture sites including the umbilicus are used: 10- or 12-mm umbilical, 5-mm right, and 5-mm left lower quadrant. The left lower quadrant puncture is the major portal for operative manipulation. The right trocar sleeve is used for retraction with atraumatic grasping forceps. When a clip is applied or a stapler is used, it is inserted through the umbilical incision and the procedure is viewed through a 5-mm laparoscope in one of the 5-mm lower quadrant sites.

Placement of the lower quadrant trocar sleeves just above the pubic hairline and lateral to the deep epigastric vessels (and thus the rectus abdominis muscle) is preferred. These vessels, an artery flanked by two veins (venae comitantes), are located lateral to the umbilical ligaments (obliterated umbilical artery) by direct laparoscopic inspection of the anterior abdominal wall. The deep epigastric vessels arise near the junction of the external iliac vessels with the femoral vessels and make up the medial border of the internal inguinal ring. The round ligament curls around these vessels to enter the inguinal canal. When the anterior abdominal wall parietal peritoneum is thickened from previous surgery or obesity, the position of these vessels is judged by palpating and depressing the anterior abdominal wall with the back of the scalpel; the wall will appear thicker where rectus muscle is enclosed, and the incision site should be chosen lateral to this area near the anterior superior iliac spine.

Vaginal preparation

Hysteroscopy with CO_2 is performed during insufflation of pneumoperitoneum. This is especially useful for myoma hysterectomies to identify the location of the fibroids (Figure 1). Following hysteroscopy the endocervical canal is dilated to Pratt number 25, and the Valtchev uterine mobilizer is inserted into the uterus.

Exploration

The upper abdomen is inspected, and the appendix is identified. If appendiceal pathology such as dilatation, adhesions or endometriosis is present appendectomy is performed after ureteral isolation by mobilizing the appendix, desiccating its blood supply, and placing three Endo-loops at the appendiceal–cecal junction after desiccating the appendix just above this juncture. The appendix is left attached to the cecum and its stump is divided later in the procedure, after opening the cul-de-sac, so that removal from the peritoneal cavity is accomplished immediately after separation.

Ureteral dissection

Immediately after exploration of the upper abdomen and pelvis, each ureter is isolated deep in the pelvis, if possible. This is undertaken early in the operation before the pelvic sidewall peritoneum becomes edematous and/or opaque due to irritation by the CO_2 pneumoperitoneum or aquadissection and before ureteral peristalsis is inhibited by surgical stress, pressure, or the Trendelenburg position. The ureter and its overlying peritoneum are grasped deep in the pelvis on the left to avoid division of the lateral rectosigmoid attachments required for high identification (Figure 2). An atraumatic

grasping forceps is used from a right-sided cannula to grab the ureter (Figure 3) and its overlying peritoneum on the left pelvic sidewall below and caudad to the left ovary, lateral to the left uterosacral ligament. Scissors or a CO_2 laser at 10–30 W superpulse or ultrapulse are used to divide the peritoneum overlying the ureter and are then inserted into the defect created and spread (Figure 4). Thereafter one blade of the scissors is placed on top of the ureter, the buried scissors blade is visualized through the peritoneum, and the peritoneum is divided. This is continued into the deep pelvis where the uterine vessels cross the ureter, lateral to the cardinal ligament insertion into the cervix (Figure 5). Connective tissue between the ureter and the vessels is separated with scissors (Figure 6). Bleeding is controlled with microbipolar forceps.

Bladder mobilization

The left round ligament is divided at its mid-portion with minimal bleeding using a spoon electrode (Electroscope) at 150-W cutting current (Figure 7). Persistent bleeding is controlled with monopolar fulguration at 80-W coagulation current or bipolar desiccation at 30-W cutting current. Thereafter scissors or a CO_2 laser are used to divide the vesicouterine peritoneal fold starting at the left side, continuing across the midline to the right round ligament. The right round ligament is divided, as was the left; with unipolar electrosurgery. The bladder is mobilized from the uterus and upper vagina using scissors.

Upper uterine blood supply

When ovarian preservation is desired, the utero-ovarian ligament and Fallopian tube pedicle are suture-ligated adjacent to the uterus with 0-Vicryl (Figure 8). When ovarian preservation is not desired, the infundibulopelvic ligaments and broad ligaments are coagulated until desiccated with bipolar forceps at 25–35-W cutting current and then divided.

Uterine vessel ligation

The broad ligament on each side is skeletonized down to the uterine vessels. Each uterine vessel pedicle is suture-ligated, with 0-Vicryl on a CT-1 needle (70 cm). The needles are introduced into the peritoneal cavity by pulling them through a 5-mm incision. The curved needle is inserted on top of the unroofed ureter where it turns medially towards the previously mobilized bladder. A short rotary movement of the Cook oblique curved needle holder brings the needle around the uterine vessel pedicle. Sutures are tied extracorporeally using a Clarke

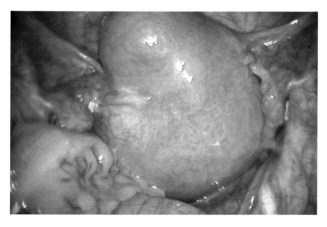

Figure 1 Large fibroid uterus fills the pelvis

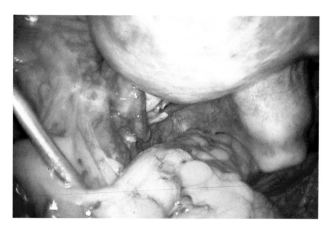

Figure 2 Left ureter is grasped from the right side. Valtchev retractor delineates junction of cervix with vagina

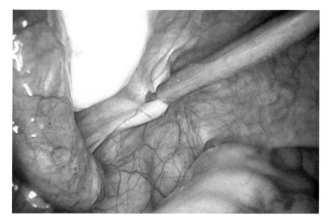

Figure 3 Close-up of grasper on left ureter

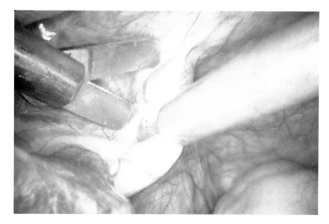

Figure 4 Scissors or CO_2 laser are used to divide peritoneum just above and lateral to ureter which has been placed on tension

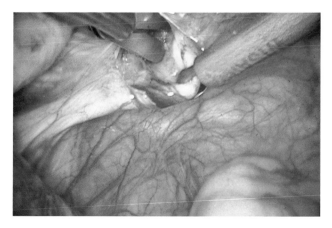

Figure 5 Dissection of left ureter continues to left uterine artery pedicle

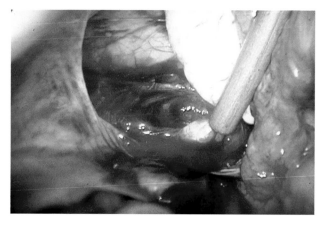

Figure 6 Uterine artery is isolated above the ureter

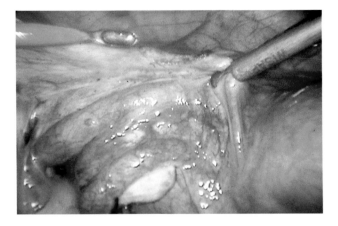

Figure 7 Round ligaments are divided with a spoon electrode at 150 W cutting current

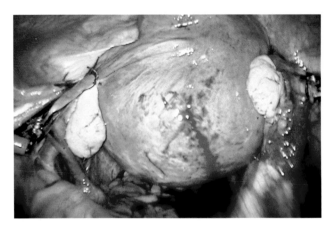

Figure 8 Utero-ovarian ligaments are suture ligated with 0-Vicryl

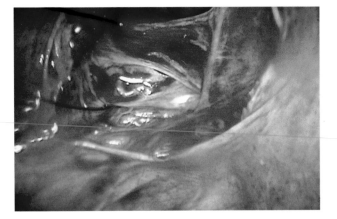

Figure 9 Suture ligature is placed around left uterine vessels with left ureter beneath

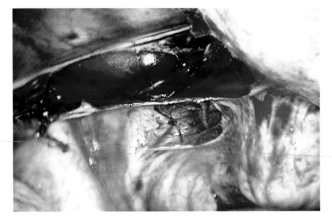

Figure 10 Left broad ligament is open to the bladder. Ligature is around left uterine artery

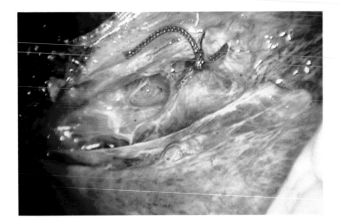

Figure 11 Close-up of ligature around left uterine artery with ureter beneath

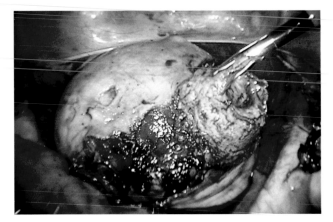

Figure 12 The uterus is free in the peritoneal cavity

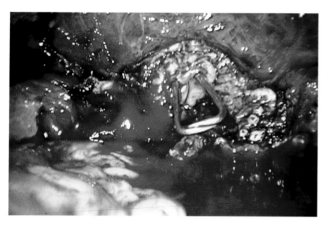

Figure 13 A single toothed tenaculum is used to pull the cervix into the vagina

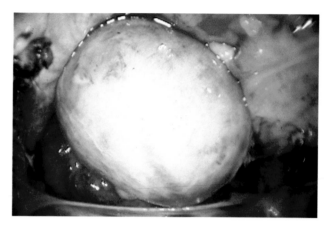

Figure 14 As the uterus is large, vaginal morcellation is required for removal

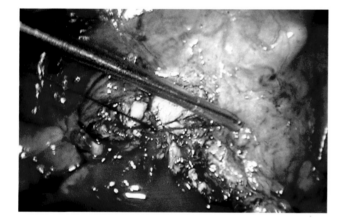

Figure 15 The uterosacral ligaments and posterior vagina are sutured together for vaginal apical support

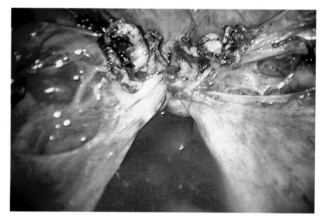

Figure 16 In the deep cul-de-sac the uterosacral ligaments are together with the ureters lateral

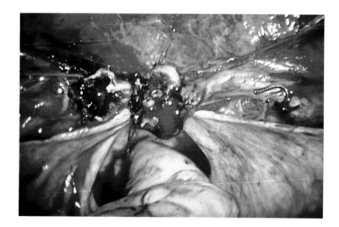

Figure 17 Excellent support of the vaginal cuff is noted with all anatomy visible

knot pusher[20]. A single suture placed in this manner on each side serves as a 'sentinel stitch', identifying the ureter for the rest of the operation (Figures 9–11).

Circumferential culdotomy (division of cervicovaginal attachments)

The cardinal ligaments on each side are divided with the CO_2 laser at high power. Control of bleeding is often necessary, using bipolar forceps. The vagina is entered posteriorly over the Valtchev retractor, which identifies the junction of cervix with vagina. A ring forceps inserted into the anterior vagina above the tenaculum on the anterior cervical lip identifies the anterior cervico-vaginal junction, which is entered using the laser. Following the ring forceps or the aquapurator tip, and using them as backstops, the operator divides the lateral vaginal fornices. The uterus is morcellated if necessary and pulled out of the vagina (Figures 12–14). Alternatively, a 4-cm diameter operative colonoscope (Richard Wolf) is used to outline circumferentially the cervicovaginal junction; it also serves as a backstop for laser work.

Laparoscopic vaginal vault closure and suspension with McCall culdoplasty

Vaginal repair is accomplished after packing the vagina. The left uterosacral ligament and posterolateral vagina are first elevated. A suture is placed through this uterosacral ligament into the vagina, exits the vagina including posterior vaginal tissue near the midline on the left, and re-enters just adjacent to this spot on the right. Finally, an opposite-sided oblique Cook needle holder is used to fixate the right posterolateral vagina to the right uterosacral ligament. This suture is tied extracorporeally and gives excellent support to the vaginal cuff apex, elevating it superiorly and posteriorly toward the hollow of the sacrum (Figures 15–17). The rest of the vagina and overlying pubocervical fascia is closed vertically with a figure-of-eight suture.

Underwater examination

At the close of each operation, an underwater examination is used to detect bleeding from vessels and viscera tamponaded during the procedure by the increased intraperitoneal pressure of the CO_2 pneumoperitoneum. The CO_2 pneumoperitoneum is displaced with 2–5 l of Ringer's lactate solution, and the peritoneal cavity is vigorously irrigated and suctioned until the effluent is clear of blood products. Any further bleeding is controlled underwater using microbipolar forceps to coagulate through the electrolyte solution, and at least 2 l of lactated Ringer's solution are left in the peritoneal cavity.

COMPLICATIONS

Complications of laparoscopic hysterectomy are the same as for hysterectomy in general: anesthetic accidents, postoperative pulmonary emboli, hemorrhage, injury to ureters, bladder and rectum, and infections, especially of the vaginal cuff[21]. Since the introduction of prophylactic antibiotics, vaginal cuff abscess, pelvic thrombophlebitis, septicemia, pelvic cellulitis, and adnexal abscesses have become rare. Abdominal wound infection is rare, but the incidence of incisional hernias after operative laparoscopy is greatly increased if trocars of > 10 mm are placed at extra-umbilical sites.

Febrile morbidity following a vaginal hysterectomy is about half as common as after abdominal hysterectomy. Laparoscopic treatment with evacuation of all blood clots and the sealing of all blood vessels after removal of the uterus should reduce the infection rate further. Morcellation during laparoscopic or vaginal hysterectomy carries a slightly increased risk of fever, especially if prophylactic antibiotics are not used.

REFERENCES

1. Bachmann, G.A. (1990). Hysterectomy: a critical review. *J. Reprod. Med.*, **35**, 839–62
2. Reich, H. (1992). Laparoscopic hysterectomy. *Surg. Laparosc. Endosc.*, **2**, 85–8
3. Liu, C.Y. (1992). Laparoscopic hysterectomy: a review of 72 cases. *J. Reprod. Med.*, **37**, 351–4
4. Liu, C.Y. (1992). Laparoscopic hysterectomy. Report of 215 cases. *Gynaecol. Endosc.*, **1**, 73–7
5. Reich, H., DeCaprio, J. and McGlynn, F. (1989). Laparoscopic hysterectomy. *J. Gynecol. Surg.*, **5**, 213–6
6. Kovac, S.R., Cruikshank, S.H. and Retto, H.F. (1990). Laparoscopy-assisted vaginal hysterectomy. *J. Gynecol. Surg.*, **6**, 185–9
7. Summit, R.L., Stovall, T.G., Lipscomb, G.H. and Ling, F.W. (1992). Randomized comparison of laparoscopy-assisted vaginal hysterectomy with standard vaginal hysterectomy in an outpatient setting. *Obstet. Gynecol.*, **80**, 895–901
8. Minelli, L., Angiolillo, M., Caione, C. and Palmara, V. (1991). Laparoscopically-assisted vaginal hysterectomy. *Endoscopy*, **23**, 64–6
9. Maher, P.J., Wood, E.C., Hill, D.J. and Lolatgis, N.A. (1992). Laparoscopically assisted hysterectomy. *Med. J. Aust.*, **156**, 316–8
10. Lyons, T.L. (1993). Laparoscopic supracervical hysterectomy. In Hunt, R.B. and Martin, D.C. (eds.) *Endoscopy in Gynecology*, Proceedings of the World Congress of Gynecologic Endoscopy, AAGL 20th Annual Meeting, Las Vegas Nevada, pp.129–31. (Baltimore: Port City Press)
11. Reich, H., MacGregor, T.S. and Vancaillie, T.G.

(1991). CO_2 laser used through the operating channel of laser laparoscopes: *in vitro* study of power and power density losses. *Obstet. Gynecol.*, **77**, 40–7

12. Reich, H. (1990). Laparoscopic extrafascial hysterectomy with bilateral salpingo-oophorectomy using stapling techniques for endometrial adenocarcinoma. Presented at the *AAGL 19th Annual Meeting*, Orlando, Florida, November 14–18

13. Reich, H., McGlynn, F. and Wilkie, W. (1990). Laparoscopic management of Stage I ovarian cancer. *J. Reprod. Med.*, **35**, 601–5

14. Canis, M., Mage, G., Wattiez, A., Pouly, J.L., Manhes, H. and Bruhat, M.A. (1990). Does endoscopic surgery have a role in radical surgery of cancer of the cervix uteri? *J. Gynecol. Obstet. Biol. Reprod.*, **19**, 921

15. Reich, H., McGlynn, F. and Salvat, J. (1991). Laparoscopic treatment of cul-de-sac obliteration secondary to retrocervical deep fibrotic endometriosis. *J. Reprod. Med.*, **36**, 516–22

16. Valtchev, K.L. and Papsin, F.R. (1977). A new uterine mobilizer for laparoscopy: Its use in 518 patients. *Am. J. Obstet. Gynecol.*, **127**, 738–40

17. Reich, H. and McGlynn, F. (1990). Short self-retaining trocar sleeves. *Am. J. Obstet. Gynecol.*, **162**, 453–4

18. Schlaff, W.D., Zerhouni, E.A., Huth, J.A., Chen, J., Damewood, M.D. and Rock, J.A. (1989). A placebo-controlled trial of a depot gonadotropin-releasing hormone analogue (leuprolide) in the treatment of uterine leiomyomata. *Obstet. Gynecol.*, **74**, 856–62

19. Freidman, A.J., Hoffman, D.I., Comite, F., Browneller, R.W. and Miller, J.D. (Leuprolide Study Group). (1991). Treatment of leiomyomata uteri with leuprolide acetate depot: a double-blind, placebo-controlled, multicenter study. *Obstet. Gynecol.*, **77**, 720–5

20. Reich, H., Clarke, H.C. and Sekel, L. (1992). A simple method for ligating in operative laparoscopy with straight and curved needles. *Obstet. Gynecol.*, **79**, 143–7

21. Woodland, M.B. (1992). Ureter injury during laparoscopy-assisted vaginal hysterectomy with the endoscopic linear stapler. *Am J. Obstet. Gynecol.*, **167**, 756–7

The place of endoscopy in malignancy: laparoscopic hysterectomy and lymphadenectomy

J. Donnez, V. Anaf, M. Berlière, S. Bassil and M. Nisolle

THE PLACE OF ENDOSCOPY IN MALIGNANCY

The indications for gynecologic endoscopic surgery have, in recent years, increased. In the case of neoplastic pathology, however, the situation remains unclear.

INDICATIONS FOR LAPAROSCOPIC PROCEDURES IN ENDOMETRIAL CANCER

The evaluation of the anatomosurgical stage is crucial in the therapeutic strategy of endometrial cancer. Lymph node involvement plays a major role in this evaluation, as an indicator of both prognosis and the need for adjuvant therapy. Lymph node metastasis is related to tumor size and grade, tumor stage and invasion of the myometrium (Table 1). In our department, bilateral laparoscopic adnexectomy followed by vaginal hysterectomy is performed in atypical hyperplasia and in cases of stage 0-1, grade I endometrial cancer. Stage 1, grade 2–3 endometrial cancer requires an additional lymphadenectomy (Table 2). Laparoscopic lymphadenectomy is also performed 2 weeks after laparoscopically assisted vaginal hysterectomy when histology reveals either a myometrial invasion of more than 2/3 the depth of the myometrium, a histological invasion of the cervix or a histological grade more severe than that suspected from the preoperative biopsy.

Stage II endometrial cancer requires laparoscopic lymphadenectomy followed by vaginal hysterectomy, as described by Schauta[1]. This technique should only be attempted by experienced surgeons who are experts in the vaginal approach. In many departments, stage II endometrial cancer is treated by a Wertheim–Meigs surgical procedure with lymphadenectomy.

In stage III and IV endometrial cancer, the role of laparoscopy is not yet clearly defined. It could be an indication for performing multiple biopsies in different sites of the peritoneal cavity.

In patients with endometrial cancer, initial laparoscopic lymphadenectomy together with a bilateral adnexectomy allows the subsequent hysterectomy to be performed either vaginally or laparoscopically[3,4]. The few studies which have been reported[3–5] suggest that more extensive studies are needed to determine the possible future role of laparoscopic surgery in the treatment of endometrial cancer.

In our department, laparoscopic bilateral adnexectomy followed by vaginal hysterectomy is the procedure of choice in the treatment of stage I endometrial cancer. Laparoscopic lymphadenectomy is also performed in cases of non-differentiated endometrial cancer.

INDICATIONS FOR LYMPHADENECTOMY IN VAGINAL CANCER

Primary carcinoma of the vagina is a malignant lesion that appears in the vagina and does not involve the cervix or vulva. It is rare, representing 1–2% of all gynecological malignancies. In an extensive review of the literature, Plentl and Friedman[6] found that 51.7% of primary vaginal cancers occurred in the upper third of the vagina and 57.6% were on the posterior wall. Tumors originating in the vagina may spread along the vaginal wall to involve the cervix or the vulva. However, if biopsies of the cervix or the vulva are positive at diagnosis, the tumor cannot be considered a primary vaginal lesion.

The lymphatic drainage of the vagina consists of an extensive intercommunicating network. The lymphatics in the upper portion of the vagina drain primarily via the lymphatics of the cervix, whereas those in the lowest portion of the vagina drain either to cervical lymphatics or follow drainage patterns of the vulva into femoral and inguinal nodes. The anterior vaginal wall usually drains into the deep pelvic nodes, including the interiliac and parametrial nodes.

The incidence of positive pelvic nodes at diagnosis varies with the stage and location of the primary tumor. Because the lymphatic system of the vagina is so complex, any of the nodal groups may be involved

Table 1 Prevalence of lymph node metastasis for tumor size and tumor grade in endometrial cancer

Tumor grade	Tumor size		
	≤ 2 cm diameter	> 2 cm diameter	Entire surface
I	0/15 (0%)	0/14 (0%)	0/3 (0%)
II	0/10 (0%)	4/12 (33%)	1/3 (33%)
III	2/10 (20%)	6/20 (30%)	3/4 (75%)

Table 2 Indications for laparoscopic procedures in endometrial cancer

Diagnosis	Proposed therapy
Atypical hyperplasia Adenocarcinoma stage 0–1; grade 1	laparoscopic adnexectomy followed by hysterectomy
Adenocarcinoma stage I; grade 2–3	laparoscopic adnexectomy followed by hysterectomy + laparoscopic lymphadenectomy
Adenocarcinoma stage II	laparoscopic lymphadenectomy followed by radical vaginal hysterectomy (Schauta)
Adenocarcinoma stage III–IV	+ multiple biopsies?

regardless of the location of the lesion. Involvement of inguinal nodes is most common, however, when the lesion is located in the lower third of the vagina. The reported incidence of clinically positive nodes at diagnosis varies from 5.1%[7] to 20.8%[6]. Radiation therapy is the preferred treatment for most carcinomas of the vagina. Surgical procedures may be reserved for the treatment of irradiation failures and for nonepithelial tumors. For tumors of the upper third of the vagina (Figures 1 and 2), surgery can be an excellent alternative, specially if the tumor is near the cervix. Here, laparoscopic lymphadenectomy (Figure 3) can be performed before radical hysterectomy and colpectomy (Figure 4).

CERVICAL CANCER

Laparoscopic surgery offers two possible options in order to avoid laparotomy in cervical cancer:

(1) A laparoscopic lymphadenectomy followed by the vaginal operative approach according to the Schauta technique[8,9].

(2) Lymphadenectomy followed by an enlarged laparoscopic hysterectomy[10,15].

The presence of lymph node metastasis is the most significant prognostic factor in cervical cancer. Squamous carcinoma of the cervix spreads principally by direct local invasion to adjacent tissue and by lymphatics, and less commonly through blood vessels. Initially, the tumor grows by direct continuity along tissue spaces of least resistance, the perineural and perivascular tissues, into the paracervical and parametrial areas and into the cardinal and uterosacral ligaments. Ultimately, lateral spread may reach the bony pelvis and obstruct one or both ureters. Direct extension may also involve the uterine cavity and vagina, with

extension into the urinary bladder and rectum, resulting in vesicovaginal and rectovaginal fistulas.

The spread of cervical cancer via lymphatics occurs relatively early in the course of the disease and is found in 25–50% of patients with stage Ib and II carcinomas. The preferential course of dissemination is via the paracervical hypogastric, and external iliac lymph nodes followed by extension to lateral sacral, common iliac, para-aortic and inguinal nodes. Isolated invasion of the sacral, external iliac, and hypogastric nodes is occasionally observed. Metastases to distant lymph nodes above the diaphragm, including the supraclavicular lymph nodes, are uncommon and are a feature of widespread disease. In these cases, cancer cells are transported from the para-aortic nodes into the mediastinum and then into the thoracic duct. Diagnosis of lymph node metastasis can be made by lymphography, computerized tomography and/or nuclear magnetic resonance (Figure 5). The low sensitivity of lymphography (< 30%)[12], computerized tomography (between 30 and 70%)[12–14], nuclear magnetic resonance and lymphoscintigraphy[8] in the detection of potentially malignant adenopathies has prompted some authors to perform retroperitoneal lymph node sampling[15,16].

The first laparoscopic lymphadenectomies were performed by Dargent[17], Reich[18], Querleu and colleagues[2,8], Canis and colleagues[10] and Nezhat and co-workers[11]. Results are very encouraging, with a 100% sensitivity rate in a series of 75 patients and a very low postoperative complication rate[2,8]. The first indication for laparoscopic lymphadenectomy in gynecological oncology is the staging of early, operable, carcinoma of the cervix[2]. The risk of 'skip' metastases to the para-aortic nodes without pelvic node involvement is very low (< 1%); this occurs almost exclusively in patients with large tumors (> 4 cm). Patients with stage IB, IIA or IIB disease and negative pathological staging may be cured by radical or abdominal surgery. However, radical hysterectomy does not seem justified when nodes are involved by metastatic disease[15–19] (Figure 6).

In stage IV carcinoma (extension into the urinary bladder) (Figure 7), laparoscopic lymphadenectomy must be carried out before performing an anterior pelvectomy.

TECHNIQUE

Laparoscopic hysterectomy

Endometrial cancer typically occurs in obese, high-risk women. The use of the laparoscope precludes an abdominal incision wound infection in these patients. Atypical hyperplasia and stage 0–I, grade I endometrial cancer do not require lymphadenectomy. Treatment may be by laparoscopically assisted vaginal hysterectomy (LAVH) or a laparoscopic hysterectomy (LH) (see Chapter 22): all maneuvers following internal vessel

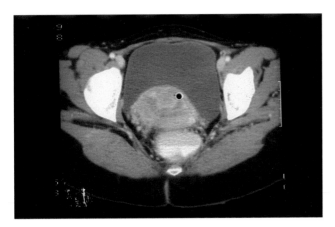

Figure 1 CT scan: cancer of the vagina located in the upper third on the posterior wall

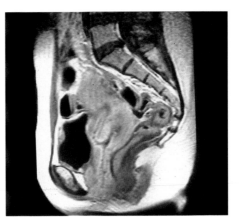

Figure 2 Magnetic resonance imaging (same patient as in Figure 1) provides an excellent view of vaginal involvement

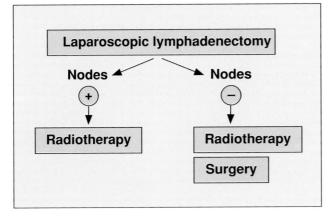

Figure 3 Proposed therapy for carcinoma of the upper third of the vagina

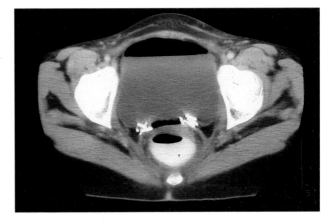

Figure 4 CT scan (a) and radiography (b) after hysterectomy and colpectomy in cases of primary carcinoma (same patient as in Figure 1)

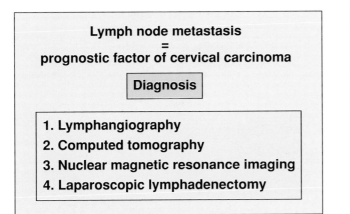

Figure 5 Diagnosis of lymph node metastasis

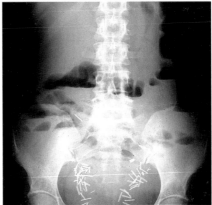

Figure 4(b) *See legend above*

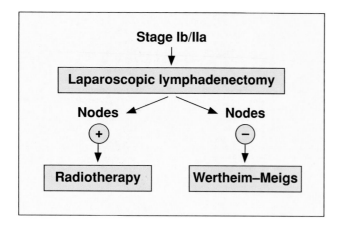

Figure 6 Proposed therapy for cervical carcinoma stage IB, IIA and IIB

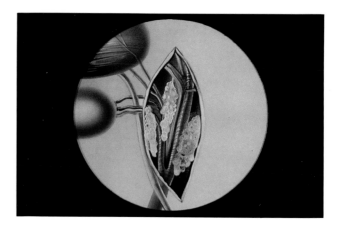

Figure 8(a)–(c) Incision of the peritoneum between the round ligament and the lomboovarian ligament. The iliac vessels are identified behind the lymph nodes and the retroperitoneal fatty tissue

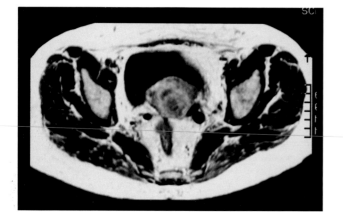

Figure 7(a) and (b) Magnetic resonance imaging of stage IV cervical carcinoma. The involvement of the urinary bladder wall is clearly seen

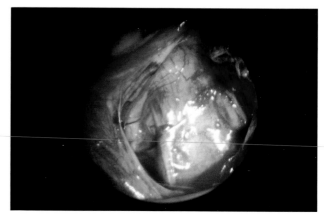

Figure 8(b) *See legend above*

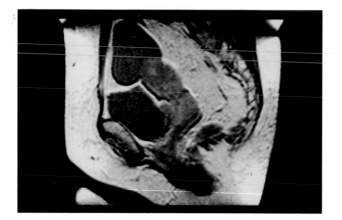

Figure 7(b) *See legend above*

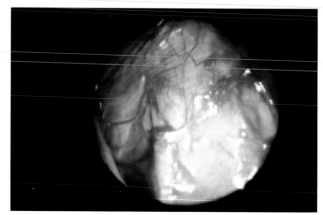

Figure 8(c) *See legend above*

ligation can be done vaginally or laparoscopically, including anterior and posterior vaginal entry, cardinal and intersacral ligament division, intact uterine removal and vaginal closure.

The adnexa are removed first. The infundibulopelvic ligament is identified and exposed by applying traction to the adnexa with an opposite forceps. The bipolar forceps is used to compress and desiccate the vessels which are then cut with scissors. Alternatively, staples or sutures may be applied. The other steps are described in Chapter 21. Ligation of the uterine vessels can also be performed by the vaginal approach. Some authors prefer suture ligation of the vascular bundle. If LAVH is being performed, the rest of the operation is done vaginally, as is suturing of the vaginal vault.

Laparoscopic lymphadenectomy

The preparation of the patient for surgery follows standard procedures. In order to avoid any possible disturbance due to an overdistended large bowel, cleansing of the digestive system must be undertaken. A pneumoperitoneum is achieved through the sub-umbilical incision. Three suprapubic incisions are made. The operation begins with a peritoneal cytology and abdominopelvic exploration. The ureters are visualized. The peritoneum is incised between the round and the lumbo-ovarian ligament. The subperitoneal space is opened using scissors and the iliac vessels are identified (Figure 8).

During the whole operation, the round ligament is grasped and kept in an elevated and medial position. This allows identification of the umbilical artery, the internal limit of node sampling. The obturator nerve is then identified, located against the pelvic wall under the iliac vessels. Node sampling can begin with the subvenous group, which is the lowest one; this ensures that any bleeding does not make further dissection more difficult.

The operation can also begin by the sampling of the supra-arterial nodes. Dissection is performed towards the origin of the external iliac vein (Figure 9) with gentle traction on the nodes. Careful lymphostasis with clips is performed throughout the dissection when a large lymphatic canal is encountered.

Once the space between the pelvic wall and the inferior side of the internal iliac vein has been treated, dissection of the internal retrocrural nodal group is begun (Figure 10). The obturator nerve is clearly seen (Figure 11). During this procedure an anastomosis between the external iliac vein and the obturator vein may be encountered: careful dissection is required to avoid venous injury.

A forceps (celioextractor)[9-17] can be used to remove nodes from the abdominal cavity without any risk of abdominal wall contamination. They can also be removed through the laparoscope trocar or through a 25 mm trocar (Figure 12) with a forceps. Analysis of suspect nodes may be indicated in order to avoid further dissection in cases of node positivity. Querleu et al.[2] reported false-negative analyses in 14 cases of cervical cancer. The duration of lymphadenectomy varies from 75 to 150 min, depending largely on the associated surgical procedures, such as hysterectomy. The number of nodes removed varies: the average number of lymph nodes has been reported as 13–22, 10, 19–34, while in our series of lymphadenectomies, the number of nodes ranged from 20 to 37.

COMPLICATIONS

Vascular injury is the major potential risk of laparoscopic pelvic lymphadenectomy, but is much less frequent than expected. Significant bleeding may occur due to injury to pelvic arteries or veins. Injury to the branches of the hypogastric artery (uterine artery, superior vesical artery or umbilical artery) is managed by direct application of vascular clips or bipolar hemostasis to the vessel. Injury to the external iliac vein or a main branch of the internal iliac veins is the most serious potential complication of pelvic lymphadenectomy because its management is more difficult than for arterial injury.

When fixed lymph nodes are encountered, any attempt at their dissection is hazardous and cytological examination (needle aspiration) must be carried out in order to prevent a vein injury[18]. If bleeding of the external iliac vein occurs, compression may be successful: a closed forceps may be firmly applied in order to compress the vessel against the pelvic sidewall. If hemorrhage persists, the use of clips or coagulation may worsen the laceration; laparotomy must be performed in order to manage an external iliac vein laceration.

The risk of accidental section of the obturator nerve is very low.

Ureteral injury during lymphadenectomy is extremely infrequent; indeed, the ureter is not in the operative field. The ureter may, however, be identified under the peritoneum and dissected free.

Lymphocyst formation is a complication of lymph node sampling. This may be prevented by using surgical clips during lymph node dissection and by drainage of the retroperitoneum. Querleu and Leblanc[18] do not, however, place preventive clips for lymphastasis nor any drain in the dissection area, and report no case of significant lymphocyst formation.

Scarring may follow peritoneal or retroperitoneal repair. The peritoneum usually heals with minimal scarring and no or minimal adhesions (Figure 13). The tissue in the retroperitoneal space heals with a dense fibrosis, making subsequent dissections difficult. If indicated, radical hysterectomy must be performed no more than 7 days after laparoscopic lymphadenectomy[9,18].

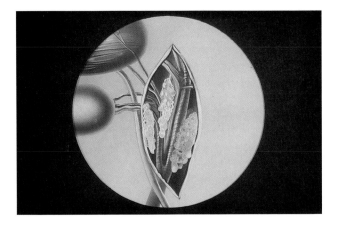

Figure 9(a)–(c) Dissection of the external and subvenous groups. Using gentle traction on the nodes, the dissection is performed. The external iliac vein is then visible

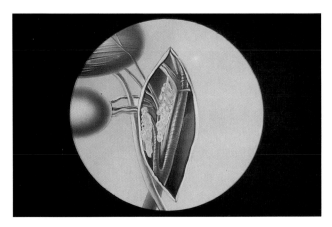

Figure 10(a)–(c) Dissection of the internal retrocrural and obturator group

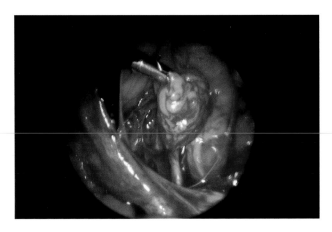

Figure 9(b) *See legend above*

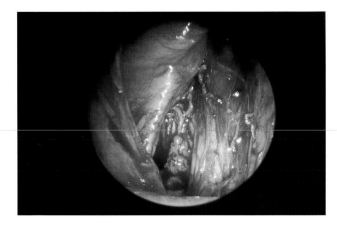

Figure 10(b) *See legend above*

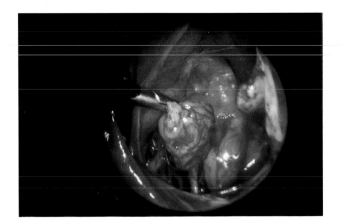

Figure 9(c) *See legend above*

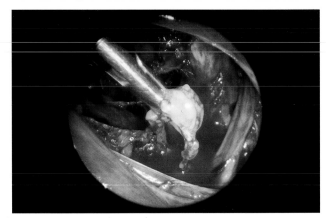

Figure 10(c) *See legend above*

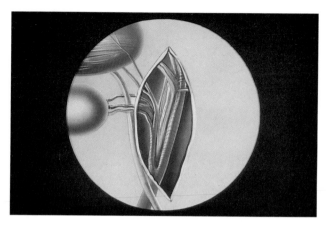

Figure 11(a)–(c) The obturator nerve is clearly identified

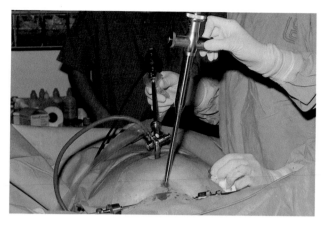

Figure 12(a) A 25-mm trocar is inserted suprapubically

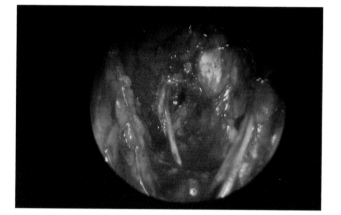

Figure 11(b) *See legend above*

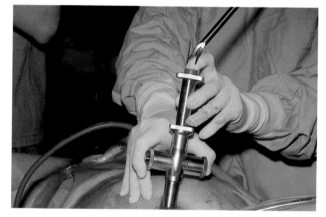

Figure 12(b) A forceps is introduced via a trocar reducer

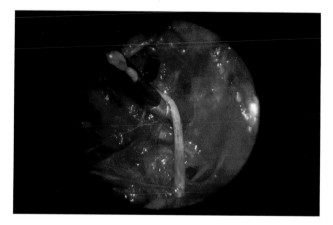

Figure 11(c) *See legend above*

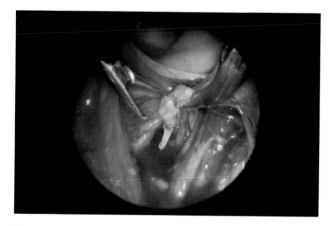

Figure 12(c)–(e) The lymph nodes are systematically removed after their dissection in order to avoid their loss in the peritoneal cavity and to determine their exact location (in cases of metastasis)

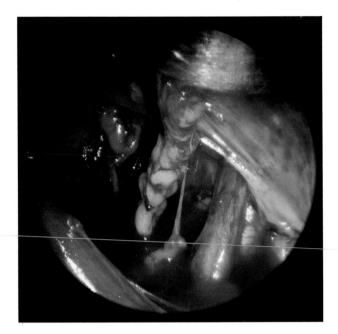

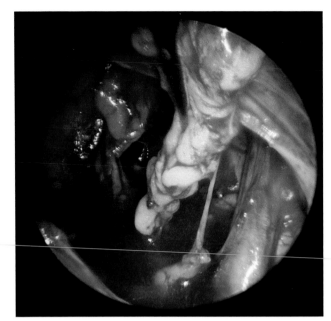

Figure 12(d)   *See legend on previous page*

Figure 12(e)   *See legend on previous page*

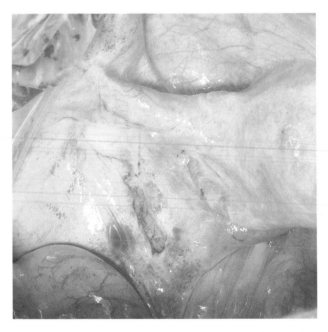

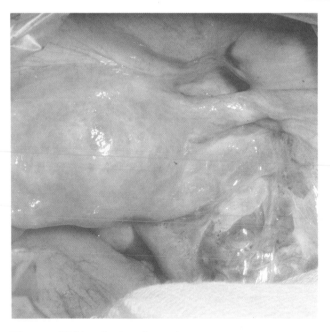

Figure 13(a) and (b) Peritoneal healing after laparoscopic lymphadenectomy

Figure 13(b)   *See legend opposite*

CONCLUSION AND DISCUSSION

The main advantage of the laparoscopic approach is that bilateral adnexectomy can be carried out laparoscopically, making a laparotomy unnecessary. Hysterectomy can then be performed either by the vaginal approach or by laparoscopy. The intraoperative advantages of this laparoscopic approach are numerous. It allows ureteral identification, complete hemostasis and evacuation of all the blood clots at the end of the procedure. Removal of blood clots and the instillation of intra-abdominal antiseptics or antibiotics may reduce the incidence of postoperative infection associated with vaginal hysterectomy, thus decreasing the postoperative hospitalization and recovery time.

The results of radical laparoscopic hysterectomy ('Wertheim' procedure) performed with lymphadenectomy are clearly less optimistic. In spite of the less painful postoperative convalescence, a significantly faster recovery of bowel movement, a less pronounced drop in the hemoglobin rate and reduced hospitalization costs[19], the procedure has several disadvantages. The relatively long operating time (6–8 h) and the rather difficult technical approach of this procedure[10,19] lead us to conclude that this technique (of which only a few cases have been published) still requires further research and evaluation, especially in oncological surgery. Continued studies involving greater numbers of women should thus demonstrate the potential advantages of laparoscopic surgery compared to laparotomy, but also its harmful effects, such as tumor dissemination due to internal trauma during uterine mobilization or lymph node removal.

All surgical maneuvers are more or less feasible by laparoscopy: the important thing to consider with regard to this new approach to radical uterine surgery is not its feasibility, but rather whether it is justifiable and safe[19].

As already stated in this chapter, lymphangiography is unable to visualize internal iliac and other medial node groups. CT scanning and magnetic resonance imaging are not sensitive if the nodes are not macroscopically enlarged. As a consequence, lymph node biopsy remains the only reliable method for appraising the status of pelvic lymph nodes.

Pelvic lymph node sampling by a retroperitoneal endoscopic approach has been described[16]. Progress in laparoscopic surgery allows a surgically satisfactory pelvic lymphadenectomy to be performed, removing the obturator, external iliac and hypogastric lymph nodes. Dargent and Salvat[16] have described a panoramic retroperitoneal approach. Querleu and Leblanc have described the technique of pelvic lymphadenectomy[2,18] and para-aortic lymphadenectomy by laparoscopy[18].

The indication for laparoscopic lymphadenectomy in gynecological oncology is the staging of carcinoma of the cervix[2]. The risk of involvement of para-aortic nodes is very low (< 1%) if the pelvic nodes are negative histologically. Stage IB-IIA-IIB cancer with negative pathological staging may be cured by radical vaginal or abdominal surgery. However, radical hysterectomy does not seem justified when metastatic nodes are present.

Pre-treatment laparoscopic staging of stage I endometrial carcinomas is not very useful since the prevalence of lymph node metastasis is low in this condition. Laparoscopic lymphadenectomy may be included in the surgical step of treatment, in association with vaginal surgery[4]. Ovarian carcinomas are best treated by laparotomy. Adequate infrarenal para-aortic node sampling can be completed by laparoscopy only in very experienced hands[20].

REFERENCES

1. Schauta, R. (1961). Techniques chirurgicales. In *Encyclopedie Medico Chirurgicale*, pp. 41–735. (Paris)
2. Querleu, D., Leblanc, E. and Castelain, G. (1991). Laparoscopic pelvic lymphadenectomy in the staging of early carcinoma of the cervix. *Am. J. Obstet. Gynecol.*, **164**, 579–81
3. Mage, G., Wattiez, A., Chapron, C., Canis, M., Pouly, J.L., Pingeon, J.M. and Bruhat, M.A. (1992). Hystérectomie per-coelioscopique: résultats d'une série de 44 cas. *J. Gynecol. Obstet. Biol. Reprod.*, **21**, 436–44
4. Donnez, J., Nisolle, M. and Anaf, V. (1993). Place de l'endoscopie dans le cancer de l'endomètre. In Dubuisson, J.B., Chapron, C. and Bouquet de Jolinière, J. (eds.) *Coelioscopie et Cancerologie en Gynecologie*, pp. 77–82. (Paris: Arnette)
5. Photopulos, G.J., Stovall, T.G. and Summitt, R.L., Jr. (1992). LAVH, bilateral salpingoophorectomy, and pelvic lymph node sampling for endometrial cancer. *J. Gynecol. Surg.*, **8**, 91–4
6. Plentl, A.A. and Friedman, E.A. (1971). *Lymphatic System of the Female Genitalia: The Morphologic Basis of Oncologic Diagnosis and Therapy*, pp. 57–74. (Philadelphia: WB Saunders)
7. Perez, C.A., Korba, A. and Sharma, S. (1977). Dosimetric considerations in irradiation of carcinoma of the vagina. *Int. J. Radiol. Oncol. Biol. Phys.*, **2**, 639–45
8. Querleu, D., Leblanc, E. and Castelain, B. (1990). Lymphadénectomie pelvienne sous contrôle coelioscopique. *J. Gynecol. Obstet. Biol. Reprod.*, **19**, 576–8
9. Dargent, D. (1987). A new future for Schauta's operation through presurgical retroperitoneal pelviscopy. *Eur. J. Gynecol. Oncol.*, **8**, 292–6
10. Canis, M., Mage, G., Wattiez, A. Pouly, J.L., Manhes, H. and Bruhat, M.A. (1990). La chirurgie endoscopique a-t-elle une place dans la chirurgie radicale du cancer du col utérin ? *J. Gynecol. Obstet. Biol. Reprod.*, **19**, 921–6
11. Nezhat, G.R., Burrel, M.O., Nezhat, F.R., Benigno, B.B. and Welander, C.E. (1992).

Laparoscopic radical hysterectomy with paraaortic and pelvic node dissection. *Am. J. Obstet. Gynecol.*, **166**, 864–5

12. Vercamer, R., Janssens, J., De P. Usewils, R.I., Baert, A., Lauwerijns, J. and Bonte, J. (1987). Computerised tomography and lymphography in the presurgical staging of early carcinoma of the uterine cervix. *Cancer*, **60**, 1745–50

13. King, L.A., Talledo, O.E., Gallup, D.G. and El Gammal, T.A.M. (1986). Computed tomography in evaluation of gynecological malignancies: a prospective analysis? *Am J. Obstet. Gynecol.*, **60**, 1055–61

14. Walsh, J.M. and Goplerud, D.R. (1981). Prospective comparison between clinical and CT staging in primary cervical carcinoma. *Am. J. Roentgenol.*, **137**, 997–1003

15. Wurtz, A., Mazman, E., Gosselin, B., Woelffle, D., Sauvage, L. and Rousseau, O. (1987). Bilan anatomique des adénopathies rétropéritonéales par endoscopie chirurgicale. *Ann. Chir.*, **41**, 258–63

16. Dargent, D. and Salvat, J. (1989). *L'envahissement Ganglionnaire Pelvien*. (Paris, Midsi/Mac Graw Hill)

17. Reich, H. (1989). New techniques in advanced laparoscopic surgery. *Clin. Obstet. Gynecol.*, **3**, 655–81

18. Querleu, D. and Leblanc, E. (1993). Laparoscopic pelvic lymphadenectomy. In Sutton, C. and Diamond, M. (eds.) *Endoscopic Surgery for Gynecologists*. p. 172–8. (London: Saunders)

19. Canis, M., Mage, G., Wattiez, A., Pouly, J.L., Chapron, C. and Bruhat, M.A. (1992). Vaginally assisted laparoscopic radical hysterectomy. *J. Gynecol. Surg.*, **8**, 103–5

20. Reich, H., McGlynn, F. and Wickie, W. (1990). Laparoscopic management of stage 1 ovarian cancer: a case report. *J. Reprod. Med.*, **35**, 601

Part 4

Complications

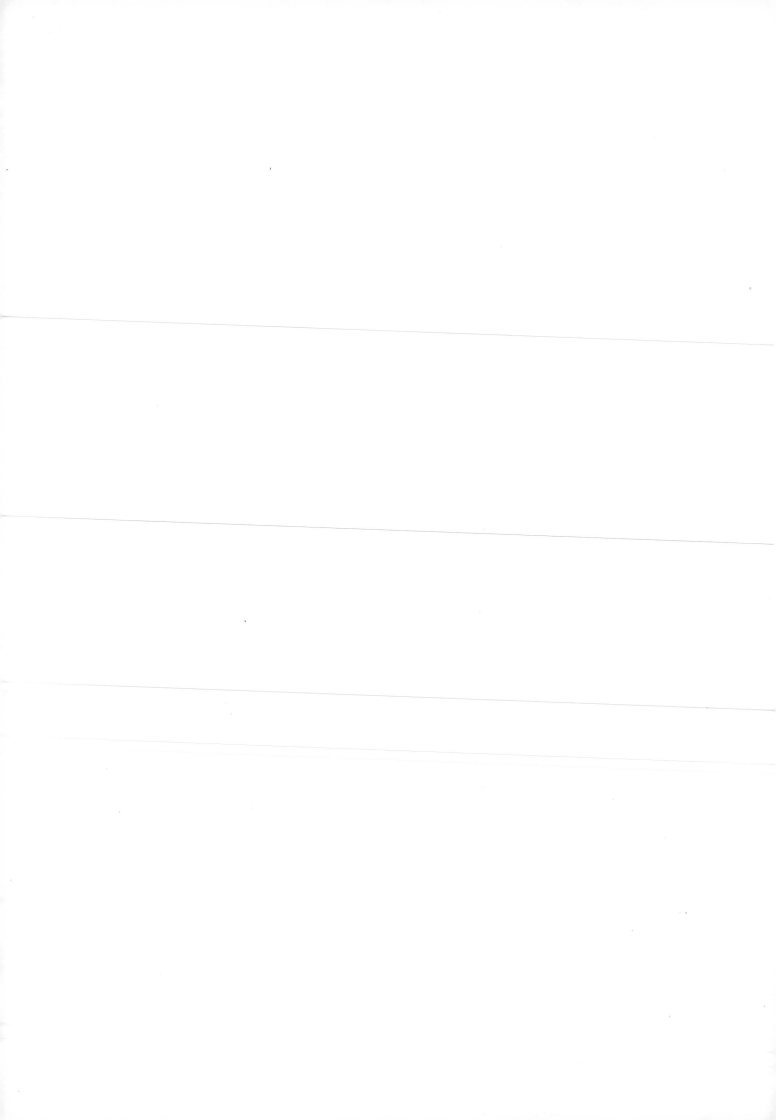

Ureteral and bladder injury during laparoscopic surgery

24

J. Donnez, S. Bassil, V. Anaf, M. Smets and M. Nisolle

The reported risks of laparoscopy include perforation of the bowel, bladder, uterus or blood vessels, in addition to the risks of general anesthesia.

In the years since 1980, tubal sterilization has become the most frequent indication for laparoscopy. The main complications of laparoscopy are hemorrhage, and perforation of the bladder and bowel by the Verres needle and trocar. Tubal sterilization by electro-coagulation carries some further specific risks, such as electrical burns and hemorrhage in the mesosalpinx. Reports of ureteral burn injuries during laparoscopic sterilization are rare. In reports prior to 1980, the incidence of burn injuries during laparoscopic sterilization by electrocoagulation was approximately two per 1 000[2-4].

The abdominal wall and bowel are the most frequently affected structures. Burns to the bowel are usually diagnosed not at the time of surgery but 3–7 days later. Assuming that the electrosurgical equipment is well calibrated, these burns are caused by inadvertent contact or by sparks during cauterization. Two develop-ments – non-conductive trocar sheaths and the bipolar coagulation technique – prevent burn injuries to a certain extent. But even with the bipolar cauterization technique, in which the current flows between the tips of the coagulation forceps, burn injuries have been described[1].

URETERAL INJURIES

This paper presents two cases of ureteral injury resulting from operative laparoscopy in a series of 12 000 cases of laparoscopic surgery. The 13 previously reported cases of ureteral injury[5] occurring at laparoscopy are reviewed. The modes of diagnosis and the methods of treating the ureteral injuries are described.

Case reports

Case 1

A 35 year-old woman presented with a 5-year history of severe dysmenorrhea. Physical examination demon-strated tenderness in the cul-de-sac consistent with endometriosis. Laparoscopy revealed stage I endome-triosis. Peritoneal black lesions were present extensively on both uterosacral ligaments. CO$_2$ laser vaporization of the endometriotic implants was performed as well as laser uterine nerve ablation (LUNA). Because of

bleeding at the level of the left uterosacral ligament, unipolar electrocoagulation was used. The ureter was well visualized and was seen 1 cm from the site of coagulation.

On postoperative day 7, the patient presented with increasing abdominal pain, peritonitis, leukocytosis and fever (39.1°C). A computerized tomographic (CT) scan revealed the presence of fluid in the retroperitoneal space (Figure 1). An intravenous pyelogram (IVP) revealed a urinoma on the left side of the pelvis (Figure 2). A JJ catheter was inserted and removed 3 months later. No complication occurred.

Case 2

A 29-year-old patient was referred for evaluation of infertility and recurrent pelvic pain. One year previously, she had undergone laparoscopy for acute salpingitis treated by antibiotics. Postoperative hystero-salpingography revealed a bilateral hydrosalpinx and a laparoscopy for salpingostomy was proposed to the patient. At laparoscopy, the ovaries were found to be fixed to the broad ligament by very dense adhesions. During left ovariolysis, bleeding encountered 1 cm beneath the ovary was controlled with bipolar coagulation. The left ureter was clearly visible about 1.5 cm from the bleeding. Because a vein of the ovarian hilus was responsible for the bleeding, there was some difficulty in achieving complete hemostasis and numerous attempts were made before cessation of the bleeding was accomplished. The patient was discharged the next day. Seven days later, she developed fever and peritonitis. An IVP revealed extravasation of urine in a left urinoma (Figure 3). Retrograde stent placement was successful; a double-J stent was inserted for 3 months. Three months after removal, IVP demonstrated a small ureteral stenosis (Figure 4), which was successfully dilated by a retrograde stent (Figure 5).

Discussion

Ureteral injuries occurring during laparoscopy were documented in a review by Grainger and colleagues[5]. Table 1 summarizes the 15 cases of ureteral injury resulting from laparoscopy that are reported in the literature. Four of these 15 cases were complications of laparoscopic sterilization procedures, and seven

237

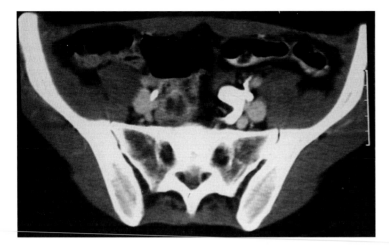

Figure 1 CT scan: presence of contrast medium in the retroperitoneal space after pyelography

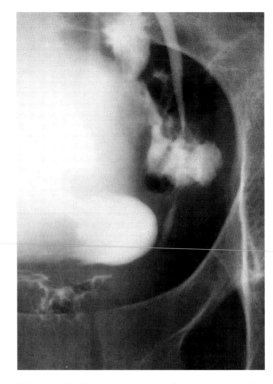

Figure 2 Intravenous pyelogram revealing a urinoma

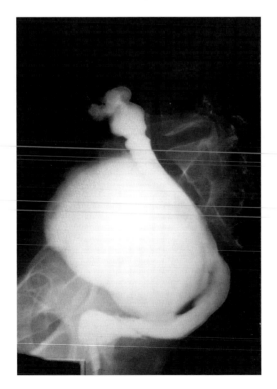

Figure 3(a) Extravasation of urine in a left urinoma after pyelography. The urinoma is clearly separated from the rectum; (b) a double-J stent was placed for 3 months

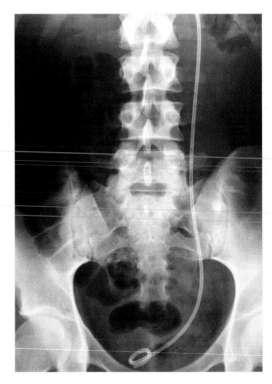

Figure 3(b) *See legend opposite*

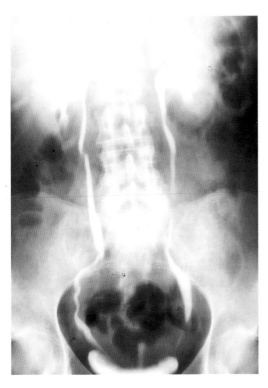

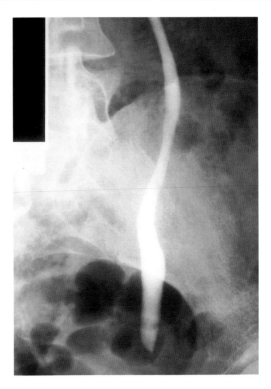

Figure 4(a) and (b) Small ureteral stenosis

Figure 4(b) *See legend opposite*

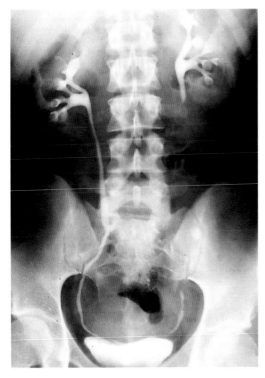

Figure 5 Final result 3 months after dilatation

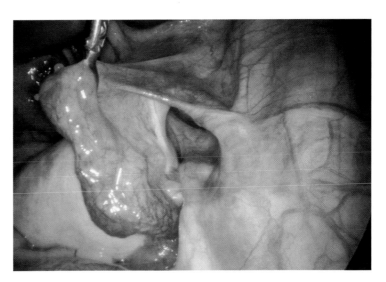

Figure 6 Ureter visualized through the peritoneum

Table 1 Summary of the 15 cases of ureteral injury resulting from laparoscopy that are reported in the literature

Case number	Time of presentation	Indication for initial procedure	Treatment modality	Method of diagnosis	Treatment
1*	7 days	endometriosis (LUNA)	CO_2 laser/unipolar cautery	IVP–CT scan	retrograde stent (double J)
2*	7 days	salpingoovariolysis	CO_2 laser/bipolar cautery	IVP	retrograde stent (double J)
3[5]	48 h	endometriosis	unipolar cautery	IVP	end-to-end anastomosis
4[5]	48 h	adhesions/endometriosis	unipolar cautery	IVP	transverse uretero–ureterostomy
5[5]	24 h	uterosacral ligament transection	unipolar cautery	repeat laparoscopy	transverse uretero–ureterostomy
6[5]	36 h	adhesions	bipolar cautery	repeat laparoscopy	end-to-end anastomosis
7[5]	48 h	endometriosis	CO_2 laser/bipolar	IVP	percutaneous stent
8[3]	5 days	endometriosis	unipolar cautery	IVP	transverse uretero–ureterostomy
9[2]	2 weeks	sterilization	bipolar cautery	IVP	Boari flap
10[4]	unknown	endometriosis	unipolar cautery	IVP	unknown
11[6]	3 weeks	sterilization	cautery (not specified)	laparotomy	ileal interposition
12[7]	3 weeks	diagnostic laparoscopy	trocar injury (?)	IVP	end-to-end anastomosis
13[8]	5 days	adhesions	cautery (not specified)	IVP	stent at laparotomy
14[1]	4 days	sterilization	bipolar cautery	IVP, repeat	retrograde stent
15[9]	5 days	sterilization	bipolar cautery	IVP	transverse uretero–ureterostomy

*, Donnez, *et al.*, present study; LUNA = laser uterine nerve ablation

complications of laparoscopic treatment of endometriosis. Although the ureter may often be visualized through the peritoneum in the upper pelvis (Figure 6), it cannot be identified reliably in the area of the uterosacral ligaments. This is particularly true in the presence of diseases such as endometriosis. The presence of uterosacral ligaments that are thickened and nodular can induce a distortion of the normal anatomy of the ureter in this area.

Electrocoagulation has been used routinely in sterilization. It is erroneously assumed that bipolar coagulation is 'safe'; five reported ureteral injuries have occurred using this method. In addition to direct tissue damage, the electrical current may damage the vascular supply to the coagulated tissue.

Time of presentation of symptoms

Ureteral injury was symptomatic soon after the procedures – between 24 h and 7 days – except for three cases, in which the diagnosis was made 2–3 weeks after endoscopic surgery. In our two cases, the ureter was precisely visualized before coagulating an artery of the uterosacral ligament (case 1) or a venous blood vessel (case 2). In both cases, the distance between the ureter and the blood vessel was at least 1.5 cm. The time lapse between endoscopic surgery and onset of symptoms was 7 days in both cases. We conclude that 7 days are required for the creation of a ureteral fistula when the cause is the propagation either of the current or of the heat. In the review by Grainger and co-workers[5], the most common symptoms were abdominal pain with peritonitis, leukocytosis and fever.

Mode of diagnosis

The diagnosis of ureteral injury is usually made by IVP, which shows that the cause of the 'retroperitoneal mass' is a urinoma, and also demonstrates the site of the fistula. Our two cases were diagnosed by the presence of a pelvic mass confirmed by echography and CT scan.

Treatment

Among the reviewed cases, management consisted of exploratory laparotomy with one of the following procedures:

(1) Reimplantation of the ureter into the bladder (one case);

(2) Anastomosis of the damaged ureter (three cases);

(3) Transureteral ureterostomy (four cases); and

(4) Interposition of an isoperistaltic loop of ileum between the ureter and the bladder (one case).

In our series, both patients avoided laparotomy for ureteral repair. The placement of a ureteral stent allowed drainage of urine, resolution of the pelvic urinoma and spontaneous healing of the injured site. The placement of these ureteral stents may be accomplished in a retrograde manner. If technically possible, this method of treatment is preferable in managing such types of ureteral injuries.

Several of the ureteral injuries occurred at the time of sterilization. These were most likely a result of the cautery forceps touching the sidewall during application of the current. It is unlikely that these injuries will occur as a result of 'arcing' of electrical energy or from burning through the peritoneum by excess heat in the coagulated tissue after the sterilization is complete. Therefore, the tube must be grasped in the bipolar forceps and moved away from the sidewall before applying the current. Bleeding in the area of the uterosacral ligaments, whether it occurs at the time of uterosacral ligament transection or ablation of endometriosis, must be carefully controlled. The advent of laparoscopically applied surgical clips may provide a greater margin of safety when controlling bleeding in this area. Other techniques that can now be applied laparoscopically include suturing, endocoagulation and electrocoagulation. The best solution remains prevention, and an increase in aquadissection and dissection of the ureter before doing a coagulation in the area of the uterosacral ligaments is suggested.

BLADDER INJURIES

The incidence of bladder injury during operative laparoscopy is unknown. In our series of 12 000 laparoscopies, three cases of such injury were reported (one was due to the second-puncture trocar and one to dilaceration during transabdominal myoma removal (Figure 7) and one to vesicouterine space dissection during the vaginal approach in laparoscopy-assisted vaginal hysterectomy). The surgeon may see or suspect a bladder injury; in our series cases 1 and 3 were suspected at the time of laparoscopy and immediately confirmed by the infusion of 500 ml of saline solution with methylene blue into the bladder by gravity drainage.

Mode of diagnosis

Urine may be seen in the pelvis, usually secondary to an extraperitoneal perforation or laceration. If an injury is suspected but no definitive urine is seen, 5 ml of indigo carmine or methylene blue can be administered intravenously and the bladder can be observed laparoscopically for leakage. Because the bladder is hidden within the true pelvis, injuries to the lateral and posterior wall may be missed visually. Therefore, if

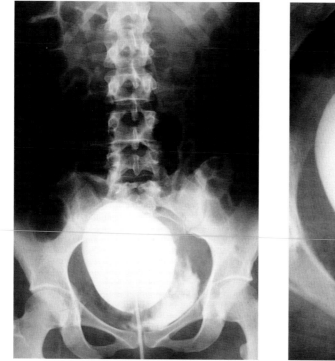

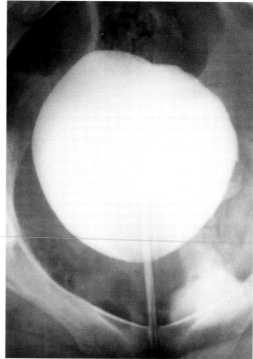

Figure 7 Cystography: (a) and (b) extravasation of contrast medium through the dilaceration site (2 days after the endoscopic procedure)

Figure 7(b)   *See legend opposite*

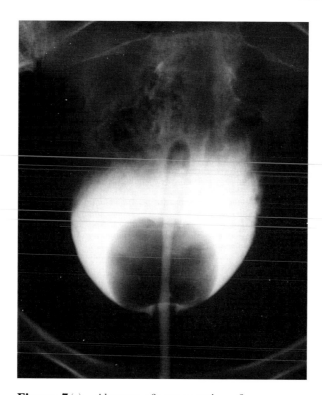

Figure 7(c)   Absence of extravasation after management with large-bore Foley catheter drainage (7 days later)

bladder damage is suspected, a gravity cystogram should be performed immediately. Approximately 250 ml of contrast medium is infused into the bladder by gravity drainage and an X-ray film obtained. If a rupture is seen, a catheter is inserted to allow gravity drainage, which starts immediately. Small bladder perforations may be seen on the lateral, oblique or drain-out films. Radiographically, intraperitoneal injuries will allow contrast medium to fill the cul-de-sac, outline loops of bowel, and extend along the pericolic gutter.

Suprapubic pain and fullness, with or without diminished urine output, may suggest bladder injury. If an intraperitoneal bladder injury has been missed, a dramatic increase in the blood urea nitrogen (BUN) due to urinary contact with the peritoneum is observed. The definitive diagnosis is made by cystography.

Thermal injuries to the bladder may not manifest themselves initially. Sudden hematuria, well into the postoperative period, may be a sign of thermal damage. A true perforation may not yet be present and therefore a negative cystogram may be misleading. Cystoscopy should be performed to identify any areas of devitalized tissue.

Treatment

There is a consensus that all large intraperitoneal bladder injuries should be repaired by open surgery at the time the diagnosis is made. In our series, two cases of bladder injury provoked by trocar were managed with large-bore Foley catheter drainage for 10 days. Usually, the bladder will heal. A gravity cystogram is performed on days 8–10 and if no extravasation is noted, the catheter is removed.

In the case of bladder laceration, open surgery is required in order to identify the lesion clearly and to close the perforation carefully in two layers using 2/0 chromic catgut. The peritoneal cavity is not drained but the space of Retzius is drained. In the cases of bladder laceration in our series, the diagnosis was made during the vaginal approach in laparoscopy-assisted vaginal hysterectomy. The closure of the laceration was performed vaginally, using 2/0 chromic catgut.

CONCLUSION

The incidence of ureteral and/or bladder injury at laparoscopy is unknown but seems to be very low in an experienced team – two (0.02%) and three (0.03%) cases, respectively, in a series of 12 000 laparoscopies. Prompt recognition and treatment will most probably result in a favorable outcome for the patient.

REFERENCES

1. Bauman, H., Jaeger, P. and Huch, A. (1988). Ureteral injury after laparoscopic tubal sterilization by bipolar electrocoagulation. *Obstet. Gynecol.*, **71**, 483–5
2. Stengel, J.N., Felderman, E.S. and Zamora, D. (1974). Ureteral injury: complication of laparoscopic sterilization. *Urology*, **4**, 341–2
3. Cheng, Y.S. (1976). Ureteral injury resulting from laparoscopic fulguration of endometriotic implant. *Am. J. Obstet. Gynecol.*, **8**, 1045–6
4. Daly, J.W. and Higgins, K.A. (1988). Injury to the ureter during gynecologic surgical procedures. *Surg. Gynecol. Obstet.*, **167**, 19–22
5. Grainger, D.A., Soderstrom, R.M., Schiff, S.F., Glickman, M., DeCherney, A.H. and Diamond, M.P. (1990). Ureteral injuries at laparoscopy: insights into diagnosis, management and prevention. *Obstet. Gynecol.*, **75**, 839–43
6. Irvin, T.T., Gligher, J.C. and Scott, J.S. (1975). Injury to the ureter during laparoscopic tubal sterilization. *Arch. Surg.*, **110**, 1501–3
7. Schapira, M., Dizerensh, H., Essinger, A., Wauters, J.P., Loup, P. and Von Niederhausern, W. (1987). Urinary ascites after gynecological laparoscopy. *Lancet*, **1**, 871–2
8. Winslow, P.H., Kreger, R., Ebbesson, B. and Oster, E. (1986). Conservative management of electrical burn injury of ureter secondary to laparoscopy. *Urology*, **27**, 60–2
9. teBrevil, W. and Boeminghaus, F. (1977). Harnleitorlasion bei laparoskopistcher lubensterilisation. *Geburts. Frauenheilkd*, **37**, 572–6

Complications of laparoscopic surgery in gynecology

25

S. Bassil, M. Nisolle and J. Donnez

INTRODUCTION

Every surgical technique is evaluated according to its short- and long-term results and its complications. Surgery by laparotomy has been well defined after several years of evaluation. For endoscopy, this evaluation is still in progress; even if endoscopy is a relatively safe procedure, as in any other, complications do occur. In endoscopic gynecology, laparoscopy was developed first as a diagnostic tool and later as an efficacious surgical technique. If the technical aspects and the surgical procedures of endoscopic surgery in gynecology are well known, there is still a lack of information concerning their complications. Most of our knowledge comes from the experience of diagnostic laparoscopy and tubal sterilization. Lessons learned in the 1970s and 1980s still apply in the 1990s, but the frequency of indications, the increasing number of surgeons using endoscopy, and the introduction of new instruments (forceps, trocars, electrocoagulation, lasers) have given rise to new types of complications. In this chapter, technical and general surgical aspects of laparoscopic complications, their management and recommendations for prevention will be discussed. Complications of anesthesia and treatment of different gynecological pathologies will not be described.

The incidence of laparoscopic complications is 2.49 to 6% for major occurrences and 1.07 to 5.2% for minor ones[1]. Each laparoscopic procedure may be divided into three steps:

(1) The first step or 'blind step' includes the induction of the pneumoperitoneum and the installation of the laparoscope.

(2) The second step or 'visual step' includes the installation of the operating trocars and surgical procedures.

(3) The third step is 'uterine cannulation'.

COMPLICATIONS OF THE FIRST STEP

The blind puncture of the abdominal wall with the insufflation needle and the laparoscope trocar must be performed with great care. If they penetrated the abdominal cavity, the needle or the trocar could injure vascular, gastrointestinal or urinary structures. Also, poor positioning of the insufflation needle may be responsible for subcutaneous emphysema.

Vascular injuries

We must distinguish 'major vascular injury' from 'minor vascular injury'. Perforation of the aorta, vena cava, common, right and left iliac arteries and veins, superior mesenteric, and inferior epigastric vessels has been reported.

Major vascular injuries

The true incidence of 'major vascular injury' is unknown, since the vast majority of cases go unreported. In 1989, Baadsgaard and colleagues[2] reported 15 cases from the literature and added their own case. In the majority of the 15 patients, the injury was caused by the pneumoperitoneum needle and only in two cases by the trocar. Characteristically, the terminal aorta near the bifurcation or the common iliac arteries were injured. In only one case was the injury as far from the aortic bifurcation as the external iliac artery.

Diagnosis A vascular injury is suspected in the presence of one of these signs:

(1) Return of blood from the open insufflating needle;

(2) Sudden deterioration in blood pressure of a previously stable patient after needle or trocar insertion, especially if the positioning of the needle was difficult;

(3) The presence of an unexplained volume of blood in the peritoneal cavity, and if this blood reappears after aspiration[3].

In over half of the cases reported in the literature[2-8], the diagnosis was made immediately and a laparotomy was performed. In other cases, the diagnosis was delayed (6–21 days) and in one case reported by Bisler and co-workers[9], a patient had a 3-month-old laparoscopic lesion and was treated on suspicion of a ruptured aortic aneurysm.

Management If vascular injury with the insufflation needle is strongly suspected, the needle is left in place to help mark the site of injury while an expeditious midline incision is made for laparotomy. A trocar injury to the major vessels is more serious and the measures described above must be applied. Usually, in the case of a major vessel injury, the retroperitoneal hematoma occupies all of the field of view and, once laparotomy is performed, the first priority is the compression of the aorta. This can be accomplished with the hand or with a vascular clamp and may reduce the bleeding until a vascular surgeon arrives. If vascular injury is not certain and blood pressure is stable, the insufflation needle is still left in place and the pneumoperitoneum can be achieved in another way. A 5-mm laparoscope is introduced through a suprapubic trocar. If bleeding is very minimal, endoscopic repair must be considered for small vessels, but laparotomy is necessary for major vessel injury. In cases of delayed symptoms, a computed tomogram and/or a magnetic resonance image are helpful for diagnosis, and management is decided upon in collaboration with vascular surgeons.

Prevention The success of the prevention of such an injury depends on the surgeon's experience, anatomical knowledge and understanding of the procedure. Important points to consider include:

(1) Thin patients are at highest risk of vascular injury; the aorta may lie less than 3 cm below the skin in these women. Introduction of an insufflation needle or trocar must be done with due consideration of this anatomy.

(2) The position of the tip of the needle must be checked before any mobilization. Many tests have been proposed for this; all depend on the principle of negative intra-abdominal pressure.

(3) In cases of malpositioning of the insufflation needle, it must be removed and the pneumoperitoneum established again. The manipulation of the needle, in an attempt to position it properly intra-abdominally, exposes the patient to a high risk of vascular injury. If blood returns from the open insufflating needle, the needle must be left fixed without any manipulation, because this may induce a wide laceration of the vascular wall.

(4) Elevation of the abdominal wall is recommended prior to needle insertion. This will increase the distance over which the needle must travel to reach the major vessels[10]. This must be done manually; attempts to elevate the abdominal wall with towel clips merely give the illusion of safety. They elevate the skin or subcutaneous space only and do nothing to the peritoneum[11].

(5) It is important to insure that an adequate pneumoperitoneum is created, prior to inserting the trocar.

(6) The use of blunt needles and trocars increases the risk of vascular injury, because blunt instruments need increased force for insertion and this may cause the trocar to slip[12].

(7) Introducing the laparoscope trocar without any pneumoperitoneum has been attempted by some authors[13-16]. They do not report any vascular injury from more than 4000 laparoscopies. We do not have any experience of this technique but it should be taken into consideration in difficult cases.

Minor vascular injury

Essentially, this concerns injury to the omentum or presacral vessels. In most cases it is unlikely that this injury can induce acute shock and the management depends on the experience of the surgeon.

Diagnosis Minor vascular injury is suspected when blood returns from the open insufflating needle, or when blood is present in the peritoneal cavity. In both cases, the blood pressure remains stable without shock. In the first case, the diagnosis can be made by visualization of the bleeding using a 5-mm suprapubic laparoscope introduced after the creation of a pneumoperitoneum in another site with another insufflation needle. In the second case, the bleeding is visualized when the laparoscope is introduced.

Management Usually, the bleeding is controlled by bipolar coagulation or with laparoscopic suture. It is rare that the bleeding necessitates a laparotomy.

Prevention The same preventative measures as for major vascular injury apply for minor vascular injury.

Gastrointestinal injury

Stomach injury

Gastric perforation by the insufflation needle or the trocar is a rare occurrence. Its incidence was evaluated as 0.027% by Loffer[17]. In the literature, more than 30 cases have been reported[18-20].

Diagnosis The main sign of gastric perforation by the insufflation needle is the occurrence of bouts of eructation. Perforation with the trocar is diagnosed by visualization of the gastric mucosa.

Management In cases of gastric perforation with the insufflation needle without any tearing, no further therapy is needed because its small diameter leaves no defect. In all other cases of such injury, a laparotomy to suture the stomach must be performed.

Prevention The most common conditions which lead to gastric injury are distortion of the abdominal anatomy by previous surgery, difficult induction of anesthesia[17,19] and aerophagia[18]. In the presence of one of these conditions some precautions are mandatory:

(1) Inserting a nasogastric or oropharyngeal tube after the induction of anesthesia;

(2) Placing the patient in a 15° Trendelenburg position prior to insertion of the insufflation needle;

(3) Lifting the abdominal wall and respecting an angle of 45° with the skin for needle insertion.

(4) Insuring that an adequate pneumoperitoneum is created to prevent injury to the stomach at the time of trocar insertion.

Bowel injuries

Inadvertent traumatic perforation of the bowel is a well-recognized potential complication of laparoscopy. This complication has been reported to occur with an incidence of 0.06 to 0.30%[21,22]. Insertion of the insufflation needle and the initial trocar into the peritoneal cavity is the most common cause of bowel perforation[23].

Diagnosis Injuries to the bowel can be treacherous because they may not be recognized at the time of surgery. Diagnosis is made immediately in the presence of stool on the tip of the needle or the trocar, if fecal material is seen in the abdominal cavity, if the surgeon notices a foul smell when introducing the laparoscope, if a hematoma is noticed on the bowel serosa, or if the laparoscope is introduced into the lumen of the intestine. In cases of delayed diagnosis, especially with through-and-through perforation of the bowel, signs of peritonitis may be present postoperatively and the diagnosis is confirmed at the time of laparotomy.

Management The treatment of bowel injury will depend on the etiology. Perforations with the insufflating needle without laceration of the intestinal wall do not require any surgical repair, and a medical approach with broad-spectrum antibiotics may be sufficient. In the case of trocar perforation or wide laceration, surgical repair is mandatory and the method of repair depends on the instrumentation available and the proficiency of the laparoscopist. Laparotomy with suture repair is probably the preferred treatment for most laparoscopists. However, laparoscopic repair is possible providing the injury is not extensive and stool contamination of the abdominal cavity is limited. In cases of delayed diagnosis with peritonitis, laparotomy is still indicated.

Prevention Certain predisposing factors, such as a dilated gastrointestinal tract or an atypical anatomical laceration secondary to adhesions will increase the risk of bowel injury. Attention must be paid in cases of:

(1) Patients with previous laparotomy; and

(2) The use of blunt instruments.

The trocar insertion technique should be standarized; with the patient in a completely horizontal position, an angle of 45° with the skin must be respected when introducing the trocar. Premature Trendelenburg positioning does nothing to avoid bowel injuries. Exploration of the anterior abdominal wall with a syringe and needle to check for the presence of bowel adhesions is a helpful test in patients with previous laparotomy. After a pneumoperitoneum has been established, a 10-ml syringe containing 3 ml of normal saline is connected to a short, 18-gauge spinal needle, which is inserted through the umbilicus. If there is adequate peritoneal space to accommodate the trocar, gas bubbles will appear in the saline. The limits of the potential space can be further confined by gradually advancing the needle. Recently, much attention has been paid to the disposable trocar, because of its sharp tip and spring-loaded safety shield[24]. Nevertheless, there have been no large-scale clinical trials to establish the advantage of these single-use trocars[12].

Urinary tract injuries

Urinary injuries can also occur as a result of inadvertent instrument insertion. Essentially, this happens with an overdistended bladder because of a lack of catheterization before the procedure. The diagnosis is made when urine comes out of the insufflating needle; no surgical repair is required in this case. A small hole may require only Foley catheter drainage[25]. Such injuries are more likely to occur with suprapubic trocars and were discussed in Chapter 24.

Subcutaneous emphysema

Subcutaneous emphysema is reported to occur during laparoscopy at a rate between 0.4 and 2%[26]. This phenomenon is a result of improper positioning of the insufflation needle. The introduction of CO_2 into the preperitoneal space will allow its dissection up along the anterior chest wall, neck and face.

Diagnosis

The diagnosis is made by the palpation of the CO_2 bubbles under the skin.

Management

After introduction of the laparoscope, the suprapubic trocar must be inserted into the preperitoneal space, with the valve in the open position. The operator must then press the skin with his hands to push the CO_2 out of the preperitoneal space.

Prevention

It is not a major complication, but the distension of the preperitoneal space could occupy the operating area and thus make the exposure of organs more difficult. Preventing this complication is easy by:

(1) Respecting the technique of introducing the insufflation needle; and

(2) Respecting the limits of the insufflating pressure.

Tests based on the negative intra-abdominal pressure may be helpful in cases of difficulties encountered when inducing the pneumoperitoneum to avoid this occurrence.

COMPLICATIONS OF THE SECOND STEP

During the second step, complications could occur while inserting the secondary trocars or during the surgical procedures. Vascular, urinary or intestinal structures may be injured with the trocars or while performing electrosurgery, laser surgery or sharp dissection.

Injuries with secondary trocars

Major vascular injury or bowel injury is diagnosed and managed as described above. Epigastric vessel perforation and bladder injury are managed differently as described further.

Epigastric vessel perforation

Perforation of the inferior and/or superficial epigastric vessels is the most common complication encountered during laparoscopic surgery (Figure 1). The inferior epigastric artery extends from the external iliac artery and lies beneath the rectus muscle and above the peritoneum. The superficial epigastric artery extends from the femoral artery near the inguinal ring and courses medially over the rectus muscle toward the midline.

Diagnosis If injured, these large vessels can produce a rapid and massive hemorrhage. While an injured inferior epigastric artery creates retroperitoneal or

intraperitoneal bleeding, the superficial epigastric vessel induces intramuscular or subcutaneous bleeding. In most cases, blood spillage around the trocar sleeve announces the injury.

Management An essential rule to keep in mind is that the sleeve cannot be removed, as it is the only mark of the vessel's location. In cases of minimal bleeding and a small hematoma, no repair is required. Sometimes the bleeding can be extremely swift, and repair using several techniques might then be necessary. Both ends of the transected vessel must be secured for an adequate hemostasis. Bipolar coagulation of the vessel through the peritoneum is the best and fastest way to ensure optimal hemostasis. This can be efficacious only when there is no hematoma in the field of view, making the vessel's identification impossible. Laparoscopic ligation of the vessel will achieve hemostasis. A large curved or straight needle can be passed through the abdominal wall and into the abdomen. The needle is then passed back through the abdominal wall and tied outside the abdominal wall, cephaled and cauded to the sleeve. At the end of the surgery, the ligature can be removed without any recurrence of bleeding. Hemostasis can also be achieved by simple compression. As soon as the swift bleeding is noticed around the sleeve, a number 12 Foley catheter is passed through the sleeve into the abdominal cavity. The Foley balloon is inflated with fluid. The sleeve is pulled out and the Foley balloon pulled up against the abdominal wall. The pressure maintained on the Foley balloon occludes the bleeding vessel. As soon as hemostasis is obtained, a second trocar is inserted and the operation can continue. In some rare cases, hemostasis cannot be achieved: the skin incision must be enlarged around the trocar sleeve and the vessel promptly secured by ligature.

Prevention An injury to the superficial and/or inferior epigastric vessels may occur during any laparoscopy, but is more likely to happen under specific circumstances. Obese women, or patients who have undergone previous abdominal surgery, are prone to having an epigastric vessel obscured by the fat paniculus or by the incisional scar. Removing and replacing trocars of different sizes and/or trying repeatedly to place the second trocar increases the risk of such injury. During the laparoscopy, a security triangle should be visualized using the obliterated umbilical arteries as the lateral sides of the triangle and the dome of the bladder as the third side of the triangle. Secondary puncture trocars must be inserted within the margins of this triangle. The epigastric vessels rarely lie within the confines of this area. Sometimes, close laparoscopic inspection of the peritoneal side of the anterior abdominal wall allows the visualization of these vessels, so that the surgeon can choose a safe location to introduce the suprapubic trocar.

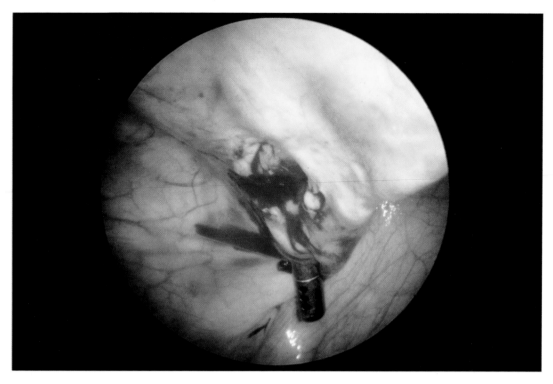

Figure 1(a) and (b)   Epigastric vessel perforation

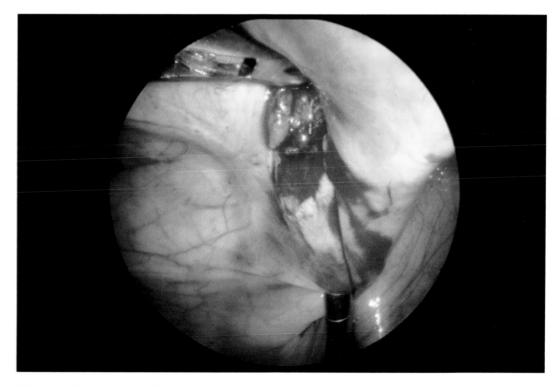

Figure 1(b)   *See legend above*

Bladder injury

Bladder injuries are more common with secondary trocars. A lack of bladder catheterization is the main reason for such injuries. Although the bladder heals rapidly, intraoperative recognition of the injury is crucial because it facilitates management and postoperative recovery. Delay in the diagnosis can result in abdominal distension and azotemia, although ascites, urinoma and vesicocutaneous fistulas are sometimes encountered.

Diagnosis Diagnosis is made intraoperatively by the recognition of the bladder muscularis separated by the trocar, or by urine spillage around the trocar sleeve. If a Foley catheter is left in place, the appearance of gas in the Foley bag or of hematuria must be investigated. In every other case, the diagnosis is made postoperatively in the presence of hematuria, decreased urinary output, anuria, abdominal swelling or peritoneal signs. In the absence of infected urine, peritoneal signs rarely occur. A retrograde cystogram localizes the leak from the bladder and abdominal sonography confirms the presence of liquid in the abominal cavity.

Management The first rule in the treatment of a bladder injury is a 12–15-day drainage. In cases of small leaks (<2 cm) or extraperitoneal damage, drainage may be sufficient. In other cases, immediate surgical repair is necessary. Prolonged manipulation of the perforating instruments increases the degree of damage. If the damage is recognized intraoperatively, the trocar is left in place and by minilaparotomy, a pursestring (two- or three-layer closure) is immediately performed[27,28]. Laparoscopic repair with a two-layer closure must be considered only by experienced laparoscopists. A patient managed in this way remained asymptomatic throughout a 1-year follow-up[29]. If the damage is suspected intraoperatively without any demonstrable leak or intraperitoneal spillage, drainage and observation may be useful[30]. In cases of delayed diagnosis, bladder injuries are handled in the same way as other traumatic ruptures. Intraperitoneal leaks are repaired and drained while extraperitoneal leaks are drained[30]. Prior to catheter removal, a cystogram is performed. If the leak persists, drainage is prolonged up to 30 days prior to repeating the cystogram.

Prevention The first step before inserting the suprapubic trocar is to check that the bladder is well catheterized. For short procedures this can be an in-and-out catheterization. For longer procedures, a Foley catheter must be drained constantly in a sterile closed system. This may be very useful when the surgeon has to replace the secondary trocar often. After emptying the bladder, the second step to prevent trocar damage is the visualization of the dome of the bladder when inserting the trocar.

Patients who have had a previous Cesarean section or who have undergone multiple pelvic surgery could present a distortion in peritoneal bladder repair; thus, trocars have to be placed taking this anatomy into consideration. In difficult cases, the insertion site can be modified.

Injuries during surgical procedures

A host of instruments have been developed for specific purposes during laparoscopic procedures. In addition to sharp and blunt dissection, performed by means of a laparoscope in a similar manner to standard open procedures, there are special laser and electrosurgical devices specifically designed for laparoscopic application. Two major complications have been described when using these devices: bowel and ureteral injury.

Bowel injury during surgical procedures

Bowel perforation could occur during laparoscopic dissection. Besides occurrences directly related to dense adhesions and the dissection plane, complications could be induced by the use of a thermal energy device[23].

Diagnosis In the majority of cases, diagnosis is delayed and patients present signs of peritonitis or bowel occlusion. Intraoperatively, diagnosis is made by the direct visualization of the damage.

Management Management of perforations of the bowel is related to the site and the extent of damage, and to when the injury is discovered. For perforations by the laser beam or an electrosurgical device diagnosed intraoperatively, a laparotomy with resection of the necrotic zone is necessary. The bowel must be repaired with two- or three-layer sutures. This type of closure is appropriate only if the damage is limited and superficial. In the presence of a significant bowel lesion or peritonitis, a timely intraoperative consultation with the general surgeon is mandatory to decide how to handle the damage.

Prevention Laser surgery must be carried out by an experienced surgeon, with adequate instruments[31]. In addition, the laser should always be placed on stand-by mode when not in use. Care must be taken when using monopolar electrosurgery to ensure that the patient's return plate is properly attached, the instruments are well insulated and the bowel is out of the field of energy application. With bipolar coagulation the forceps must not come into contact with the bowel when activated or immediately after inactivation.

Ureteral injury during surgical procedures

Ureteral injuries are a major concern for the laparoscopic surgeon. Although only 13 cases of ureteral injury in laparoscopy-related procedures have been reported in the literature, extreme care must be taken when dissecting within the pelvis[32]. All of the injuries reported were caused by cautery or CO_2 laser. These 13 cases occurred during gynecology-related procedures involving sterilization and endometriosis.

Diagnosis In none of the cases described in the literature was the diagnosis made intraoperatively. Usually patients tend to present 48–72 h postoperatively with abdominal pain and peritonitis, leukocytosis and fever. Flank tenderness or hematuria are rarely described. Sometimes an evaluation of the drained abdominal fluid including levels of urea and creatinine is helpful. The presence of ascites and/or a pelvic mass is constant on sonography, and the diagnosis is confirmed by intravenous pyelography.

Management The repair of ureteral injuries must be performed with the collaboration of the urological surgeon. Percutaneous or cystoscopic techniques can probably be used to manage most such injuries[32]. Exploratory laparoscopy and/or laparotomy are used for surgical repair in cases of end-to-end reanastomosis, reimplantation of the ureter to the bladder, transureteral ureterostomy and other techniques.

Prevention Unfortunately, direct visualization of the ureter is difficult at the time of pelviscopy. Although the ureter may be visualized through the peritoneum in the upper pelvis, it cannot be identified reliably in the area of the uterosacral ligaments. This is particulary true in the presence of endometriosis or pelvic adhesions. Also, some procedures such as laparoscopic hysterectomy, lymphadenectomy and laparoscopic uterine nerve ablation (LUNA) increase the risk of ureteral injuries[33]. Specific guidelines are unavailable to prevent this serious complication. Several general points must be considered:

(1) The operator must understand the anatomy of the pelvic ureter and appreciate its proximity to the cervix in cases of endometriosis or when performing LUNA or other risky procedures. Sometimes the dissection of the ureter may be helpful. Some have advocated using 'hydrodissection' or 'hydroprotection' to protect retroperitoneal structures[31,34]. This technique involves making a small incision on the lateral parietal peritoneum and inserting fluid into the retroperitoneal space. Hydroprotection is useful when using the laser.

(2) Electrocauterization must always be done under strict visual control of the structures lying under and around the field of application. Bipolar coagulation is preferred over monopolar coagulation[35]. However, it is erroneously assumed that bipolar coagulation is completely safe; in fact, it is safe only when the bipolar forceps is correctly positioned without touching the ureter, and when an appropriate coagulating time is calculated[32,36]. A lengthy coagulation induces a diffusion of thermal energy and the current may damage the vascular supply around the coagulated tissue leading to delayed tissue necrosis[37,38]. The operator must check the energy unit that he is using and ensure that it functions correctly. It appears that burn injuries are related to faults in the electrocoagulation equipment and its use. Faulty insulation of the cautery device may cause burns[39]. Also, the use of a hyperfrequenced electrocautery unit is preferable to other high-energy, spark-gap-type generators[40,41].

DISCUSSION

The increased use of laparoscopy as a therapeutic method necessitates a reappraisal of the risks involved. Complications frequently described include injuries to the large and small bowel, uterus, bladder, ureters and blood vessels. These risks, in addition to the risk of general anesthesia, have been increased by the addition of new devices and instruments for operative laparoscopy. Each complication has a specific etiology that is usually preventable or treatable if recognized in time. Usually complications of the first (blind) and second (visual) steps are recognized intraoperatively and treated, with a simple postoperative recovery. Complications of surgical procedures, specifically thermal injuries, are diagnosed postoperatively.

This is still a major problem with operative laparoscopy because delayed diagnosis worsens the prognosis and increases morbidity. Also this type of injury often requires repair by laparotomy. The exact percentage of laparoscopic complications is unknown. In Table 1, data of different studies are summarized. The complication rate requiring laparotomy varied from 0.7 to 2.7%. The likelihood of laparotomy being required

Table 1 Frequency of complications of laparoscopic surgery necessitating laparotomy

Authors	Year	n	Laparotomy n	Laparotomy (/1000)
Henry-Suchet *et al.*[42]	1984	9 662	14	(1.4)
Von Theobald *et al.*[43]	1990	1 429	03	(2.0)
Peterson *et al.*[44]	1990	36 928	96	(2.6)
Bruhat *et al.**	1991	7 604	21	(2.8)
Donnez and Nisolle*	1991	12 000	08	(0.7)

*, Personal data

Table 2 Complications of endoscopic surgery (laparoscopy, $n = 12\,000$)

Venous gas embolism	4
Subcutaneous emphysema	4
Pneumothorax	4
Bowel injuries	
perforation by the trocars	6
mesenteral hematoma	1
rectal perforation by the laser	2
(recto-vaginal endometriosis	
Ureteral injuries (delayed)	2

was directly related to the degree of complexity of the laparoscopic surgical procedure, and to the experience of the surgeon. Intestinal or ureteral injuries represented more than 60% of complications requiring laparotomy and in more than 50% of these cases the diagnosis was delayed. Major vessel injury or bladder injury occurred more commonly with trocars. Bowel and ureteral injury occurrences were more frequently caused by surgical procedures, and complications with thermal energy represented about 40% of these cases. According to data now available, there are numerous possible complications directly related to surgical laparoscopy. However, major complications are relatively rare when there are no technical complications (Table 2); technical complications are avoidable with experience. The rate of complications of the surgical procedure itself does not seem to be higher than that occurring during surgery by laparotomy[10,23].

CONCLUSIONS

With thousands of gynecological operative laparoscopies and hysteroscopies having been performed around the world, it has been shown that both procedures are extremely safe and effective. However, the possibility of complications must be kept in mind. Understanding these complications and how to assess them is the only way to avoid them in the future. Gynecological surgeons are now dealing with a host of new instruments and devices. As well as the anatomical knowledge required in their surgical training, a minimum of technical knowledge of the new instrumentation is recommended. For this purpose, the following are required:

(1) Didactic lectures on both laparoscopic and hysteroscopic procedures and their complications;

(2) Hands-on experience with live laboratory animals; and

(3) Preceptorship with experienced operators, or special residency training.

Respecting these conditions will enhance endoscopic surgery results and minimize the rate of complications.

REFERENCES

1. Kane, M.G. and Krejs, G.L. (1984). Complications of diagnostic laparoscopy in Dallas: A 7 year prospective study. *Gastrointest. Endosc.*, **30**, 237
2. Baadsgaard, S.E., Bille, S. and Egeblad, K. (1989). Major vascular injury during gynecologic laparoscopy. *Acta Obstet. Gynecol. Scand.*, **68**, 283
3. Lynn, C.S., Katz, R.A. and Ross, J.P. (1982). Aortic perforation sustained at laparoscopy. *J. Reprod. Med.*, **27**, 217
4. Rust, M., Buquoy, F. and Bonke, S. (1980). Retroperitoneale Gefäßverletzung bei gynäkologischen Laparoskopien. *Anästh. Intensivether. Notfallmed.*, **15**, 356
5. Heinrich, P., Jahn, R. and Neumann. A. (1985). Iatrogene Gefäßschäden im Beckenbereich. *ZbL. Gynäkol.*, **107**, 432
6. Erkrath, K.D., Weiler, G. and Adebahr, G. (1979). Zur Aortenverletzung bei Laparoskopie in der Gynäkologie. *Geburts. Frauenheilk.*, **39**, 687
7. Shin, C.S. (1982). Vascular injury secondary to laparoscopy. *NY State J. Med.*, 935
8. McDonald, P., Rich, N., Collins, G. Jr, Anderson, C. and Kozloff, L. (1978). Vascular trauma secondary to diagnostic and therapeutic procedures: laparoscopy. *Am. J. Surg.*, **135**, 651
9. Bisler, H., Sinde, J., Alemany, J. and Kunde, H.J. (1980). Verletzungen der großen Gefäße bei gynäkologischen laparoskopien. *Geburts. Frauenheilk*, **40**, 553
10. Bergqvist, D. and Bergqvist, A. (1987). Vascular injuries during gynecologic surgery. *Acta Obstet. Gynecol. Scand.*, **66**, 19
11. Corson, S.L. (1980). Major vessel injury during laparoscopy. *Am. J. Obstet. Gynecol.*, **138**, 589
12. Oshinsky, G.S. and Smith, A.D. (1992). Laparoscopic needles and trocars: an overview of designs and complications. *J. Laparoendosc. Surg.*, **2**, 117
13. Dingfelder, J.R. (1978). Direct laparoscope trocar insertion without prior pneumoperitoneum. *J. Reprod. Med.*, **21**, 45
14. Saidi, M.H. (1986). Direct laparoscopy without prior pneumoperitoneum. *J. Reprod. Med.*, **31**, 684
15. Copeland, C., Wing, R. and Hulka, J.F. (1983). Direct trocar insertion at laparoscopy: an evaluation. *Obstet. Gynecol.*, **62**, 655
16. Borgatta, L., Gruss, L., Barad, D. and Kaali, S. (1990). Direct trocar insertion versus Veress needle use for laparoscopic sterilization. *J. Reprod. Med.*, **35**, 891
17. Loffer, F.D. and Pent, D. (1975). Indications, contraindications and complications of laparoscopy. *Obstet. Gynecol. Surv.*, **30**, 407
18. Endler, G.C. and Moghissi, K.S. (1976). Gastric perforation during pelvic laparoscopy. *Obstet. Gynecol.*, **47** (Suppl.), 40S

19. Edgerton, W.D. (1974). Laparoscopy in the community hospital: safety, performance, control. *J. Reprod. Med.*, **12**, 239

20. Hirt, P.S. and Morris, R. (1982). Gastric bleeding secondary to laparoscopy in a patient with salpingitis. *Obstet. Gynecol.*, **59**, 655

21. Birns, M.T. (1989). Inadvertent instrumental perforation of the colon during laparoscopy: nonsurgical repair. *Gastrointest. Endosc.*, **35**, 54

22. Levy, B.S., Soderstrom, R.M. and Dail, D.H. (1985). Bowel injuries during laparoscopy, gross anatomy and histology. *J. Reprod. Med.*, **30**, 168

23. Krebs, H.B. (1986). Intestinal injury in gynecologic surgery: a ten year experience. *Obstet. Gynecol.*, **155**, 509

24. Corson, S.L., Batzer, F.R., Gocial, B. and Maislin, G. (1989). Measurement of the force necessary for laparoscopic trocar entry. *J. Reprod. Med.*, **34**, 282

25. Evans, M.R., Hulbert, C.J. and Reddy, K.P. (1992). Complications of laparoscopy. *Semin. Urol.*, **10**, 164

26. Kalhan, S.B. and Reaney, J.A. (1990). Pneumomediastinum and subcutaneous emphysema during laparoscopy. *Cleve. Clin. J. Med.*, **57**, 639

27. De Cherney, A.H. (1988). Laparoscopy with unexpected viscus penetration. In Nichols, D.H. (ed.) *Clinical Problems, Injuries and Complications of Gynecologic Surgery*, p.63. (Baltimore: Williams and Wilkins)

28. Peters, P.C. (1989). Intraperitoneal rupture of the bladder. *Urol. Clin. N. Am.*, **16**, 279

29. Reich, H. and McGlynn, F. (1990). Laparoscopic repair of bladder injury. *Obstet. Gynecol.*, **76**, 909

30. Corriere, J.N. Jr and Sandler, C.M. (1989). Management of extraperitoneal bladder rupture. *Urol. Clin. N. Am.*, **16**, 275

31. Donnez, J. (1989). Instrumentation and operational instructions. In Donnez, J. (ed.) *Laser Operative Laparoscopy and Hysteroscopy*, p.15. (Leuven: Nauwelaerts Printing)

32. Grainger, D.A., Soderstrom, R.M., Schiff, S.F., Glickman, M.G., De Cherney, A.H. and Diamond, M.P. (1990). Ureteral injuries at laparoscopy: insights into diagnosis, management and prevention. *Obstet. Gynecol.*, **75**, 839

33. Woodland, M.B. (1992). Ureter injury during laparoscopy-assisted vaginal hysterectomy with the endoscopic linear stapler. *Am. J. Obstet. Gynecol.*, **167**, 756

34. Nezhat, C. and Nezhat, F.R. (1989). Safe laser endoscopic excision or vaporization of peritoneal endometriosis. *Fertil. Steril.*, **52**, 149

35. Seiler, J.C., Gidwana, G. and Ballard, L. (1986). Laparoscopic cauterization of endometriosis for fertility. A controlled study. *Fertil. Steril.*, **46**, 1098

36. Bauman, H., Jaeger, P. and Huch, A. (1988). Ureteral injury after laparoscopic tubal sterilization by bipolar electrocoagulation. *Obstet. Gynecol.*, **71**, 483

37. Schwimmer, W.B. (1974). Electrosurgical burn injuries during laparoscopy sterilization. Treatment and prevention. *Obstet. Gynecol.*, **44**, 526

38. Jaffe, R.H., Willis, D. and Bachem, A. (1929). The effect of electric currents on the arteries. A histologic study. *Arch. Pathol.*, **7**, 244

39. Irvin, T.T., Goligher, J.C. and Scott, J.S. (1975). Injury to the ureter during laparoscopic tubal sterilization. *Arch. Surg.*, **110**, 1501

40. Levinson, C.J., Schwartz, S.F. and Saltzstein E.C. (1973). Complication of laparoscopic tubal sterilization: small bowel perforation. *Obstet. Gynecol.*, **41**, 253

41. Corson, S.L. and Bolognese, R.J. (1974). Electrosurgical hazards in laparoscopy. *J. Am Med. Assoc.*, **927**, 1261

42. Henry-Suchet, J., Tort-Grumbach J. and Loysel F. (1984). Complications des coelioscopies colligées par le Club Gynéco-informatique en 1980-1982. *Contr. Fertil. Sex.*, **12**, 901

43. Von Theobald, P., Marie, G., Herlicoviez, M. and Levy, G. (1990). Morbiditié et mortalité de la coelioscopie: étude rétrospective d'une série de 1429 cas. *Rev. Fr. Gynecol. Obstet.*, **85**, 611

44. Peterson, H.B., Hulka, J.F. and Phillips, J.M. (1990). American Association of Gynecologic Laparoscopists 1988: Membership survey on operative laparoscopy. *J. Reprod. Med.*, **35**, 587

Complications and precautions in operative laparoscopy

26

L. Van Obbergh and B. Gribomont

INTRODUCTION

Venous air embolism is one of the most commonly encountered iatrogenic mishaps. Although it has been described most frequently in relation to posterior fossa neurosurgery performed in the sitting position, there are many other situations in which it can occur[1-5]. The incidence of venous air embolism during gynecological endoscopy is, in fact, very low. The reported figures vary from 1/63 000 to 1/7500[6,7]. This event is so rare that it does not even get a mention in the present standard reference book on anesthesia[8]. However, during the last year we have seen four cases of venous air embolism, one of which was fatal. Although this does not seem to constitute an abnormal rate (roughly 1/8000), it has none the less caused great concern in our institution. We have thoroughly re-examined the whole problem and have since completely changed our monitoring policy, among other things.

Effects of air embolism

In the arterioles, the air causes an obstruction to blood flow and produces segmental arteriolar spasm. The most common way for air to enter the circulation, however, is through the venous system. The effect depends first on the rate of entry and second on the total volume[8,9].

Experimental slow infusion of air

When air slowly enters into the venous system, its bubbles collect in the right atrium, then pass into the right ventricle where they are churned into foam before being ejected into the pulmonary artery.

If the patient is not fully paralyzed by muscle relaxants and is breathing spontaneously, the first symptom of air embolism is a characteristic gasp. This gasp consists of a small cough, immediately followed by a brief expiration and then a long forced inspiration that is held for several seconds. This gasp reflex can cause a large bolus of air to be sucked into the still open vein, leading to death. In these circumstances controlled ventilation appears to be less dangerous. The gasp reflex is mediated via receptors in the lung and is abolished by cocaine nebulized through the endotracheal tube.

Right pulmonary arterial pressure increases markedly with a small venous air embolism but reaches a plateau which it does not exceed. Central venous pressure increases and can reach a maximum of almost 20 times the control values. Heart rate increases and blood pressure falls gradually, while peripheral resistance decreases markedly. Stroke volume can increase by 80%.

Experimental bolus infusion of air

In the case of a bolus infusion of air, there is no gasp, but there is a sudden rise in central venous pressure and a decrease in arterial blood pressure; at a later stage, an increase in heart rate can be expected. The cardiovascular collapse is due primarily to an air lock in the right side of the heart. The head-down position has been shown to have a protective effect[3,9]. There is a dramatic reversal of shock with aspiration of air from the atrium.

Nitrous oxide, which is 30 times more soluble than nitrogen, diffuses quickly into the bubbles, considerably increasing their size. However, the diffusion capacity of nitrous oxide is lower than that of CO_2, and thus nitrous oxide is not likely to increase the size of CO_2 bubbles. This is one of the reasons why air should never be used for inflation during gynecological procedures.

CO_2 is also five times less lethal than air. Following experiments on dogs it has been calculated that in humans, 1 l of CO_2 can be given intravenously before cardiac output is profoundly reduced.

MONITORING TECHNIQUES

Early in the 1970s it was demonstrated that a precordial ultrasonic Doppler device was extremely sensitive in detecting air embolism during neurosurgery[10]. However, Michenfelder[10] pointed out that precordial Doppler failed to detect air embolism in some cases; nevertheless, it was proved by air aspiration from the right side of the heart. The Doppler technique cannot be considered to be completely reliable in this situation. In heavy-breasted women, locating and securing the transducer on the right side of the sternum is practically impossible. During laparoscopy, the Trendelenburg position and the surgeon's compression and rubbing movements displace the transducer and produce artificial sound changes. Moreover, the noise produced by the device can prove to be almost intolerable for the surgeon. This monitor can not thus be considered an appropriate early warning system.

Recently, transesophageal echocardiography has been found to be as sensitive as precordial Doppler ultrasound in detecting experimental air embolism[11,12]. This technique offers the additional advantage of detecting left-sided air. However, transesophageal echocardiography, as well as Doppler, cannot quantify the size of the venous air embolism. In any case, the highly prohibitive price of transesophageal echocardiography makes it impracticable for routine gynecological endoscopy[13].

Following close behind precordial Doppler and transesophageal echocardiography comes the monitoring of pulmonary artery pressure[14], end-tidal CO_2 and transcutaneous O_2[15]. All of these are equally able to detect venous air embolism when definite changes in hemodynamics have already occurred but well before total cardiovascular collapse. Moreover, they are able to quantify the size of the venous air embolism and provide information on the cessation of air entrapment as the result of the treatment[16]. An esophageal stethoscope will help to eliminate false positives[17]. In cases of severe venous air embolism there is always a change in heart sounds. Clinical signs, such as blood pressure, heart rate, arrhythmias and central venous pressure, come too late to be useful as warning signals (Table 1).

Surgical procedures performed during hysteroscopy are more often associated with venous air embolism because of the high insufflation pressure (up to 150 mmHG), the high CO_2 output (up to 80 ml/min) and the relatively large surgical wound compared to the very small size of the uterine cavity[18]. However, during laparoscopy, the quantity of air which can pass into a vein is much greater. In certain difficult circumstances, such as in obese patients in whom high pressures are needed, the risk of venous air embolism is seriously increased.

In gynecological procedures, venous air embolism is usually sudden and therefore it is crucial to detect it immediately. Any delay in exsufflation and treatment can prove to be fatal.

Routine monitoring during anesthesia for gynecological laparoscopy and hysteroscopy should include the following:

(1) An esophageal stethoscope;

(2) A continuous end-tidal CO_2 analyzer;

(3) The close observation of pressure in the abdomen or the uterus which must be kept within predetermined limits; and

(4) In obese patients undergoing surgical laparoscopy, it could be wise to insert a catheter through the internal jugular vein into the right atrium prior to the procedure, as an extra precaution.

During laparoscopy, as soon as the end-tidal CO_2 drops, the abdominal pressure must be immediately reduced. If this maneuver is not followed by an increase in end-tidal CO_2 or if there is any sign of cardiovascular problems, a venous air embolism must be considered to have occurred and appropriate measures must be taken. The mechanical impairment of ventilation by overdistention reduces the output of CO_2 and is indeed a common false-positive sign of venous air embolism (Figures 1 and 2).

Differential diagnosis is provided by the esophageal stethoscope; if a mill-wheel murmur is heard, venous air embolism has occurred. But in all cases of cardiovascular impairment such as dysrhythmias or hypotension, venous air embolism is highly probable.

TREATMENT

It must be emphasized that the currently available monitoring techniques detect venous air embolism only at a rather late stage when impairment of circulation has already occurred. We can not afford any delay in diagnosis and treatment following a decrease in end-tidal CO_2.

Table 1 Methods of monitoring air embolism, and their characteristics

Method	Sensitivity	Detection delay	Comments
Precordial Doppler	before physiological changes	none	noisy, difficult to secure
Transesophageal echocardiography	before physiological changes	none	too expensive
Pulmonary pressures	early physiological changes	short	too invasive for minor surgery
Sudden reduction of end-tidal CO_2	early physiological changes	short	easy and non-invasive, to be combined with esophageal stethoscope
Esophageal stethoscope	with definite air embolism	depends on size of venous air embolism	very useful in making the differential diagnosis of reduction of end-tidal CO_2
Electrocardiogram	questionable	too late	electromechanical dissociation always possible

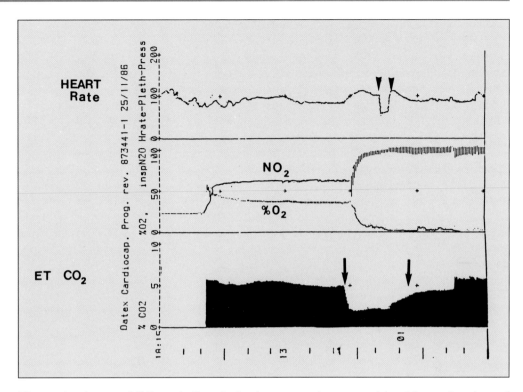

Figure 1   A case of CO_2 embolism during hysteroscopic surgery: (a) sudden and prolonged decrease in end-tidal CO_2 (arrows); (b) a severe bradycardia (arrowheads) was noted and was attributed to myocardial ischemia due to the passage of gas into the coronary arteries

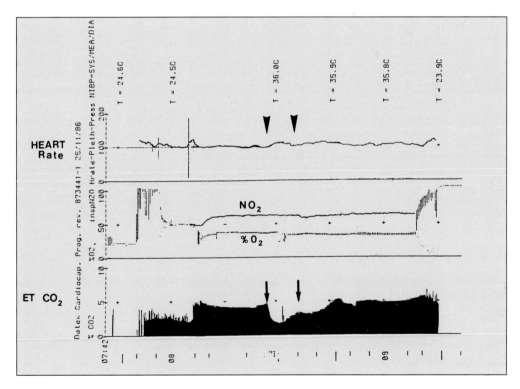

Figure 2   A case of ventilation impairment due to abdominal overdistention: (a) end-tidal CO_2 decrease but a more rapid recovery after abdominal exsufflation (arrows); (b) the heart rate remained unchanged (arrowheads)

When venous air embolism is considered probable, the patient should immediately be ventilated with 100% oxygen to prevent any hypoxemia. The Trendelenburg position should possibly be maintained as it has been shown experimentally to have a protective effect against shock[3,9]. A large catheter, always immediately available, is quickly fed into the right atrium via the internal jugular vein. Aspiration of gas confirms the embolism and produces dramatic relief from the symptoms of cardiovascular collapse. Standard cardiovascular supportive measures are also immediately taken.

As a large bolus results in a sudden cardiac arrest or at least in an asphygmia (an electromechanical dissociation), diagnosis can be established very rapidly and air can be aspirated quickly, probably making the treatment more successful.

Unfortunately, in approximately 30% of patients, a passage remains open between the right and the left sides of the heart. Air is thus able to pass into the aorta, the coronary arteries and the cerebral arteries and this can aggravate an already critical situation, making cardiac resuscitation even more difficult[19].

CONCLUSIONS

Surgical gynecological laparoscopy and hysteroscopy should not be considered trivial procedures. We can not say at present that laser surgery on its own increases the risk of venous air embolism, but it remains a possible complication even if severe cases are extremely rare. For the sake of our patients' safety, we must become more aware of the risks involved, instead of ignoring this rare eventuality. Sooner or later, it will occur.

Only teams well aware of the problems and well prepared to cope with them will be able to spare their patients any permanent damage. In surgical gynecological laparoscopy and hysteroscopy, we strongly recommend the routine monitoring of end-tidal CO_2. This monitoring is, in any case, well on its way to becoming standard procedure during anesthesia. In the meantime, the first available capnographs in an operating area should be used during these mostly elective procedures.

REFERENCES

1. Root, B., Levy, M.N., Pollack, S., Lubert, M. and Pathak, K. (1978). Gas embolism death after laparoscopy delayed by 'trapping' in portal circulation. *Anesth. Analg.*, **57**, 232–7
2. Naulty, J.S., Meisel, L.B., Datta, S. and Ostheimer, G.W. (1982). Air embolism during radical hysterectomy. *Anesthesiology*, **57**, 420–2
3. Yacoub, O.F., Cardona, I., Covelier, L.A. and Dodson, M.G. (1982). Carbon dioxide embolism during laparoscopy. *Anesthesiology*, **57**, 533–5
4. Albin, M.S. (1983). Venous air embolism is not restricted to neurosurgery! *Anesthesiology*, **59**, 151
5. Shupak, R.C., Shuster, H. and Funch, R.S. (1984). Airway emergency in a patient during CO_2 arthroscopy. *Anesthesiology*, **60**, 171–2
6. Wadhwa, R.K., McKenzie, R., Wadhwa, S.R., Katz, D.L. and Byers, J.F. (1978). Gas embolism during laparoscopy. *Anesthesiology*, **48**, 74–6
7. Yacoub, O.F., Cardona, I., Coveler, L.A. and Dodson, M. (1982). Carbon dioxide embolism during laparoscopy. *Anesthesiology*, **57**, 533–5
8. Schapiro, H.M. (1986). Neurological anesthesia and intracranial hypertension. In Miller, R. (ed.) *Anesthesia*, p.1563, 2nd edn. (New York)
9. Adornato, D.C., Gildenberg, P.L., Ferrario, M., Smart, J. and Frost, E.A.M. (1978). Pathophysiology of intravenous air embolism in dogs. *Anesthesiology*, **49**, 120–7
10. Michenfelder, J.D., Miller, R.H. and Gronert, G.A. (1972). Evaluation of an ultrasonic device (Doppler) for the diagnosis of venous air embolism. *Anesthesiology*, **36**, 164–7
11. Furuya, H., Suzuki, T. Okumura, F., Kishi, Y. and Uefuji, T. (1983). Detection of air embolism by transoesophageal echardiography. *Anesthesiology*, **58**, 124–9
12. Martin, R.W. and Colley, P.S. (1983). Evaluation of transoesophageal Doppler detection of air embolism in dogs. *Anesthesiology*, **58**, 117–23
13. Albin, M.S. (1983). The sights and sounds of air. *Anesthesiology*, **58**, 113–14
14. Marshall, W.K. and Bedford, R.F. (1980). Use of a pulmonary-artery catheter for detection and treatment of venous air embolism: a prospective study in man. *Anesthesiology*, **52**, 131–4
15. Glenski, J.A. and Cucchiara, R.F. (1986). Transcutaneous O_2 and CO_2 monitoring of neurosurgical patients: detection of air embolism. *Anesthesiology*, **64**, 546–50
16. English, J.B., Westenskow, D., Hodges, M.R. and Stanley, T.H. (1978). Comparison of venous air embolism monitoring. Methods in supine dogs. *Anesthesiology*, **48**, 425–9
17. Glenski, J.A., Cucchiara, R.F. and Michenfelder, J.D. (1986). Transoesophageal echocardiography and transcutaneous O_2 and CO_2 monitoring for detection of venous air embolism. *Anesthesiology*, **64**, 541–5
18. Gomar, C., Fernandez, C., Villalonga, A. and Nalda, M.A. (1985). Carbon dioxide embolism during laparoscopy and hysteroscopy. *Ann. Fr. Anesth. Reanim.*, **4**, 380–2
19. Hagen, P.T., Scholz, D.G. and Edwards, W.D. (1984). Incidence and size of patent foramen ovale during the first 10 decades of life: an autopsy study of 965 normal hearts. *Mayo Clin. Proc.*, **59**, 17–20

Section II

Operative hysteroscopy

Instrumentation

27

J. Donnez and M. Nisolle

Hysteroscopy was first reported by Pantaleoni in 1969[1]. He used a 12 mm diameter straight tube that was inserted into the uterine cavity with a concave mirror to reflect light into the uterus.

HYSTEROSCOPES

Rigid endoscopes

There are three main types of rigid endoscopes in use today: the panoramic hysteroscope, the contact hysteroscope and the microcolpohysteroscope.

The panoramic hysteroscope

This basically consists of a telescope and an outer sheath of stainless steel. The telescope contains an optical system for transmitting the image and an illumination system. The outer sheath contains side channels for the introduction of media or instruments. The telescopes range from 4 to 6 mm in diameter, the metallic sheaths from approximately 5.2 to 8 mm in diameter. The optical systems are designed to give a direct view (0 degree) or a range of oblique views, for which the 30° lens is most versatile.

The contact hysteroscope

The instrument consists of an optical glass stem that serves both as a conductor of light to the object being examined and as the conduit for the returning image, which is magnified. These hysteroscopes range from 4 mm to 6 or 8 mm[2,3] in outer diameter. The light source is ambient light from the room or from directed light collected by the translucent light collector on the hysteroscope. The 4 mm endoscope requires no cervical dilatation but the principal disadvantage of this instrument is a decrease in the visual field, preventing panoramic examination.

The microcolpohysteroscopes

The Hamou microcolpohysteroscope (Figure 1) utilizes a 4 mm telescope and a 5.2 mm outer sheath. The original instrument was capable of four magnifications: 1x, 30x, 60x, and 150x. The first two settings were designed for panoramic hysteroscopy and the last two for microscopic examination. Ancillary equipment required includes a cold-light source of 150 W, a flexible fiberoptic cable for light transmission, and a hysteroflator for CO_2 distension of the endometrial cavity for panoramic hysteroscopy. Microcolpohysteroscopy using the Hamou endoscope can be carried out to examine the squamocolumnar junction[4]. The procedure involves the use of 2% Lugol's solution applied to the exocervix followed by colposcopic examination with the endoscope using the 20x magnification. The microhysteroscope is then switched to the 60x magnification, and cytologic examination of the squamous epithelium is completed after staining with Waterman blue solution pH5.

Flexible endoscopes

Flexible endoscopes (Figure 2), which can be guided and deflected to observe the lateral portions of the uterus, particularly the uterotubal cones, can also deliver flexible instruments, catheters, or fibers that are directed or deflected by an operator-controlled steering mechanism. Such instruments are available in different sizes: 4 mm outer diameter for diagnostic purposes and 5 mm in diameter with an operating channel. The flexibility of the distal end permits the introduction of the instrument and inspection of the lateral areas of the uterus. The small-diameter endoscope permits the insertion of fibers that can deliver laser energy to areas which are difficult to reach with rigid instruments. This is particularly helpful for ablation of the endometrium or for the treatment of laterally located lesions such as intrauterine adhesions, which are difficult to reach using rigid ancillary instruments with currently available hysteroscopes[5,6].

An innovative approach to the examination of the uterine cavity, particularly the first portion of the intramural Fallopian tubes, involves the use of small flexible optical catheters from 1 to 3 mm in outer diameter, which can be inserted atraumatically without cervical dilatation and can be illuminated with portable battery-operated units. Furthermore, these catheters could be used as a mini-endoscope delivered through the standard hysteroscope.

Office hysteroscopes

A self-contained apparatus for office hysteroscopy incorporates in a single easily portable unit, the endoscope, a cold light source, and a CO_2 insufflator. This instrument was designed by Parent and colleagues in 1985[7] and is manufactured by the Richard Wolf Company.

The telescope is a 4 mm diameter forward-oblique endoscope. The gas comes from a cartridge or pellet that fits laterally into the instrument and contains 4 l of pressurized CO_2. The operator regulates the pressure of gas delivered by rotating the gadget from position zero to positions one and two. The gas delivery unit has a specially encased self-protection valve to vent the CO_2 in case of failure or excessive pressure.

Light is provided by a miniature projector equipped with a halogen microlamp weighing less that 50 g. The projector is connected by a cord to the power source, which consists of three rechargeable cadmium–nickel batteries.

Operative hysteroscopes

Several instruments are used in operative hysteroscopy, including biopsy and grasping forceps, miniature scissors, electrodes, probes, and catheters. New hysteroscopes have been developed that have double channels for inflow and outflow (Figure 3). These new continuous flow hysteroscopes (CFH) are equipped with completely separate in- and outflow channels for the distending medium. They are especially suitable for use with low viscosity fluids, which cannot be employed with single flow hysteroscopes. Indeed, with single flow hysteroscopes, there is a high risk of fluid overload[8,9]. The CFH provides constant irrigation of the uterine cavity, thus ensuring an optimal view. This is particularly important in patients with uterine bleeding. The CFH may be particularly useful in allowing simultaneous surgery and washing or aspiration and may prove to be of great value in laser ablation of the endometrium and other operative laser procedures. The modified urologic resectoscope has been used extensively with the coagulating loop (Figure 4). The use of video cameras for direct observation during diagnostic and operative procedures has already become a routine practice for many endoscopists (Figure 5). With new computerized units, the problem of less than optimal resolution and reliability has been resolved so that videosurgery through the hysteroscope can now be used more extensively, particularly in teaching situations, to allow assistants and participants to better observe this essentially dynamic procedure.

DISTENDING MEDIA

Rubin first introduced the use of CO_2 gas as a distending agent[10]. Other agents that have been frequently employed are dextran 70 (Hyskon) and low viscosity fluids.

Carbon dioxide

CO_2 insufflation of the uterine cavity was first achieved using a cervical suction cup to minimize egress of the gas. Suction cups are, however, not necessary. With CO_2 as the cervical dilator, the hysteroscope is slowly advanced, under direct vision, into the uterus. The continuous flow of CO_2 compensates for loss of gas through the Fallopian tubes and by absorption. Use of CO_2 as the distension medium provides excellent visibility of the uterine cavity and is conducive to photographic recording of findings. However, troublesome gas bubbles can form and obscure the view if there is fluid or mucus within the uterine cavity. In addition, surgical manipulation is more difficult using CO_2, as bleeding rapidly becomes a significant hindrance.

Use of CO_2 as a distension medium for hysteroscopy is safe. No change occurs in electrocardiograms, pCO_2, or pH in patients during CO_2 hysteroscopy[11]. However, intravasation is a potential risk. Bubbles of gas have been observed moving about in the vessels of the infundibulo-pelvic ligament in patients having simultaneous laparoscopy.

In experiments on dogs, increasing the flow to more than 400 ml/min results in the appearance of tachypnea and arrhythmias, and a flow of 1000 ml/min for 60 s is lethal[12]. These complications should not occur clinically when using the instruments developed for hysteroscopy, but certain conditions such as uterine tuberculosis, proximal tubal obstruction, or submucous leiomyomata are predisposed to these complications. Gallinot and Lueken[13] have developed a smoke evacuator for continuous gas circulation.

Dextran 70

Dextran 70 (Hyskon) was introduced as a distension medium for hysteroscopy by Edström and Fernström[14]. Hyskon is composed of 32% dextran (molecular weight 70 000) in 10% dextrose. This mixture is optically clear, electrolyte free, non-conductive, biodegradable, and immiscible with blood.

Hysteroscopic procedures employing Hyskon for uterine distension are usually performed under general anesthesia, because many procedures combine operative hysteroscopy and laparoscopy. A typical diagnostic hysteroscopy with no pathological findings requires 10–15 min and 50–100 ml of Hyskon. Operative hysteroscopy procedures take 15–30 min and frequently require as much as 200 ml of Hyskon.

The greatest advantage of Hyskon as the distension medium is its immiscibility with blood. For this reason, it has become the medium of choice when surgical hysteroscopy is perfomed. The use of dextran 70 is commonly associated with dilatation of the cervical canal: this can introduce artefacts because strips of

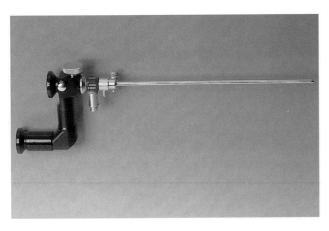

Figure 1 The 'Hamou' microcolpohysteroscope with Hopkins forward-oblique telescope 30°. Diameter 4 mm

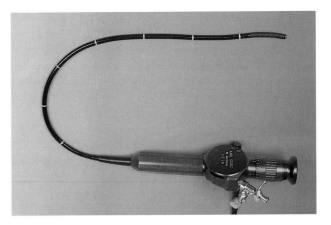

Figure 2 Flexible fiberoptic hysteroscope. Instrument channel, 1.2 mm; direction of view, 0°; viewing angle, 100°; working length, 530 mm; outer diameter, 4.4 mm

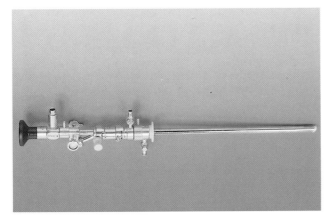

Figure 3(a) Continuous flow hysteroscope equipped with completely separate in and out outflow channels

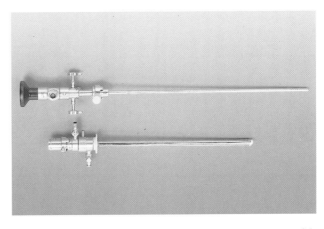

Figure 3(b) Continuous flow hysteroscope, with working element (above) and double sheath with two separate channels (below)

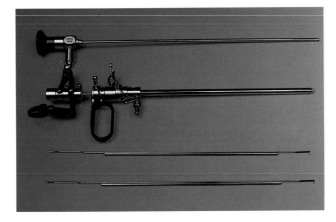

Figure 4 Myoma resectoscope. Working element, motion by means of a spring cutting loop

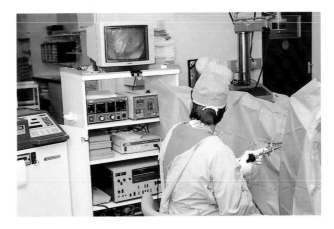

Figure 5 Use of video cameras. Videosurgery through the hysteroscope can be used in teaching situations

endometrium can become dislodged. When these dislodgements are anchored at one pole, they can easily be confused with polyps. In fact, studies comparing the diagnostic use of CO_2 versus dextran 70 as a distending medium have shown a high incidence of false-positive results with the latter, probably due to the cervical dilatation procedure. Hyskon is, therefore, recommended for surgical hysteroscopy under anesthesia, whereas CO_2 is preferred for office diagnostic hysteroscopy.

The use of Hyskon is associated with potential complications. Anaphylactic reactions to dextran have been described in patients after intravenous injection. Their estimated incidence is very low, only 1/10 000 cases[15]. Such anaphylactic reations could be due to the presence of IgG antibodies generated previously in response to beet sugars. Alternatively, these rare occurrences may in some cases be due to unidentified air emboli or be anesthesia-related phenomena rather than an anaphylactic response to Hyskon.

Liquid distension media such as Hyskon may introduce endometrial tissue into the peritoneal cavity[16]. Although the potential for this tissue to initiate endometriosis is unclear, intraperitoneal implantation is one of the classic theories about the pathogenesis of this disease.

Another disadvantage of Hyskon is its high viscosity, and its stickiness upon drying can cause jamming of instruments if they are not thoroughly cleaned in warm water after each use.

Low viscosity fluids

Low viscosity fluids such as 5% or 10% dextrose in water, 4% or 6% dextran, and 1.5% glycine provide adequate distension of the uterine cavity. The fluid is placed in a plastic container wrapped in a blood pressure cuff inflated to 80–120 mmHg in order to maintain a constant pressure and flow of the fluid into the uterine cavity. Approximately 250 ml is used in 10 min.

The view is initially clear, but the field becomes obscured rapidly due to egress of fluid through the cervix. In addition, because dextrose is miscible with blood, the view becomes impaired, and constant rinsing is necessary. A simple procedure to clean the uterine cavity is to introduce a fine polyethylene catheter through the operating channel of the endoscope. This catheter is attached to a 20 ml syringe containing the distension medium.

In our department, 1.5% glycine solution was chosen for its excellent optical and non-hemolytic properties during endoscopic hysteroscopic surgery. This electrolyte-free solution is widely used by urologists during transurethral resections. When electrical energy is used inside the uterine cavity, it is essential to use a distension fluid which is electrolyte-free and does not conduct electricity. Excessive absorption of such an electrolyte-free solution can be associated with

hyponatremia and hemolysis[9,10,17]. Glycine is metabolized in the body to urea, creatinine, serine, pyruvate and glutamine with production of ammonia. Ammonium toxicity may be an important cause of ecephalopathy in some patients[10].

The advantages of low viscosity fluids are numerous. These fluids are less expensive, readily available, cause less pain, and the risks of media intravasation are reduced. However, there is a potential risk of anaphylactic reactions when dextran is used.

In our department, glycine solution is used as the distending medium in the operating room while CO_2 is used as medium in outpatient diagnostic hysteroscopy.

Saline solution

Normal saline solution (0.9% NaCl) is optically clear, cheap and easily available. The concentration of electrolytes is similar to that of blood and it is metabolically inert. Normal saline solution is miscible with blood. If the view becomes impaired, rinsing is necessary. Continuous flow hysteroscopes provide a constant irrigation of the uterine cavity so that saline solution can be used even when there is bleeding in the uterine cavity. Saline cannot be used if electrical instruments are employed, but can be used concomitantly with the Nd : YAG laser. Excess intravasation is not associated with any major electrolyte or metabolic disturbances and any fluid overload can rapidly be reversed with diuretic therapy alone[10].

Nd : YAG LASER HYSTEROSCOPY

Both the electrical current of the resectoscope and the energy of the Nd : YAG laser have proved to be effective tools in the destruction of endometrial tissue to sufficient depth to avoid regeneration. The resectoscope has a possible disadvantage, however, since it is a unipolar electrical instrument. There is, therefore, the potential for damage to the bowel or bladder from the current transmitted through the uterine wall or by actual penetration of the uterine wall with the cutting loop. In addition, there is the risk of bleeding if major uterine vessels are transected by cutting too deeply into the uterine wall. On the other hand, the resectoscope has an advantage over the laser in that the equipment is readily available in most operating rooms. It does not, therefore, require the major capital investment needed for a laser.

Laser energy has some advantages in precision of tissue destruction that are not shared by the electrical energy used in the resectoscopes. The most popular laser in gynecology has been the CO_2 laser, so it is natural that an effort has been made to adapt this for hysteroscopic use[18]. However, several features of the CO_2 laser make it impractical for hysteroscopic use.

First, the CO_2 beam must be reflected through a series of mirrors into the uterine cavity, which is awkward and difficult. Light guides to direct the CO_2 laser beam are still in a developmental stage. Second, the tissue effect of the CO_2 laser beam is primarily one of vaporization. Here, precise vaporization is not required, since the purpose of endometrial ablation is to destroy large areas of tissue to a depth of 4–5 mm. Third, the CO_2 laser beam is absorbed by fluids; therefore only a gaseous distending medium can be used during hysteroscopy. Finally, because a gaseous distending medium is employed, evacuating the plume from CO_2 laser vaporization becomes problematic, since even a minute pressure imbalance will cause the uterus to contract and the intrauterine view to be lost.

There are three reasons why the Nd:YAG laser is readily adaptable for hysteroscopic endometrial ablation:

(1) Its ability to transmit the beam of energy easily into the uterine cavity by means of a flexible quartz fiber;

(2) Its ability to transmit laser energy to the tissue surface through a liquid distending medium;

(3) Its ability to penetrate tissue to a controlled depth (Table 1).

Argon and KTP 532 lasers have some of the same advantages for hysteroscopic work; both can be carried by fiberoptic light guides and can penetrate water. However, neither has the ability to penetrate tissue as well as the Nd:YAG laser.

Table 1 Nd:YAG laser: physics

1064/1318 nm (infrared)
Absorption in tissue protein
Mechanism coagulation
High penetration of tissue (4–6 mm)
Fiberoptic delivery system
Transmissible through fluid

Tissue effects of the Nd:YAG laser

The ability of this laser to penetrate the uterine wall and cause damage to the bowel and bladder is limited, since tissue destruction occurs to a depth of only about 5 mm. Although some energy from the laser beam may penetrate more deeply into the uterine musculature and potentially even further, it does little more than cause a slight temperature rise in that tissue. The temperature does not rise enough to denature the enzyme system and therefore does not lead to necrosis. The depth at which tissue destruction occurs can be controlled by varying the power used.

Another study that demonstrated the safety of the Nd:YAG laser for endometrial ablation used extirpated uteri with thermocouples placed 1 cm below the surface of the endometrium[19]. The laser beam was set at 55 W and directed for 5 s at the tissue over the thermocouples. A temperature of less than 50°C was measured 1 cm below the endometrial surface. The uterine wall, which is, on average, 1.5 cm in thickness, and other deep structures are therefore safe.

Hysteroscopic equipment

The quartz fiber used to carry the laser beam is surrounded by a thin plastic jacket, beyond which the tip of the fiber extends for several millimeters. The fiber is gas sterilized or wiped with alcohol or cidex prior to use. The laser power is generally set between 50 and 75 W.

There are several hysteroscopic instruments available for endometrial ablation. The first instrument used was a cystoscope designed for the Nd:YAG laser. It has a deflecting arm, which stabilizes the quartz fiber, and an integrated bundle that screws into a compatible operative port. The advantages of this instrument are that there is no leakage of fluid at the junction of the fiber and the hysteroscope and that the fiber can be manipulated within the uterine cavity. The disadvantage of this instrument is its inability to aspirate the interior of the uterine cavity to remove debris during the procedure. In order to clean the uterine cavity, a standard hysteroscope with or without a deflecting mechanism may also be used (Figure 6a). These instruments allow the removal of debris through an outflow tube. The disadvantage of this instrumentation is that the laser fiber and the outflow catheter cannot be used concomitantly. The deflecting arm is not of particular value, since the interior of the uterine cavity is not large enough to allow the fiber to be flexed at right angles to the uterine wall. There is now a hysteroscopic bridge available (Storz) (Figure 6b) using the standard telescope and sheath; it has two operating channels, allowing the quartz fiber to be placed down one channel and held in place at the end of the hysteroscope, and the outflow catheter (Figure 7) to be inserted through the second channel for cleaning out blood, bubbles and debris, which would otherwise obscure vision.

The technique used by the author to provide constant uterine distension involves attaching two 3000 ml plastic bags of glycine solution to dual blood infusion tubing[20]. Each bag is then wrapped in a pressure infusion cuff similar to that used to infuse blood under pressure. The tubing is connected to the hysteroscope. As soon as one bag begins to empty, the nurse notifies the surgeon that the bag will have to be changed. The outflow catheter cannot be opened during this time, because this will cause the uterine pressure to drop and bleeding to occur.

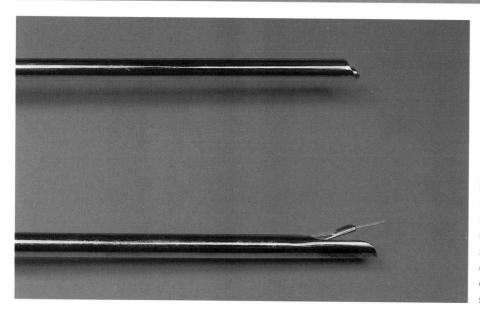

Figure 6(a)   Deflecting arm; (b) the hysteroscopic bridge (Storz) and the operating sheath allow concomitant use of the laser fiber and the outflow catheter, and connection of tubing for uterine distension using 1.5% glycine solution

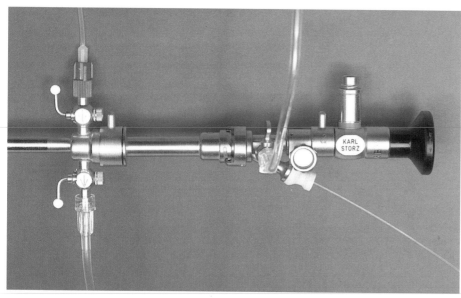

Figure 6(b)   *See legend above*

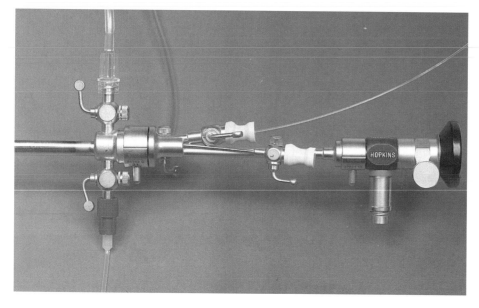

Figure 7   Hysteroscopic bridge (Storz) with two operating channels allowing the quartz fiber to be placed down one channel and the outflow catheter (or another flexible instrument, such as biopsy forceps) to be inserted through the second channel

REFERENCES

1. Pantoleoni, D. (1969). On endoscopic examination of the cavity of the womb. *Med. Press Circ.*, **8**, 26

2. Baggish, M.S. (1979). Contact hysteroscopy. A new technique to explore the uterine cavity. *Obstet. Gynecol.*, **54**, 350

3. Barbot, J., Parent, B. and Dubuisson, J.B. (1980). Contact hysteroscopy: another method of endoscopic examination of the uterine cavity. *Am. J. Obstet. Gynecol.*, **136**, 721

4. Hamou, J. (1981). Microhysteroscopy: a new procedure and its original applications in gynecology. *J. Reprod. Med.*, **26**, 375

5. Cornier, E. (1984). Intérêt de la fibroscopie utérine souple. *Contracept. Fertil. Sexual.*, **12**, 891

6. Cornier, E. (1984). La fibro-hystéroscopie opératoire souple: technique, indications, premiers résultats. *Gynécologie.*, **35**, 281

7. Parent, B., Guedj, H., Barbot, J. *et al.* (1987). *Panoramic Hysteroscopy*. Translated edition. (Baltimore: Williams & Wilkins)

8. Donnez, J. (1989). Instrumentation. In Donnez, J. (ed.) *Laser Operative Laparoscopy and Hysteroscopy*, pp.207–21. (Leuven: Nauwelaerts Printing)

9. Van Boven, M., Singelyn, F., Donnez, J. and Gbibolont, B. (1989). Dilutional hyponatremia associated with intrauterine endoscopic laser surgery. *Anesthesia*, **71**, 449–50

10. Rubin, I.C. (1925). Uterine endoscopy, endometroscopy with the aid of uterine insufflation. *Am. J. Obstet. Gynecol.*, **10**, 313

11. Hulf, J.A., Corall, I.M. Knights, K.M. *et al.* (1979). Blood carbon dioxide tension changes during hysteroscopy. *Fertil. Steril.*, **32**, 193

12. Lindemann, H.J., Mohr, J., Gallinat, A. *et al.* (1976). Der Einfluss von CO_2-gas während der Hysteroscopie. *Geburtshilfe Frauenheilk.*, **36**, 153

13. Gallinot, A. (1993). Hysteroscopic treatment of submucous fibroids using the Nd‑YAG laser and modern electrical equipment. In Lucken, R.P. and Gallinot, A. (eds.) *Endoscopic Surgery in Gynecology*, pp.72–88. (Berlin: Demeter Verlag GmBH)

14. Edström, K. and Fernström, I. (1970). The diagnostic possibilities of a modified hysteroscopic technique. *Acta Obstet. Gynaecol. Scand.*, **49**, 327

15. Borten, M., Seibert, C.P. and Taymor, M.L. (1983). Recurrent anaphylactic reaction to intra-peritoneal dextran 75 used for prevention of postsurgical adhesions. *Obstet. Gynecol.*, **61**, 755

16. Nagel, T.C., Kopher, R.A., Tagatz, G.E. *et al.* (1984). Tubal reflux of endometrial tissue during hysteroscopy. In Siegler, A.M. and Lindermann, H.J. (eds.) *Hysteroscopy; Principles and Practice*, p.145. (Philadelphia: J.B. Lippincott)

17. Nisolle, M., Grandjean, P., Gillerot, G. and Donnez, J. (1991). Endometrial ablation with the Nd‑YAG laser in dysfunctional bleeding. *Min. Invasive Ther.*, **1**, 35–9

18. Tadir, Y., Raif, J. *et al.* (1984). Hysteroscope for CO_2 laser application. *Lasers Surg. Med.*, **4**, 153

19. Goldrath, M.H., Fuller, T. and Segal, S. (1981). Laser photovaporization of endometrium for the treatment of menorrhagia. *Am. J. Obstet. Gynecol.*, **140**, 14

20. Loffer, F.D. (1987). Hysteroscopic endometrial ablation with the Nd‑YAG laser using a non-touch technique. *Obstet. Gynecol.*, **69**, 679

Hysteroscopy in the diagnosis of specific disorders

28

J. Donnez, M. Nisolle, A. Charles, M. Berlière and M. Smets

A wide variety of conditions can be diagnosed hysteroscopically, and hysteroscopy has become a diagnostic gold standard against which other methods are assessed. Conditions amenable to hysteroscopic diagnosis include abnormal uterine bleeding, infertility and recurrent abortion, uterine and cervical cancer, location of intrauterine devices, complicated abortion, and fetal examination. Physiological studies are also possible.

INFERTILITY

Hysteroscopy is becoming an important tool in the evaluation of infertility in women[1]. Evaluation of the endometrial cavity by either hysterosalpingography or hysteroscopy should be performed early. Hysteroscopic abnormalities are common in infertile patients; intrauterine abnormalities have been detected in 19–62% of infertile women in some studies[2]. Abnormal findings include intrauterine synechiae, Müllerian fusion defects (arcuate, septate, or bicornuate uterus), endometrial polyps, and submucous myomas.

Müllerian anomalies

Müllerian anomalies may be associated with normal fertility, infertility, or recurrent abortion. The extent of the anomaly can range from complete agenesis of the Müllerian system to minimal deformities of the uterine form. Diagnosis usually requires combined hysteroscopy and laparoscopy. The presence of a uterine filling defect at hysterosalpingography or at hysteroscopy should be further evaluated by laparoscopy. The defect may represent a uterine septum (Figure 1), a bicornuate uterus, or a submucous myoma. Rudimentary uterine horns, another form of Müllerian anomaly, can be detected laparoscopically and their relationship with the main cavity evaluated hysteroscopically.

Intrauterine synechiae

Traumatic intrauterine adhesions (Asherman's syndrome) (Figure 2) usually result from manipulation of the endometrial cavity following pregnancy. Curettage performed postpartum or following an abortion may cause scarring and synechiae secondary to the destruction of the basal layer of the endometrium. Patients may present with hypomenorrhea, amenorrhea, infertility, or spontaneous pregnancy loss. Recurrent abortion and abnormalities of implantation and placental development have also been described in association with this condition.

Intrauterine synechiae can be diagnosed by hysterosalpingography or hysteroscopy. The hysterosalpingogram shows a small, fragmented and distorted uterine cavity. The hysteroscopic image consists of pale endometrial patches and fibrotic strands, crossing the endometrial cavity. The adhesions are paler than the surrounding endometrium.

A hysteroscopic diagnosis of intrauterine adhesions is essential, as the disease can be missed or mistakenly diagnosed by hysterosalpingography. Hysteroscopy also permits a better assessment of the extent of the adhesions, an important factor in determining therapy and prognosis.

Submucous myomas

Uterine myomas can be found in a variety of locations. Those protruding into the uterine lumen are a common cause of abnormal uterine bleeding and may lead to infertility. Submucous myomas cause infertility by a variety of mechanisms related to embryo implantation. They can also cause preterm or dysfunctional labor. Submucous myomas are suspected in patients with enlarged uteri and those in whom filling defects are detected by hysterosalpingography. The hysterosalpingographic suspicion of the lesions should be confirmed by hysteroscopy. At hysteroscopy, the tumor is seen to protrude into the uterine cavity (Figure 3) and is covered with pale endometrium. Submucous myomas can be distinguished from endometrial polyps. In addition to providing definitive diagnosis, hysteroscopy can reveal more accurately the localization of the tumor and permit a better assessment of its size. The degree of intramural involvement cannot be determined.

Tubal disease

Involvement and occlusion of the intramural portion of the Fallopian tubes may be detected hysteroscopically. The significance of these lesions and their relationship to infertility has not been clearly established. Transuterine evaluation of tubal status prior to tuboplasty has been recommended[3]. The value of this method is debatable, however, as it is difficult to perform and the same information can be obtained by a simple hysterosalpingogram.

Endometritis

Endometritis. is a potential cause of infertility and recurrent pregnancy loss.

Sperm migration test

Hysteroscopy has been used to assess the survival of spermatozoa in the upper genital tract. Using a CO_2 hysteroscope, spermatozoa are obtained from the uterine cavity and the tubal ostia following intercourse and their motility is assessed.

Gamete intrafallopian transfer and zygote intrafallopian transfer

Because the hysteroscope provides an excellent means of delivering instrumentation or substances to the Fallopian tubes from the uterine side, several techniques of intratubal manipulation have been attempted, such as tubal insemination and the postcoital test. More recently, hysteroscopy has been used with the techniques of gamete intrafallopian transfer (GIFT) and zygote intrafallopian transfer (ZIFT) to transfer the gametes or the zygote into the Fallopian tubes from the uterine side, rather than from the fimbriated end by laparoscopy or minilaparotomy.

It is possible that, with experience and simplification of the out-patient hysteroscopy, this may become a routine study for candidates for in vitro fertilization to evaluate the maturity or dysmaturity of the endometrium and predict the likelihood of implantation[4]. Furthermore, the transfer of the early embryo could be accomplished under visual control.

Abortion

In cases of abortion, hysteroscopy is useful to check the presence or absence of trophoblastic tissue (Figure 4). Echography, computerized tomography, magnetic resonance imaging and hysteroscopy can help in the diagnosis of a suspected hydatidiform mole.

ABNORMAL UTERINE BLEEDING

The common causes of abnormal uterine bleeding differ with age. In the early pubertal years, abnormal bleeding is usually dysfunctional and only rarely associated with an organic lesion. Dysfunctional bleeding often responds favorably to hormonal manipulation, and hysteroscopy is not usually needed. On occasion, however, persistent or severe bleeding may signal uterine pathology, such as endometrial polyps (Figure 5), myomas or adenomyosis

(Figure 6). In the reproductive years, pregnancy-related complications are the most common cause of abnormal bleeding. Hysteroscopy is of value in some patients with retained products of conception following a spontaneous or induced abortion, which can be difficult to locate by dilatation and curettage. Uterine myomas and endometrial and cervical polyps are also a common cause of abnormal bleeding in this age group. Polyps tend to move with the flow of the distension medium, whereas submucous myomas, which may have a similar appearance, do not. Evaluation should consist of endometrial sampling, hysterosalpingography and hysteroscopy.

In postmenopausal women with abnormal uterine bleeding, uterine and cervical neoplasia must be excluded. Hysteroscopy can serve as an adjunct to other diagnostic methods in patients in whom abnormal bleeding persists. Atrophic endometrium, another common cause of bleeding in this age group, can easily be diagnosed at hysteroscopy. Endometrial polyps can sometimes also be detected in these patients.

Historically, dilatation and curettage (D & C) has been used as a diagnostic and, often, therapeutic tool. The diagnostic accuracy of D & C has been scrutinized in efforts to determine the sensitivity and specificity of the technique. The advantages of the hysteroscope in the evaluation of abnormal uterine bleeding include, most notably, the ability to see lesions and to evaluate the endometrial cavity more objectively[5]. Indeed, comparisons have been made between the results of hysteroscopically directed biopsy and D & C in treating patients. Valle[5], Mohr[6] and Gimpelson[7] all concluded that panoramic hysteroscopy, especially with directed biopsy, is superior to D & C in patients with uterine bleeding. Alternatively, Goldrath and Sherman combined out-patient panoramic hysteroscopy with suction curettage and suggested the superiority of this technique to D & C in terms of diagnostic accuracy, cost, safety and convenience[8].

Endometrial and cervical cancer

Hysteroscopy for abnormal bleeding can detect suspicious areas in the uterus and the cervix. The hysteroscopic appearance of endometrial carcinoma consists of exophytic or endophytic lesions. Polypoid or whitish areas may indicate necrosis within the tumor. The concern about cancer spread secondary to the hysteroscopic procedure has been addressed by various authors, and no evidence for its occurrence has been found[9,10]. Hysteroscopic examination has been found to be reliable, particularly when difficulties are encountered in assigning the tumor to stage I or II.

The instrument may also be used in detecting premalignant endometrial lesions, such as polypoid or adenomatous lesions with dystrophic or dyplastic hyperplasia. The microhysteroscope can be of great

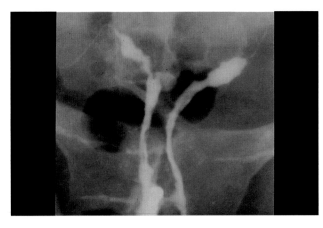

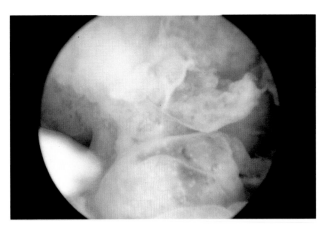

Figure 1 Müllerian anomalies: (a) hysterography reveals the presence of a complete uterine septum. Note the presence of fistula between the two cervical canals and of endometrial polyps

Figure 1(b) Hysteroscopy confirms the diagnosis of both septum and polyps

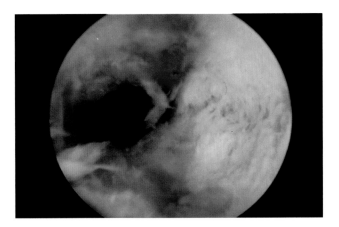

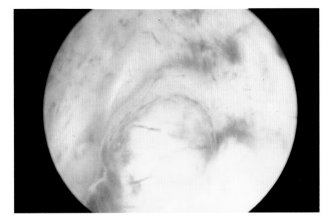

Figure 2 Intrauterine adhesions

Figure 3 Submucous myoma

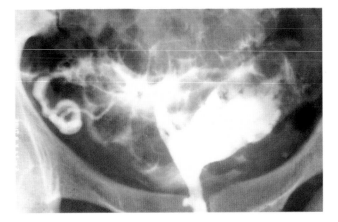

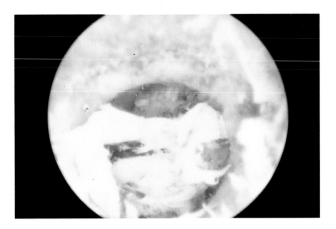

Figure 4 Uterine septum with residual trophoblastic tissue in the left horn. (a) Hysterography; (b) hysteroscopy

Figure 4(b) *See legend opposite*

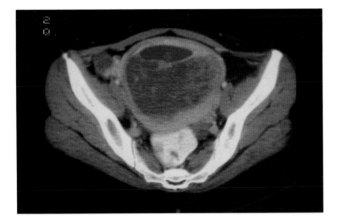

Figure 5 Hydatidiform mole: (a) computerized tomography; (b) magnetic resonance imaging; (c)–(e) hysteroscopy

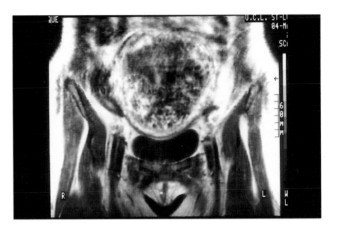

Figure 5(b)   *See legend opposite*

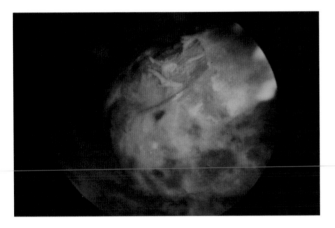

Figure 5(c)   *See legend above*

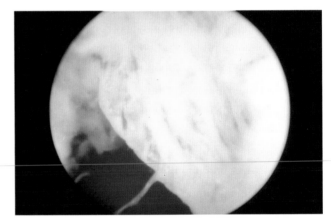

Figure 5(d)   *See legend above*

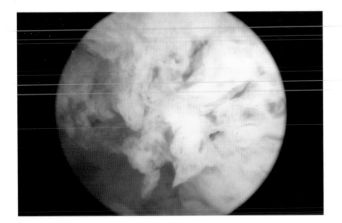

Figure 5(e)   *See legend above*

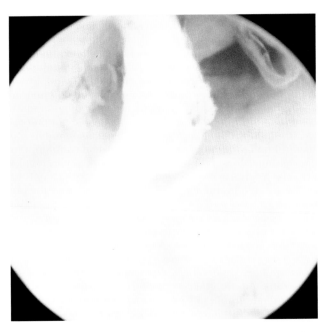

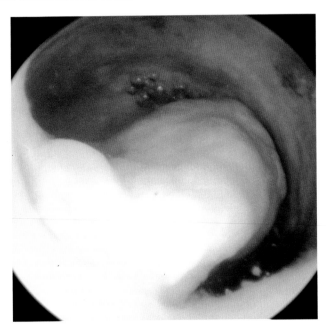

Figure 6(a) Small endometrial polyp in the left uterine horn

Figure 6(b) Larger polypoid structure

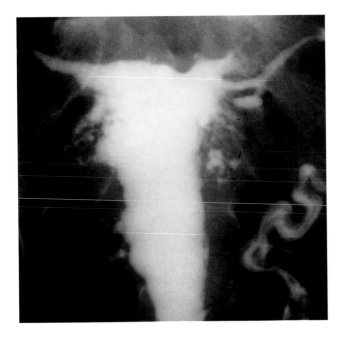

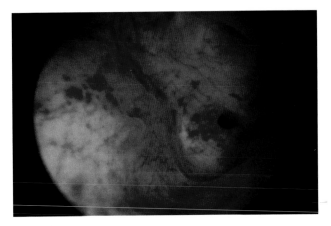

Figure 7(b) *See legend opposite*

Figure 7 Adenomyosis: (a) hysterography; (b) hysteroscopy reveals holes in the uterine cavity

value in detecting such early changes in patients with a known high risk of endometrial cancer, such as diabetics and obese individuals. Hysteroscopy can also provide an excellent view of the cervical canal and can thus be used in the diagnosis of cervical neoplasia[11].

Assessing the extent of involvement

Joelsson and co-workers in 1971 used hysteroscopy to try to distinguish cervical infiltration by tumors[12]. Clearly, if a tumor is seen growing within the endocervix, the endocervix is involved. However, the diagnosis of stage II carcinoma of the endometrium should be based on the histological contiguity of the endometrial carcinoma to normal cervical tissue (glands and stroma). This is not difficult if cervical glands or even the cervical squamous epithelium is contiguous to the cancer. However, this may be difficult if there is only stromal tissue with cancer or if there is only cancer and no cervical tissue at all. To make a diagnosis of stage II endometrial cancer in both these cases, the specimen must come from the endo-cervix. Such a biopsy requires experience rather than direct visualization of the biopsy site because the small cup of even the Storz instrument will not yield sufficiently deep tissue. The most tantalizing aspect of this problem is that the more anaplastic adeno-carcinomas and serous uterine papillary tumors may infiltrate the stroma of the endocervix, but the endo-cervical canal may look quite normal. A deep endocervical biopsy may be better than the hysteroscope for detecting such cases of endometrial cancer. In patients with superficial infiltration of the upper endocervix by endometrial cancer, hysteroscopy will certainly provide a precise topographic description of the lesion. The final diagnosis, however, still needs to be histological. Furthermore, such early superficial spread to the endocervix probably carries no worse a prognosis than a stage I lesion. Deep cervical infiltration is a danger signal for deep myometrial invasion and lymph node involvement[13].

The danger of tumor cell dissemination by the Hyskon or saline solution or even by the flow of CO_2 into the uterine veins is probably not great. Data from hystero-graphies showed that there was no greater frequency of metastases among patients who had undergone hystero-graphy than among those who had not[9].

INTRAUTERINE FOREIGN BODIES

Until recently foreign bodies within the uterine cavity were not uncommon. The most common offender is still the intrauterine device (IUD), which often becomes misplaced, making retrieval desirable. Several papers have described the usefulness of hysteroscopy in locating displaced IUDs[14–16].

Four patients with retained intrauterine fetal bones examined hysteroscopically have been described[17]. The bones were removed with hysteroscopic instruments in all patients. Other uncommon uses of the hysteroscopic approach include the removal of a Heyman capsule[18] and the broken tip of a plastic suction curette[19].

REFERENCES

1. Taylor, P.J. (1983). Correlations in infertility: symptomatology, hysterosalpingography and hyster-oscopy. *J. Reprod. Med.*, **8**, 339
2. Lindemann, H.J. (1971). Hysteroscopy for the diagnosis of intrauterine causes of sterility. *Proceedings of the 8th World Congress on Fertility and Sterility*, Kyoto, Japan, October
3. Quinones, G.R., Alvarado, D.A. and Aznar, R.R. (1974). Tubal catheterization: applications of a new technique. *Am. J. Obstet. Gynecol.*, **114**, 674
4. Bordt, J., Belkien, L., Vancaillie, T. *et al.* (1984). Ergebnisse diagnosticher Hysteroskopien in einem IVF/ET Program. *Geburtsch. Frauenheilk.*, **44**, 813
5. Valle, R.F. (1981). Hysteroscopic evaluation of patients with abnormal uterine bleeding. *Surg. Gynecol. Obstet.*, **153**, 521
6. Mohr, J.W. (1978). Hysteroscopy as a diagnostic tool in postmenopausal bleeding. In Philips, J.M. (ed.) *Endoscopy in Gynecology*, p.347. (Downey, CA: American Association of Gynecologic Laparoscopists)
7. Gimpelson, R.J. (1984). Panoramic hysteroscopy with directed biopsies vs. dilatation and curettage for accurate diagnosis. *J. Reprod. Med.*, **29**, 575
8. Goldrath, M.H. and Sherman, A.I. (1984). Office hysteroscopy and suction curettage: can we eliminate the hospital diagnostic dilatation and curettage. *Am. J. Obstet. Gynecol.*, **152**, 220
9. Johnson, J.E. (1973). Hysterography and diagnostic curettage in carcinoma of the uterine body. *Acta Radiol. (Suppl.)*, **326**, 1
10. Sugimoto, O. (1975). Hysteroscopic diagnosis of endometrial carcinoma: a report of fifty-three cases examined at the Women's Clinic of Kyoto University Hospital. *Am. J. Obstet. Gynecol.*, **121**, 105
11. Hamou, J. (1981). Microhysteroscopy: a new procedure and its original applications in gynecology. *J. Reprod. Med.*, **26**, 375
12. Joelsson, I., Levine, R.U. and Moberger, G. (1971). Hysteroscopy as an adjunct in determining the extent of carcinoma of the endometrium. *Am. J. Obstet. Gynecol.*, **111**, 696
13. Anderson, B. (1980). Hysterography and hystero-scopy in endometrial cancer. In Sciara, J.J. and Buchsbaum, H.J. (eds.) *Gynecology and Obstetrics*. (New York: Harper & Row)

14. Siegler, A.M. and Kemmann, E. (1976). Location and removal of misplaced or embedded intra-uterine devices by hysteroscopy. *J. Reprod. Med.*, **16**, 139

15. Taylor, P.J. and Comming, D.C. (1979). Hysteroscopy in 100 patients. *Fertil. Steril.*, **31**, 301

16. Valle, R.F., Sciarra, J.J. and Freeman, D.W. (1977). Hysteroscopic removal of intrauterine devices with missing filaments. *Obstet. Gynecol.*, **49**, 55

17. Chervenak, F.A., Amin, H.K. and Neuwirth, R.S. (1982). Symptomatic intrauterine retention of fetal bones. *Obstet. Gynecol.*, **59**, 585

18. Zipkin, B. and Rosenfeld, D.L. (1979). Hysteroscopic removal of a Heyman radium capsule. *J. Reprod. Med.*, **22**, 133

19. Sciarra, J.J. and Valle, R.F. (1977). Hysteroscopy: a clinical experience with 320 patients. *Am. J. Obstet. Gynecol.*, **127**, 340

Müllerian duct anomalies

M. Nisolle and J. Donnez

29

Three main principles govern the practical approach to malformations of the genital tract:

(1) The Müllerian and Wolffian ducts are so closely linked embryologically that gross malformations of the uterus and vagina are commonly associated with congenital anomalies of the kidney and ureter.

(2) The development of the gonad is separate from that of the ducts. Normal and functional ovaries are therefore usually present when the vagina, uterus and Fallopian tubes are absent or malformed.

(3) Müllerian duct anomalies are usually not associated with anomalies in the sex chromosome make-up of the individual.

EMBRYOLOGY

Gonadal development will not be examined in this chapter, which is limited to Müllerian and Wolffian duct development.

Late in the fifth or sixth week of embryonic life, at the level of the third thoracic somite, a precise area of the celomic epithelium invaginates at several points on the lateral surface of the urogenital ridge, and coalesces to form a tube, termed the Müllerian or paramesonephric duct. The duct extends caudally to the urogenital ridge, immediately lateral to the Wolffian duct. The paired Müllerian ducts give rise to the Fallopian tubes, uterus, cervix, and upper vagina. For proper Müllerian duct migration to occur, it is essential that the Wolffian duct is present[1].

Each Müllerian duct is guided by the respective Wolffian duct, migrates and develops independently of the other, and one usually descends ahead of the other. Defects in the development of the Wolffian duct lead to Müllerian anomalies. At first lateral to the Wolffian ducts, the Müllerian ducts cross over to lie medial to them as they enter the pelvis. By the end of the seventh week of embryonic life, the Müllerian ducts fuse to form a single structure between the two Wolffian ducts. The two Müllerian ducts penetrate the posterior wall of the urogenital sinus, between the orifices of the Wolffian ducts, on a mound called Müller's tubercle. It is important that the point where the tip of the Müllerian duct abuts on the posterior wall of the urogenital sinus is within the patch of mesoderm inserted into the wall of the sinus by the Wolffian ducts. This point defines the site of the future vaginal orifice, the hymenal membrane (Figure 1).

Two solid epithelial evaginations (sinovaginal bulbs) grow posteriorly from Müller's tubercle to meet the two solid tips of the fused Müllerian ducts. This epithelial proliferation of sinovaginal bulbs and the caudal ends of the Müllerian ducts form the solid vaginal plate. The vaginal plate and the adjoining Müllerian ducts elongate, canalize, and migrate from pelvic to perineal locations. At the same time the urogenital sinus exstrophies into the vestibule, the urethra elongates and the plate canalizes. The hymen remains as a membrane between the urogenital sinus and the canalized vaginal plate. The vaginal plate is first seen distinctly when the embryo is about 60–75 mm long, and its formation is complete at about 140 mm. Finally, when the cells of the plate desquamate, the vaginal lumen is formed[2] (Figure 2).

Felix[3] and Frazer[4] believed that canalization occurred in the bulbar and vaginal components of the plate and that the hymen demarcated the junction between the Müllerian and urogenital structures. In 1933, Koff[5] proposed that the sinovaginal bulbs formed the entire plate, that the plate canalized predominantly in a caudocranial direction giving rise to the hymen, and that the hymen and the caudal fifth of the vagina were formed from the plate and were therefore of urogenital sinus origin.

Witschi[6] believed that the hymen was formed from sinus and Müllerian epithelia with lateral contributions from the Wolffian ducts. He histologically identified Wolffian duct structures in the walls of the vaginal plate down to the urogenital sinus.

Frazer[4] observed the termination of the Wolffian ducts between the two layers of the hymen and the Müllerian contribution to the length of the vagina. These observations support the findings of Witschi: firstly, that the hymen marks the junction of the canalized vaginal bulbs of the urogenital sinus and the Müllerian ducts at the introitus, and secondly, that the Wolffian duct itself guides and mediates the caudal migration of the vaginal plate from pelvis to perineum. Having guided the Müllerian ducts to their destination and participated in the development of the vaginal plate, the Wolffian ducts become atrophic.

As early as the end of the first trimester[7], there is a mesenchymal thickening around that portion of the fused Müllerian duct, that is destined to become the endocervix. This mesenchymal thickening includes the Wolffian ducts, so that remnants of the latter, which persist into adulthood, are found within the body of the cervix. At all other levels of the genital canal, remnants of the Wolffian ducts are external to the wall of the adult Müllerian derivative.

Smooth muscle appears in the walls of the genital canal between 18 and 20 weeks, and, by approximately 24 weeks, the muscular portion of the uterine wall is well developed[7]. Vaginal, uterine and tubal muscular walls develop around the Müllerian duct alone, so that the Wolffian duct remnants are external to the true wall of the canal.

Cervical glands appear at about 15 weeks and rudimentary endometrial glands by 19 weeks, but the endometrium is not well developed even at term in most infants.

CLINICAL AND PATHOLOGIC IMPLICATIONS OF THE EMBRYOLOGIC DEVELOPMENT

The genital ducts and external genitalia develop as a result of hormones circulating *in utero*[8]. A non-steroidal compound, termed Müllerian-inhibiting factor (MIF), secreted by the fetal testes, inhibits the development of the Müllerian ducts and potentiates the development of the Wolffian ducts. The fetal testes also secrete androgens that stimulate the development of the external genitalia, as well as the central nervous system. If the fetal gonads are ovaries, MIF is not produced, and therefore the Müllerian ducts develop and the Wolffian ducts regress. In the absence of androgens, the indifferent external genitalia differentiate in a female direction.

Other congenital abnormalities, unrelated to the action of hormones, arise from a faulty morphogenesis and result in genital tract malformations, such as accessory tubal orifices, bicornuate uterus, or vaginal septa. These anomalies result from the lack of fusion of the Müllerian ducts or a lack of degeneration of the solid vaginal plate. Urinary tract abnormalities are also frequently associated with Müllerian duct anomalies. Improper development of the Wolffian ducts results in failure of proper migration of the Müllerian ducts. Thus, the urinary tract anomaly is primary, and the genital tract anomaly is secondary[1]. Patients who are found to have Müllerian duct-related abnormalities should, therefore, undergo an intravenous pyelogram, performed in order to assess the status of the urinary tract.

The anatomical abnormalities induced by *in utero* diethylstilbestrol exposure can be understood on the basis of the embryological development of both the lower and upper genital tract[9-11]. Diethylstilbestrol inhibits the development of the vaginal plate, resulting in the Müllerian duct component of the vagina being lower in the adult canal than is normally the case. This results in the presence of columnar, Müllerian-type epithelium as far down the vagina as the hymenal ring in extreme cases. Diethylstilbestrol also disorganizes the stromal differentiation, which is responsible for the overall structure of the cervix, uterus and tubes. This accounts for the gross structural anomalies of the cervix, such as the cervical collar, pseudopolyp, and hood, as well as the uterine deformities that may be encountered, such as the T-shaped endometrial cavity (Figure 3).

CLASSIFICATION OF MÜLLERIAN DUCT ANOMALIES

Development anomalies (Table 1)

Absence of both Müllerian ducts

Complete failure of development of the Müllerian ducts results in an absence of the Fallopian tubes, uterus and most of the vagina. In such cases the vulva is likely to be normal and there may be a depression of variable depth representing the lower (urogenital sinus) part of the vagina. It is usual to find such a depression covered with a normal hymen[12,13] (Figure 4).

Table 1 Classification of Müllerian duct anomalies

Development anomalies
Absence of both Müllerian ducts
Absence of one Müllerian duct
Incomplete development of both Müllerian ducts
Incomplete development of one Müllerian duct

Fusion anomalies
(1) Lateral fusion anomalies
  arcuate uterus
  uterus subseptus and uterus septus
  uterus bicornis
  uterus didelphys
  septate and subseptate vagina

(2) Vertical fusion anomalies
  cervical atresia
  vaginal atresia
  transverse vagina septum

The Mayer–Rokitansky–Küster–Hauser syndrome affects one in every 4000–5000 females and is the second most common cause of primary infertility after gonadal dysgenesis. Although familial aggregates have been described, the defect usually appears sporadically[14].

Absence of one Müllerian duct

Absence of one Müllerian duct (Figure 5) results in a unicornuate uterus with only one Fallopian tube. The cervix and vagina may be normal in appearance and function, but they strictly represent only one half of the fully developed organs. A true unicornuate uterus is rare

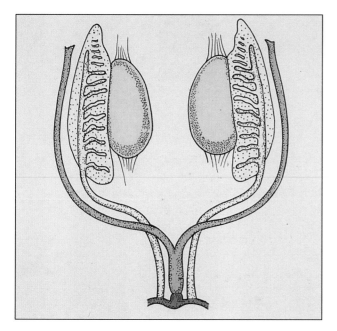

Figure 1 The genital ducts in the female at the end of the second month of development. Note the Müllerian tubercule and the formation of the uterine canal

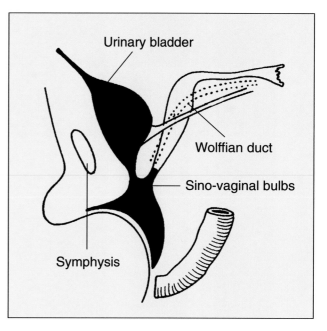

Figure 2(a) and (b) Sagittal sections showing the formation of the uterus and vagina at various stages of development

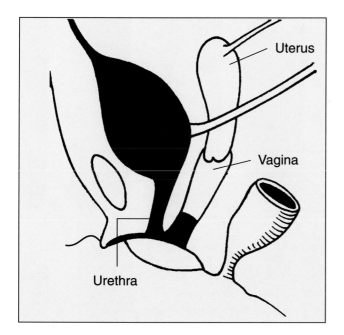

Figure 2(b)   *See legend above*

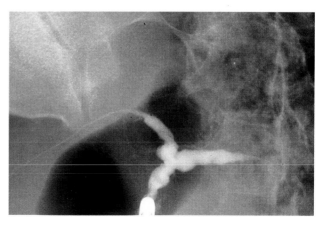

Figure 3   *In utero* diethylstilbestrol exposure: T-shaped endometrial cavity

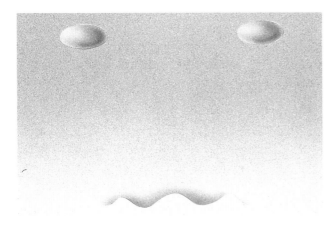

Figure 4 The Mayer–Rokitansky–Küster–Hauser syndrome: (a)–(c) development of internal genital tract; (d) and (e) external genital tract

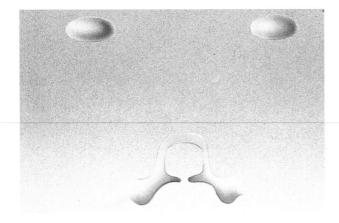

Figure 4(b)   *See legend above*

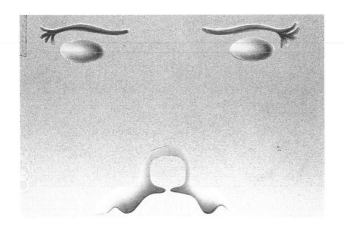
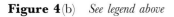

Figure 4(c)   *See legend above*

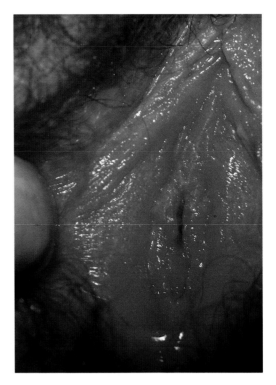

Figure 4(d)   *See legend opposite*

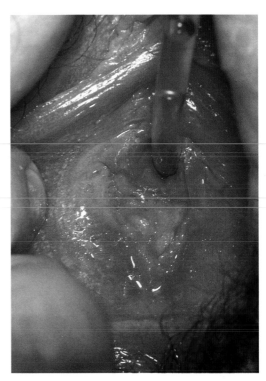

Figure 4(e)   *See legend above*

and is usually associated with an absence or gross malformation of the renal tract on the side of the missing Müllerian duct.

Incomplete development of both Müllerian ducts

Poorly formed ducts of full length result in hypoplasia of the whole genital tract. Incomplete development some-times affects the lower parts of the ducts only. Thus, well-formed abdominal ostia may be associated with hypoplasia or absence of the remainder of the tubes, of the uterus and of the vagina (Figure 4). It is possible for the tubes and uterus to be present and the vagina absent, rudimentary or imperforate. The converse is not true because the ducts grow downwards; a well-formed uterus is never associated with absence of Fallopian tubes.

Incomplete development of one Müllerian duct

Incomplete development of one Müllerian duct (Figure 6) gives rise to the more common apparent unicornuate malformation; this is distinguished by the discovery of a Fallopian tube and round ligament, rudimentary though they may be, on the affected side. In this condition, two kidneys are usually present although, occasionally, the one on the affected side may also be hypoplastic and not apparent on intravenous pyelography.

Fusion anomalies (Table 1)

Lateral fusion anomalies

The anomalies result from a failure of lateral fusion of the two Müllerian ducts, a condition which may be obstructive or non-obstructive. Failure of fusion of the Müllerian ducts occurs in varying degrees. If minor degrees affecting uterine shape are taken into consideration, this type of malformation is extremely common. The different nomenclatures and classifications of the resulting deformities are confusing.

(1) *Arcuate uterus* (Figure 7a). This is a flat-topped uterus in which the fundal bulge has not developed after fusion of the ducts.

(2) *Uterus subseptus and uterus septus* (Figure 7b). The uterus is outwardly normal but contains a complete or incomplete septum, which reflects a failure in the breakdown of the walls between the two ducts. The cervical canal may be single or double, and the vagina whole or septate.

(3) *Uterus bicornis* (Figure 7c). In this condition only the lower parts of the ducts fuse, leaving the cornua separate. The cervix and vagina may be single or double.

(4) *Uterus didelphys* (Figure 7a). If the two Müllerian ducts remain separate, the two halves of the uterus remain distinct and each has its own cervix. Some distinguish between uterus didelphys and uterus pseudodidelphys according to the degree of separation between the two ducts.

(5) *Septate and subseptate vagina* (Figure 8). A sagittal septum with a crescentic lower edge may be present in the upper vagina or throughout its length. It can occur alone or in conjunction with a septate or bicornuate condition of the uterus, and may have one or two cervices opening into it. This condition arises either because late fusion of the Müllerian ducts gives rise to two Müllerian tubercles, or because of a failure of proper canalization of the two sinovaginal bulbs.

In some cases, the hemivagina is not patent, taking the form of a blind vaginal pouch. The obstructed hemivagina is associated with either a functioning double uterus (Figure 9) or a degenerate remnant of the paramesonephric duct. This uterine remnant is lined with ciliated columnar cells with occasional papillary projections. It may also contain patches of endometrial and/or glandular epithelium that produce a mucoid and/or menstrual discharge. In childhood, an obstructed hemivagina is usually asymptomatic unless distended by mucus. In this case, a simple incision and resection of the vaginal septum will allow continued drainage. With menstruation, the resulting hematocolpos may be evacuated after a complete resection of the septum. Obstructed hemivagina and a double uterus are almost always associated with ipsilateral renal agenesis[15,16].

Vertical fusion anomalies – incomplete canalization

The Müllerian buds have solid tips behind which canalization takes place progressively. The Müllerian and sinovaginal bulb tissue which forms the vagina is also lumenless at first. Failure to canalize results in either solid organs or membranes of varying thickness obstructing the genital canal. Thus a rudimentary uterus sometimes lacks a cavity and the vagina may be represented by an uncanalized column of tissue. Atresia may affect only one Müllerian duct, so that one horn of a bicornuate uterus may fail to communicate with the cervical canal, or one half of a septate vagina may be a closed cavity. Unilateral hematocolpos, mucocolpos and pyocolpos are not common.

(1) *Cervical atresia* (Figure 10). Congenital atresia of the cervix of an otherwise normal uterus or of a bicor-nuate uterus is rare. When it does occur, a reason-ably normal vagina is invariably present. It is more common to encounter apparent cervical atresia in association with an absence of the lower vagina.

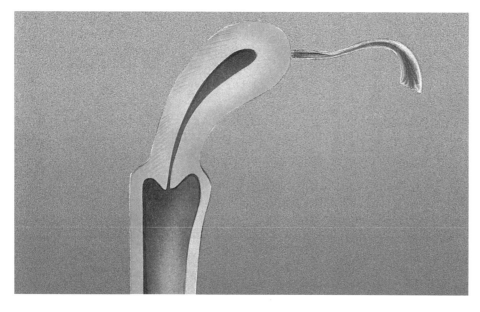

Figure 5(a) Absence of one Müllerian duct: unicornuate uterus; (b) view on hysterography; (c) view on laparoscopy

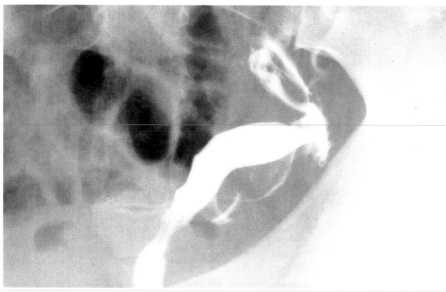

Figure 5(b) *See legend above*

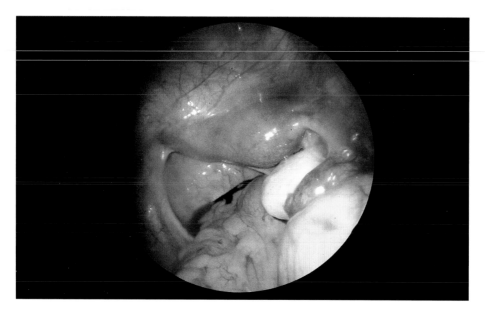

Figure 5(c) *See legend above*

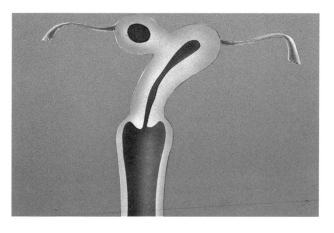

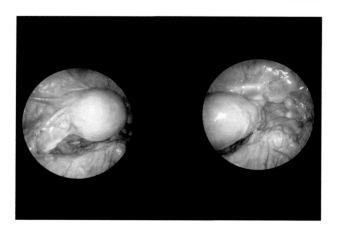

Figure 6(a) Incomplete development of one Müllerian duct; (b) laparoscopic view. The rudimentary horn is visible on the right side

Figure 6(b) *See legend opposite*

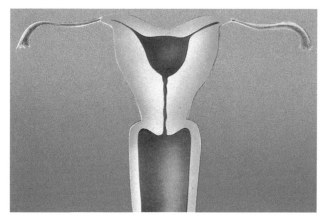

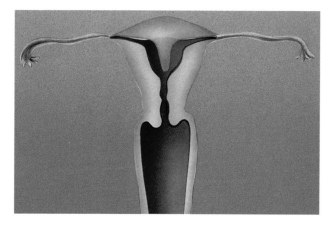

Figure 7 Lateral fusion anomalies: (a) arcuate uterus; (b) uterus septus; (c) uterus bicornis; (d) uterus didelphys

Figure 7(b) *See legend opposite*

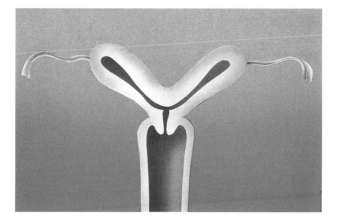

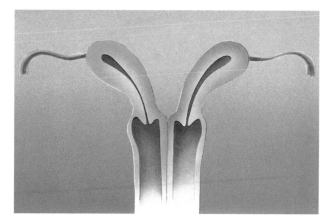

Figure 7(c) *See legend above*

Figure 7(d) *See legend above*

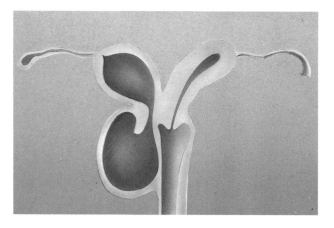

Figure 8 Septate vagina. The obstructed hemivagina is associated with a functioning double uterus

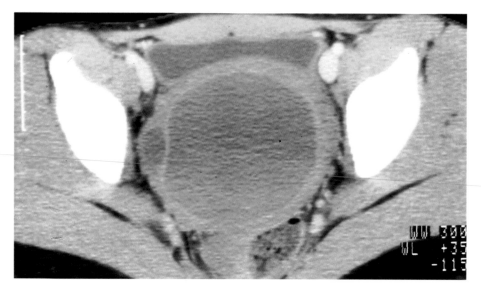

Figure 9 Computerized tomography of the completely obstructed hemivagina. Note the presence of both hematocolpos and hematometria

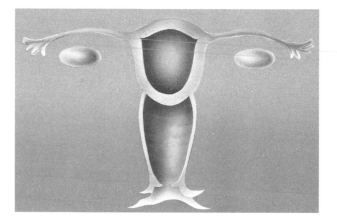

Figure 10 Cervical atresia

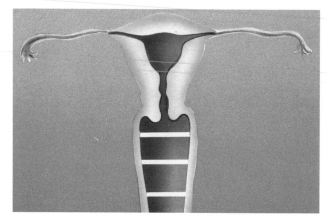

Figure 11 Transverse vaginal septum showing the three types: high transverse vaginal septum; transverse septum of the middle third of the vagina; transverse septum of the lower third of the vagina

(2) *Vaginal atresia – transverse vaginal septum* (Figure 11). Disorders of vertical fusion result from defects in the union between the downward progressing Müllerian tubercles and the up-growing derivative of the urogenital sinus. Similar defects may also occur secondary to a failure in the canalization of the solid vaginal tube, either because of abnormal proliferation of paravaginal mesoderm or because of some form of intrauterine infection. Transverse vaginal septae are relatively rare, affecting approximately one in every 80 000 females. The septum consists of a central fibromuscular plate or ring of varying thickness. When the obstruction is complete, the outer surface is covered with stratified squamous epithelium, while the inner aspect is composed of glandular columnar epithelium. The interruption can occur at any level of the vagina, and may be multiple. The middle and lower zones of the vagina may be imperforate over a length of 0.5–6.0 cm. More frequently, the vagina is obstructed by a thinner membrane situated in the vagina, just above the hymen. Transverse vaginal septae usually go unnoticed in children unless a mucocolpos has developed or vaginal patency is tested. A rim of hymenal tissue will help distinguish the low transverse septa from an imperforate hymen. Distension of the septum as seen vaginally will depend on its thickness and location. As in the imperforate hymen, the vulva may be very engorged and swollen.

Obstruction of menstrual flow and subsequent endometriosis may result in infertility. In a study of 15 teenage patients with pelvic pain and endometriosis, six (40%) were found to have obstructive anomalies of the genitalia[17]. Goldstein *et al.* reported endometriosis in 52% of 140 adolescents evaluated laparoscopically for pelvic pain[18]. Of these cases, only 5% of patients had obstructive uterine anomalies.

REFERENCES

1. Marshall, F.F. and Beisel, D.S. (1978). The association of uterine anomalies. *Obstet. Gynecol.*, **51**, 559

2. O'Rahilly, R. (1977). The development of the vagina in the human. *Birth Def.*, **13**, 123–36

3. Felix, W. (1912). The development of the urogenital organs. In Keibel, F. and Mall, F.P. (eds.) *Manual of Human Embryology*, p. 979. (Philadelphia: Lippincott)

4. Frazer, J.E. (1931). *A Manual of Embryology: The Development of The Human Body*, pp. 431–40.

(London: Ballière, Tindal and Cox)

5. Koff, A.K. (1933). Development of the vagina in the human fetus. *Contrib. Embryol. Carneg. Inst.*, **24**, 61–91

6. Witschi, E. (1951). Embryogenesis of the adrenal and the reproductive glands. *Rec. Prog. Horm. Res.*, **6**, 1

7. O'Rahilly, R. (1973). The embryology and anatomy of the uterus. In Norris, H. and Hertig, A. (eds.) *The Uterus*. (Baltimore: Williams-Wilkins)

8. Jost, A. (1971). Embryonic sexual differentiation (morphology, physiology, abnormalities). In Jones, H. Jr and Scott, W.W. (eds.) *Hermophroditism, Genital Anomalies and Related Endocrine Disorders*, 2nd edn., p.16. (Baltimore: Williams Wilkins)

9. Kaufman, R.H., Adam, E., Binder, G.L. and Gerthoffer, E. (1980). Upper genital tract changes and pregnancy outcome in offspring exposed *in utero* to diethylstilbestrol. *Am. J. Obstet. Gynecol.*, **137**, 299

10. Robboy, S.J. (1983). A hypothetic mechanism of diethylstilbestrol (DES)-induced anomalies in exposed progeny. *Hum. Pathol.*, **14**, 831

11. Robboy, S.J., Taguchi, O. and Cunha, G.R. (1982). Normal development of the human female reproductive tract and alterations resulting from experimental exposure to diethylstilbestrol. *Hum. Pathol.*, **13**, 190

12. Nisolle, M. and Donnez, J. (1989). Malformations and maldevelopments of the Müllerian ducts. In Donnez, J. (ed.) *Laser Operative Laparoscopy and Hysteroscopy*, pp.231–48. (Leuven: Nauwelaerts)

13. Nisolle, M. and Donnez, J. (1992). Vaginoplasty using amniotic membranes in cases of vaginal agenesis or after vaginectomy. *J. Endosc. Surg.*, **8**, 25–30

14. Carson, S.A., Simpson, J.L., Malinak, L.R. *et al.* (1983). Heritable aspects of uterine anomalies II. Genetic analysis of müllerian aplasia. *Fertil. Steril.*, **40**, 86

15. Woolf, R.B. and Allen, W.M. (1953). Concomitant malformations. *Obstet. Gynecol.*, **2**, 236

16. Fekete, C.N. and Nisolle, M. (1988). Anomalies de fusion ou d'accolement des canaux de Müller. *Revue médico-Chirurgicale de l'Hôpital des Enfants Malades*, Paris, p. 1

17. Schifrin, B.S., Erez, S. and Moore, J.G. (1973). Teenage endometriosis. *Am. J. Obstet. Gynecol.*, **116**, 973

18. Goldstein, D.P., Decholnoky, C., Emans, S.J. and Leventhal, J.M. (1980). Laparoscopy in the diagnosis and management of the pelvic pain in adolescents. *J. Reprod. Med. Obstet. Gynecol.*, **24**, 251

Vaginoplasty using amniotic membranes in cases of vaginal agenesis

30

M. Nisolle and J. Donnez

Malformations of the vagina are an uncommon but serious problem. Their severity ranges from complete vaginal agenesis (Figure 1), with or without a functional uterus, to vaginal shortening.

The treatment of certain gynecological malignancies, such as vaginal adenocarcinoma or severe vaginal dysplasia induced by diethylstilbestrol, requires vaginectomy, which makes coitus impossible. In some instances, radical hysterectomy for severe cervical dysplasia is accompanied by vaginectomy because of associated vaginal dysplasia. Vaginal construction or reconstruction has become well established as a method of permitting or restoring sexual function, and a variety of procedures have been described. The most popular method involves the lining of a surgically created space either with a partial thickness skin graft[1] or with amnion[2-11].

In 1934, Brindeau used human amnion to construct a vagina in a patient with Müllerian agenesis[2]. Between 1939 and 1947, Burger[3] used amnion more extensively for the same purpose. In 1973, Trelford and colleagues[4-6] successfully used fetal amnion to reconstruct the vagina during anterior exenteration. We report our experience with the use of amniotic membranes to line artificially constructed vaginas. Amniotic membranes were obtained immediately postpartum from an HIV- and HB_S-seronegative patient who had delivered 3–6 h before the vaginoplasty. She was afebrile and her membranes had been ruptured for less than 6 h. Delivery was vaginal in all cases. Elective Cesarean section was not a condition for use of the membranes.

Membranes were rinsed in sterile saline solution to remove all the blood and stored at 4°C in saline without antibiotics. Amnion was not stripped from the chorion before use.

SURGICAL PROCEDURE

Under general anesthesia, the patient is placed in the lithotomy position and vaginal dissection is performed (Figure 2). A vaginal pouch is created by blunt dissection, with the help of scissors. At the same time, a laparoscopy is performed to confirm the diagnosis and check the blunt dissection. When hemostasis has been achieved, a rigid vaginal mold (Figure 3) is selected, just large enough to ensure firm application of the amniotic membranes, with which it is covered (Figure 4). The labia majora are approximated with silk sutures to keep the mold in place. Laparoscopy is not necessary for the

dissection, but when performed to ascertain the diagnosis permits the visualization of the top of the mold between the bladder and the rectum (Figure 5). A Foley catheter is inserted before the blunt dissection and left in place for 48 h. Two rudimentary horns are sometimes clearly visible at the time of laparoscopy (Figure 6). When the patient is suffering from pelvic pain and dysmenorrhea, echography often reveals small areas of hematometria. In this case, during the same procedure, both rudimentary horns are removed laparoscopically.

Electrocoagulation of the isthmic portion of the Fallopian tube, the utero-ovarian ligament and the uterine artery is subsequently performed (Figure 6). The uterine horns are then easily removed, either through the pouch of Douglas or transabdominally, with the help of a forceps. The macroscopic view after transection of the horn (Figure 7) reveals blood in the rudimentary uterine cavity. The entire procedure is completed in 20 min. All patients receive antibiotics for 6–7 days postoperatively.

The mold is removed under light sedation 7 days later, and the newly constructed vagina is inspected and cleaned. The amniotic membranes are found to be adherent to the vagina. A flexible mold (Figure 3) is then inserted and the patient discharged the following day, having been advised to refrain from sexual activity for an additional 2 weeks and to use the mold at night during this period. Dienoestrol cream is used as a lubricant. The patient is then encouraged to have sexual intercourse. All patients are reviewed at 2 weeks and 1 month postoperatively and then at monthly intervals.

PATIENTS AND RESULTS

Between 1986 and 1992, amniotic membranes were used in 11 patients (aged 14–59 years) undergoing vaginoplasty for vaginal agenesis. None of them had undergone an anterior vaginoplasty. All patients found the mold uncomfortable postoperatively, but all were mobile and required mild analgesia only for the mold change on day 7. Routine urinary catheter insertion was performed in all cases for 48 h. All patients received prophylactic antibiotics, penicillin and metronidazole. No patients developed a urinary tract infection. At the mold change, the amniotic membranes could be seen as a distinct layer applied to the vaginal wall. At the end of 7 days, the vaginal tunnel was covered with a smooth lining, with extensive but small areas of congestion.

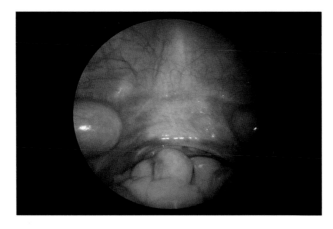

Figure 1(a)   Vaginal agenesis in Rokintansky–Hauser syndrome, laparoscopic aspect; (b) and (c) in some cases, rudimentary horns are visible

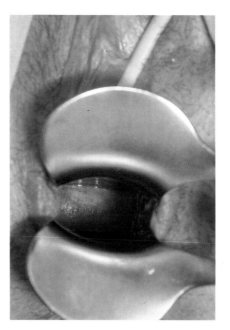

Figure 2   Dissection of the vesico-rectal space

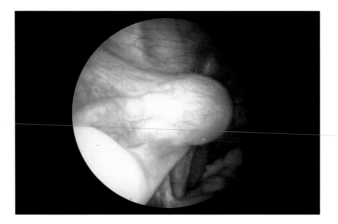

Figure 1(b)   *See legend above*

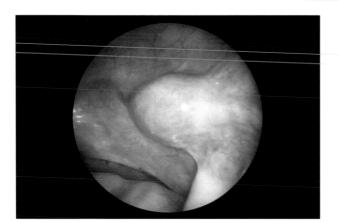

Figure 1(c)   *See legend above*

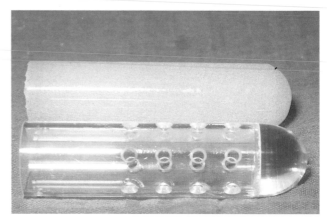

Figure 3   Top: non-rigid mold (diameter: 3.5 cm; length: 10 or 12 cm). Bottom: rigid vaginal mold (diameter: 3.5 cm; length: 10 or 12 cm). The holes allow the drainage of vaginal exudations. Two small holes allow the mold to be fixed

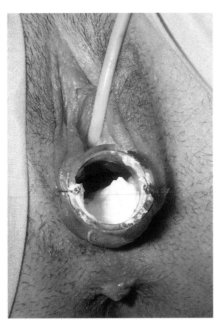

Figure 4 A rigid mold wrapped in amniotic membranes is introduced into the vaginal pouch

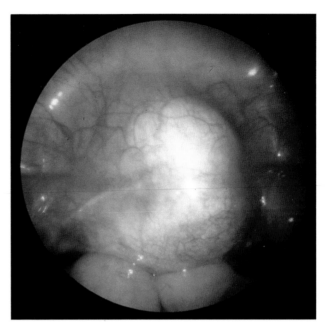

Figure 5 Laparoscopic view after blunt dissection and introduction of a rigid mold

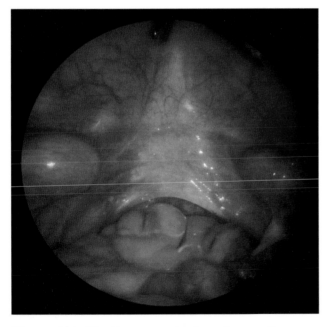

Figure 6(a)–(h) Laparoscopic view of two rudimentary horns in a case of Rokitansky–Küster–Hauser syndrome. Electrocoagulation of the isthmic portion of the Fallopian tube, the utero-ovarian ligament and the artery

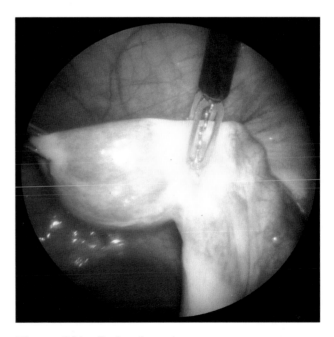

Figure 6(b) *See legend opposite*

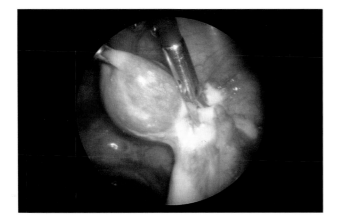

Figure 6(c)   *See legend on previous page*

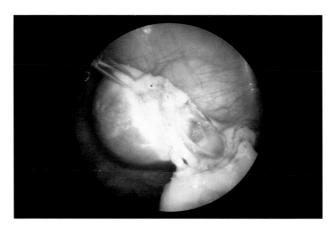

Figure 6(d)   *See legend on previous page*

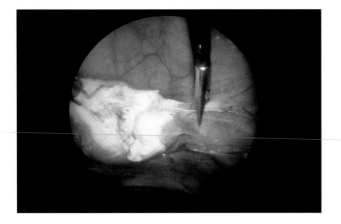

Figure 6(e)   *See legend on previous page*

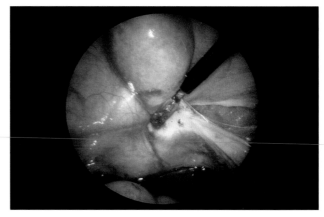

Figure 6(f)   *See legend on previous page*

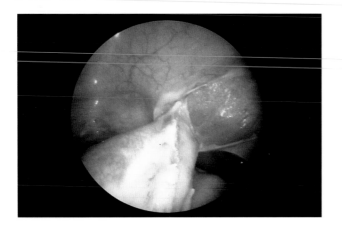

Figure 6(g)   *See legend on previous page*

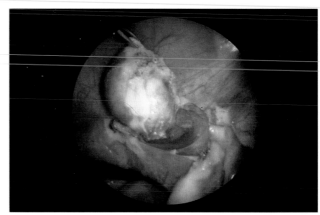

Figure 6(h)   *See legend on previous page*

By the fourth week postoperatively, healthy pink vaginal epithelium was visible with, in some cases, only small areas of granulation tissue. Initial epithelialization was excellent. At the end of 8 weeks the vagina was found to be well formed and was of normal depth and caliber. There was no exudate, adhesions, drying or scarring. Constant use of the mold produced no inflammatory reaction or formation of granuloma in unmarried patients.

The rectum was not entered in any patient during vaginal dissection.

All patients were reviewed at 2 weeks and at 1 month postoperatively and then at monthly intervals. Vaginal smears at 8 weeks postoperatively showed numerous squamous epithelial cells. In all but one patient with vaginal agenesis, epithelialization was complete, as proved by biopsy, which showed early epithelialization (at week 4–6) and mature vaginal epithelium by the end of 8–10 weeks (Figure 8). In one patient, granulation tissue was found: this patient had not used vaginal estrogen cream.

The anatomic and functional results are summarized in Table 1. The length of the vagina varied from 7 to 8 cm. All patients had greatly improved vaginal length and capacity as a result of this treatment. Excellent results were achieved in all cases. The vaginal tissue remained supple, with no evidence of fibrous tissue formation. Chronic granulation tissue was not observed and vaginal shrinkage did not occur.

The final result was directly related to the motivation of the patient and her postoperative use of the mold. No long-term complications have been observed so far: follow-up extends from 3 months to 5 years.

DISCUSSION

Various treatments have been described for vaginal agenesis. Frank[12] reported graduated vaginal dilatation but this technique has given good results in less than 50% of patients. Williams[13] described the method of a turned-in labial flap. Although the procedure required no graft, no satisfactory results were reported. The vaginal axis was often badly placed and difficulties with micturition and repeated urinary tract infections were observed.

Creating a tunnel for congenital absence of the vagina is a step common to all surgical procedures. The need for the use of a graft, and the best tissue to use (skin, intestine or amnion), is debatable. The use of cecal or sigmoid bowel segments was reported by Baldwin in 1904[14]. Though some authors claimed good results, this method is a major surgical procedure with significant morbidity and mortality. Turner-Warwick and Kirby[15] have recently reported successful reconstruction of the vagina with colocecum, with no serious surgical complication. However, profuse secretions, persistent unpleasant odour and ulceration of the mucosal surface could be major side-effects.

Wharton[16] devised an operation based on the remarkable regenerative potential of granulation tissue in the vaginal canal. To keep the space patent, a condom-covered mold was used. McIndoe and Bannister[1] modified Wharton's operation by the additional step of transplanting a split thickness skin graft into the newly formed vaginal cavity, held in place by a vaginal mold. Great variations in success rate, a high incidence of postoperative infection, necrosis of the skin graft and scarring make this technique less acceptable. The patient also suffers considerable discomfort from the donor skin site, which may remain visible.

Myocutaneous flaps have been used by several surgeons. The gracilis myocutaneous flap has become very popular in recent years[17-20], but a serious disadvantage is the precarious vascularity of the flaps. In McCraw's series of 22 patients[21], six suffered catastrophic loss of the flap. The rectus abdominis flap is another popular flap, but creates a large abdominal donor site defect[22] and requires a long operative procedure. The neurovascular pudendal thigh flap procedure can be used reliably to reconstruct the vagina[23]. All flap techniques, however, are reported to suffer from an unacceptable failure rate due to partial flap loss and necrosis. Such dissections also cause major scars and can only be indicated for vaginal reconstruction after pelvectomy for pelvic cancer, when subsequent irradiation must be carried out.

In order to overcome these difficulties, amnion alone, with the clean mesenchymal surface placed towards the host, has been used by several surgeons[2-6,9]. Dino and co-workers[24] suggested sterilization of amniotic membranes. Trelford and colleagues[4-7] found that membranes stored at 4°C in 0.5% normal saline with antibiotics were

Table 1 Postoperative functional results after vaginoplasty for vaginal agenesis due to Rokitansky–Kuster–Hauser syndrome ($n = 11$)

Vaginal length (cm)		Functional
Preoperative	Postoperative	results
1	7	+++*
1	7	+++
1	7	+++
1	8	+++
1	7	+++
1	7	+++
1	7	+++
1	7	+++
1	7	+++*
1	7	+++
3	8	+++

*, No sexual intercourse. Only the mold is used.
+++ normal vaginal capacity

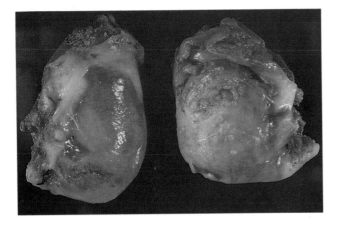

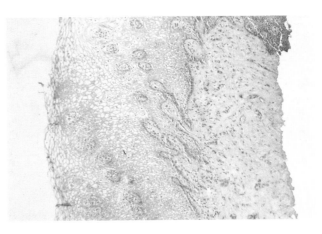

Figure 7 Macroscopic view of the removed rudimentary horns: (a) external view; (b) transection reveals the presence of collected blood

Figure 8 Vaginal biopsy taken from the newly formed vaginal cavity, 8 weeks after surgery (Gomori's trichrome, × 25) shows mature vaginal epithelium

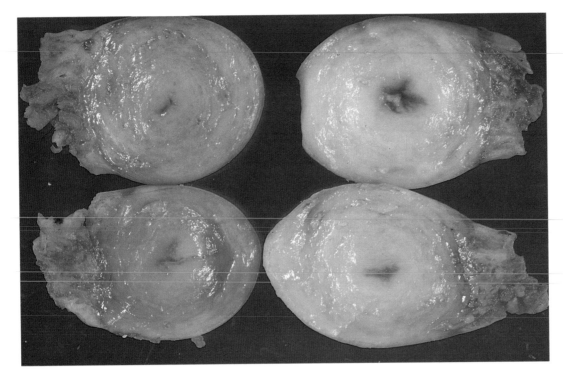

Figure 7 (b)   *See legend above*

sterile at the end of 48 h. In our study[11], amniotic membranes were taken immediately postpartum (<6h). Saline solution with antibiotics was never used. Membranes were only rinsed in sterile physiological solution (NaCl 0.9%).

Faulk and colleagues[25] have demonstrated microscopic evidence of new vessel formation and suggested that an angiogenic factor is produced by amnion. There is no problem with immune rejection because amnion does not express histocompatibility antigens and Akle and associates[26] found no evidence of tissue rejection when amnion was implanted subcutaneously in volunteers.

Tancer and co-workers[8], Dhall[9] and Ashworth and colleagues[10] have reported the successful use of amnion as a graft in vaginoplasties. Removal of the more antigenic chorion has been suggested to contribute to the successful use of the amnion. In the study of Nisolle and Donnez[11], however, the amnion was not stripped from the chorion. Our results showed the vagina to be well formed and of normal depth and caliber. There was no problem of immune rejection. Sexual intercourse was reported to be satisfactory in all cases. Vaginal smears and vaginal biopsy specimens were taken at follow-up visits. Vaginal epithelium was present by 8–10 weeks.

In conclusion, amniotic membranes are readily available, easily stored, and inexpensive, and can be used without a sterilization procedure as a graft for vaginal reconstruction. The amniotic membranes adhere firmly, protect the underlying granulation and facilitate epithelialization. Hospitalization is considerably reduced and major skin defects occurring after myocutaneous flap reconstruction are avoided. No postoperative dilatation is needed once normal sexual intercourse is resumed.

REFERENCES

1. McIndoe, A.H. and Bannister, J.E. (1938). An operation for the cure of congenital absence of the vagina. *J. Obstet. Gynaecol. Br. Empire*, **45**, 490
2. Brindeau, A. (1934). Creation d'un vagin artificiel à l'aide des membranes ovulaires d'un oeuf à terme. *Gynecol. Obstet.*, **29**, 385
3. Burger, K. (1947). Weitere Erfahrungen über die kunstliche Scheidenbildung mit Eihäuten. *Zentralbl. Gynäkol.*, **69**, 1153
4. Trelford, J.D., Hanson, F.W. and Anderson, D.G. (1973). Amniotic membrane as a living surgical dressing in human patients. *Oncology*, **28**, 358
5. Trelford, J.D., Anderson, D., Hanson, F. and Mendel, V. (1973). Amniotic membrane used for radical vulvectomies. *Obstet. Gynecol. Observ.*, **12**, 1
6. Trelford, J.D., Hanson, F.W. and Anderson, D.S. (1973). The feasibility of making an artificial vagina at the time of anterior exenteration. *Oncology*, **28**, 398
7. Trelford-Sauder, M., Telford, J.D. and Matolo N.M. (1977). Replacement of the peritoneum with amnion following pelvic exenteration. *Surg. Gynecol. Obstet.*, **145**, 699
8. Tancer, M.L., Katz, M. and Veridiano, N.P. (1979). Vaginal epithelialization with human amnion. *Obstet. Gynecol.*, **54**, 345
9. Dhall, K. (1984). Amnion graft for treatment of congenital absence of the vagina. *Br. J. Obstet. Gynaecol.*, **91**, 279
10. Ashworth, M.F., Morton, K.E., Dewhurst, J., Lilford, R.J. and Bates, R.G. (1986). Vaginoplasty using amnion. *Obstet. Gynecol.*, **67**, 443
11. Nisolle M. and Donnez, J. (1992). Vaginoplasty using amniotic membranes in cases of vaginal agenesis or after vaginectomy. *J. Gynecol. Surg.*, **8**, 25–30
12. Frank, R.T. (1938). The formation of an artificial vagina without operation. *Am. J. Obstet. Gynecol.*, **35**, 1053
13. Williams, E.A. (1964). Congenital absence of the vagina — a simple operation for its relief. *J. Obstet. Gynaecol. Br. Commonw.*, **71**, 511
14. Baldwin, J.F. (1904). The formation of an artificial vagina by intestinal transplantation. *Ann. Surg.*, **40**, 398
15. Turner-Warwick, R. and Kirby, R.S. (1990). The construction and reconstruction of the vagina with the colocecum. *Surg. Gynecol. Obstet.*, **170**, 132
16. Wharton, L.R. (1938). A simple method of constructing a vagina. *Ann. Surg.*, **107**, 842
17. Heath, P.M., Woods, J.E., Podratz, K.C., Arnold, P.G. and Irons, G.B. (1984). Gracilis myocutaneous vaginal reconstruction. *Mayo Clin. Proc.*, **59**, 21
18. Lagasse, L.D., Berman, M.L., Watring, W.G. and Ballon, S.C. (1978). The gynecologic oncology patient: restoration of function and prevention of disability. In McGowan, L., (ed.) *Gynecologic Oncology*, p.398. (New York: Appleton-Century-Crofts)
19. Lacey, P.M. and Morrow, C.P. (1986). Myocutaneous vaginal reconstruction. In Morrow, C.P. and Smart, G.E. (eds.) *Gynecologic Oncology*, p.255 (Berlin: Springer-Verlag)
20. Wheeless, C.R. (1981). Vulvar-vaginal reconstruction. In Coppleson, M. (ed.) *Gynecologic Oncology: Fundamental Principles and Clinical Practice*, Vol 2, p.933. (Edinburgh: Churchill Livingstone)
21. McCraw, J.B., Massey, F.M., Shanklin, K.D. and Horton, C.E. (1976). Vaginal reconstruction with gracilis myocutanuous flaps. *Plast. Reconstr. Surg.*, **58**, 176
22. Gordon, R.T. and Thomas, G.D. (1988). Vaginal and pelvic reconstruction with distally based rectus abdominis myocutaneous flaps. *Plast. Reconstr. Surg.*, **81**, 71
23. Wee, T.K. and Joseph, V.T. (1989). A new technique of vaginal reconstruction using

neurovascular pudendal-thigh flaps: a preliminary report. *Plast. Reconstr. Surg.*, **83**, 701

24. Dino, B.R., Eufemio, G.G. and De Villa, M.S. (1966). Human amnion: the establishment of an amnion bank and its pactical applications in surgery. *J. Philippine Med. Assoc.*, **42**, 357

25. Faulk, W.P., Matthews, R., Stevens, P.J. *et al.* (1980). Human amnion as an adjunct in wound healing. *Lancet*, **1**, 1156

26. Akle, C.A., Adinolfi, M., Welsh, K.I., *et al.* (1980). Immunogenicity of human amniotic epithelial cells after transplantation into volunteers. *Lancet*, **2**, 1003

Müllerian fusion defects: septoplasty and hemihysterectomy of the rudimentary horns

31

M. Nisolle and J. Donnez

SEPTOPLASTY

In the past, whenever a patient presented with a Müllerian fusion defect that was thought to be the cause of recurrent pregnancy loss, a Jones, Strassman, or Tompkins procedure would be performed by laparotomy. These procedures required lengthy anesthesia. Surgery could be complicated by infection or hemorrhage, necessitating antibiotic treatment and blood transfusions. Also, because the full thickness of the uterine fundus was surgically damaged, the patient would require Cesarean section for future deliveries. Some women became infertile as a result of adhesions or tubal occlusion, developing secondary to the procedure itself. Many Müllerian fusion defects are, however, amenable to hysteroscopic treatment.

Operative technique and management

The endoscopic technique for the management of uterine septa was first proposed by Edström and Fernström in 1970[1], but the method has only become widely used in recent years. Several different procedures have been adopted, with more or less similar results. The basic concept involves the transcervical observation of the uterine septum by means of hysteroscopy, followed by its resection. The use of operative hysteroscopes permits the passage of surgical instruments. Several authors[2,3] use liquid distension media in the uterine cavity, while others prefer CO_2[4]. We use a liquid medium for all hysteroscopic surgical procedures.

The traditional liquid distension medium has been dextran 70 or a solution of 5% dextrose; glycine is now preferred by most authors. This medium is not viscous, permits a clear visual field and is not a conductor of electricity. If electricity is not used, saline or Ringer's lactate can be employed. These are well tolerated when absorbed into the system.

Various instruments can be used for the resection of the septum. Miniature scissors were formerly used for the incision, but did not cut efficiently because they were non-rigid. Semi-rigid miniature scissors can be used for this type of surgery; they permit the required pressure, but are small enough to pass through the hysteroscopic operating sheath and along the cervical canal with no difficulty or risk. The blades can be opened wide enough to allow resection of even thick septa. Other surgeons[5,6] prefer to use the resectoscope, with cutting currents

ranging from 30 to 40 W/s. The resectoscope has several advantages: it is inexpensive and readily available in most operating rooms, as well as being simple to operate and highly efficient at removing the septum. Hamou reported the use of true electric knives, consisting of a miniature electric probe that is passed along the hysteroscopic operating sheath. He also uses an electric cutting current, although high frequency electric sources are advised for safety reasons. Finally, others[8–10] have suggested the use of lasers for this type of hysteroscopic surgery.

Partial uterine septum

Whatever the instrument used, the surgeon begins with resection of the septum (Figure 1), continuing until it has been resected almost flush with the surrounding endometrium. Regardless of the type of medium employed, the surgeon must be able to see the right and left cornual regions completely and keep the septum in view at all times. Concurrent laparoscopy at the time of hysteroscopic resection is recommended to confirm the diagnosis.

Querleu and co-workers[11] removed uterine septa using scissors without the help of hysteroscopy. Peroperative echography was performed in order to distinguish the septum from the myometrium. De Cherney and colleagues[5] advanced the loop of the resectoscope with cutting currents ranging from 30 to 40 W/s. The septum thus melts away. Care must be taken, however, to ensure that the laparoscopic observer constantly advises the hysteroscopist that the uterus is free of all contact with the bowel, bladder and other organs. Argon, krypton, KTP 532 and Nd : YAG lasers have all been successfully employed in the resection of uterine septa; however, certain limiting factors must be taken into consideration. First, Hyskon should not be used because caramelization can prove troublesome and may damage the laser fiber, resulting in delay while fibers are replaced or repaired. Second, the surgeon must be thoroughly acquainted with the physics of the particular laser being used. Third, only bare fibers should be used: CO_2-conducting fibers may cause bubbling of the medium which may lead to gas embolism, cardiovascular compromise and even death. In our department, the resection of uterine septa is systematically carried out using the Nd : YAG laser. The septum is cut using the 'touch technique' (Figure 2). The hysteroscope with the laser fiber is advanced and melts away the septum, while visual contact is maintained with the right and left uterine ostia. The mean time of hysteroscopic resection is < 15 min. The risk of fluid overload is therefore minimal.

The most delicate part of the procedure is probably deciding exactly when the resection is sufficient, and when continuing would cause damage to the myometrium and immediate complications such as perforation, or more delayed complictions such as uterine rupture during pregnancy. Almost all surgeons stop resection when the area between the tubal ostia is a line (Figure 2). Simultaneous laparoscopic control is extremely useful for this purpose, especially for beginners or when electricity is used. Querleu and associates[11] use echography to distinguish the septum from the myometrium, and thus the decision to stop the resection is easily made.

Complete uterine septum

For many years, only partial septal defects were treated hysteroscopically and wide (> 2 cm) or complete septal defects were corrected via an abdominal metroplasty. Donnez and co-workers[10] have described a method that will allow even complete septal defects to be managed hysteroscopically (Figure 3). Rock and colleagues[12] proposed the use of the resectoscope for the lysis of a complete uterine septum by means of a new method which makes it possible to leave the cervical septum intact, thus avoiding any subsequent cervical incompetence. For treating a complete uterine septum, they described a one-stage method where the other cervical os is occluded with the balloon of a Foley catheter, in order to prevent loss of the distending medium. They believe that it is better not to remove the cervical canal, since this might lead to subsequent cervical incompetence. We do not agree with this hypothesis, and all complete uterine septa are removed using the following surgical procedure, usually in two steps.

In some cases, not only may a double cervical canal be observed, but a vaginal sagittal septum may also be present in the upper vagina or throughout its length. In the first step, the vaginal septum (if present) is resected using a CO_2 laser. The cervical septum is then incised with a CO_2 laser connected to a colposcope, until the lower portion of the uterine septum is seen. The second step is performed 2 months after the first operation, when the aspect of the external cervical os is completely normal (Figure 4). Nd:YAG laser resection of the uterine septum is then carried out. The hysteroscope is advanced while visual contact is maintained with the right and left uterine ostia. Because the septum is poorly vascularized, bleeding is usually minimal. Hysterosalpingography (Figure 5) demonstrates the presence of a normal, single cervical canal 2 months after the first step and a normal uterine cavity 2 months after the second step.

No patients in our department presented any subsequent cervical incompetence. Prophylactic cerclage was never performed after resection of a complete cervical and uterine septum. Following hysteroscopic metroplasty Cesarean section should be performed only for obstetric reasons.

Pre- and postoperative management

Following excision of very wide septa, the surgeon's vision may be obscured by pieces of resected tissue and, at times, by uterine bleeding. The Nd:YAG laser produces no debris and carries a reduced risk of bleeding. Several authors have suggested preoperative treatment with danazol or LHRH agonists; others[7] inject a solution of pitressin into the cervix. Neither pitressin nor hormone administration is required with laser therapy. Although preoperative hormonal therapy causes atrophy of the endometrium and reduces vacularization and intraoperative bleeding, it also reduces the depth of the myometrium and therefore increases the risk of perforation and/or myometrial damage.

Postoperatively, a broad-spectrum antibiotic is administered for 3–4 days. In order to avoid the risk of synechiae, an intrauterine device (IUD; Multiload®) is inserted into the uterine cavity. Hormone replacement therapy with estrogens (100–200 μg of ethinylestradiol) and progestogens (5–15 mg Lynestrenol) is given for 3 months. DeCherney and co-workers[5], however, use neither hormone replacement therapy nor IUDs. Formerly, Perino and associates[13] administered both estrogens and medroxyprogesterone and inserted IUDs, but they have recently abandoned these measures and now administer no postoperative therapy. Hamou[7] performs a hysteroscopic procedure 1 month after surgery in order to separate synechiae, if necessary.

Almost all authors agree that a follow-up examination should be performed 1–2 months after the operation, irrespective of the postoperative management. Inspection can be made either by means of hysterosalpingography or hysteroscopy. Hamou performs a hysteroscopic inspection 1 month after resection of the septum; in his opinion, this is early enough to prevent the development of synechiae.

In our department, the postoperative morphology of the uterine cavity is systematically evaluated 4 months after the resection. One month after the removal of the IUD, a hysterosalpingography is carried out (Figure 5); the morphology of the uterine cavity almost always resembles an arcuate uterus. Indeed, it is preferable not to resect the septum too much, but to leave a sufficient depth of myometrium at the top of the uterus. A hysteroscopy is also performed to confirm that re-epithelialization of the resected endometrial area has occurred.

Results

DeCherney and associates[5] reported the successful use of the urologic resectoscope in 72 out of 103 women, with

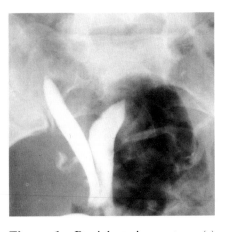

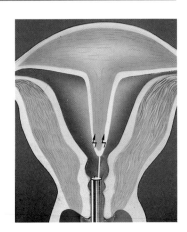

Figure 1 Partial uterine septum: (a) hysterography; (b) illustration; and (c) hysteroscopic view

Figure 2(a)–(c) Resection of the uterine septum is carried out with the help of the ND : YAG laser

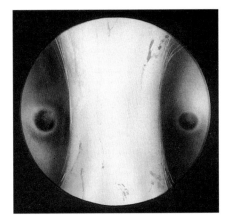

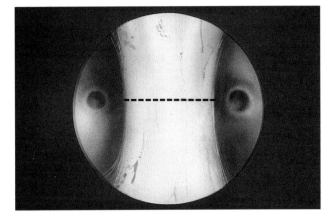

Figure 1(b)   *See legend above*

Figure 2(b)   *See legend above*

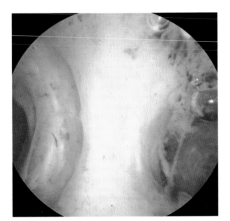

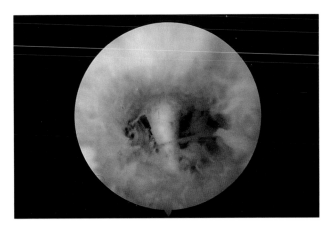

Figure 1(c)   *See legend above*

Figure 2(c)   *See legend above*

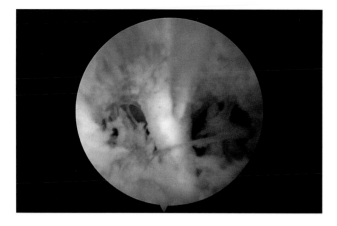

Figure 2(d)–(g) The septum is cut using the touch technique. The hysteroscope with the laser fiber is advanced. The septum is melted away by a simple advancement of the bare fiber

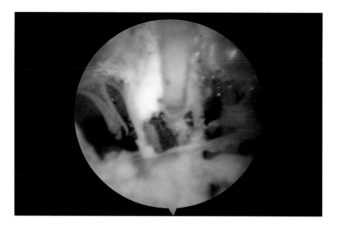

Figure 2(e) *See legend opposite*

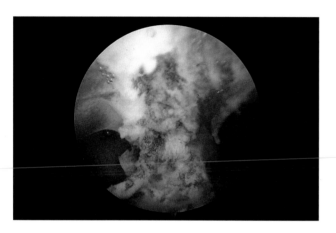

Figure 2(f) *See legend above*

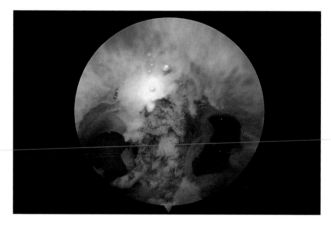

Figure 2(g) *See legend above*

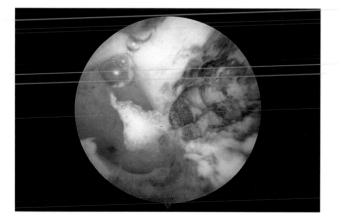

Figure 2(h) Visual contact with uterine ostia

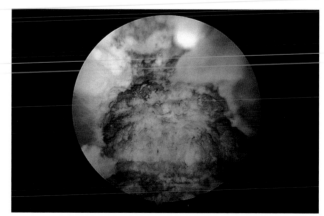

Figure 2(i) Final view

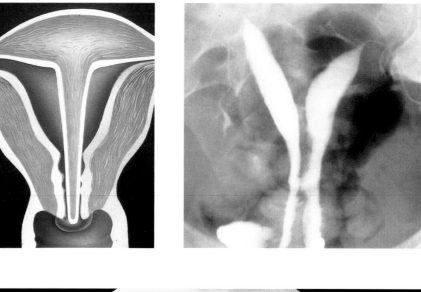

Figure 3(a) and (b) Complete uterine septum (utero-cervical septum)

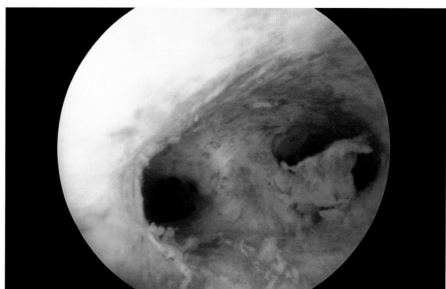

Figure 4 Two months after resection of the cervical septum, the aspect of the cervical canal is completely normal and the uterine septum is clearly seen

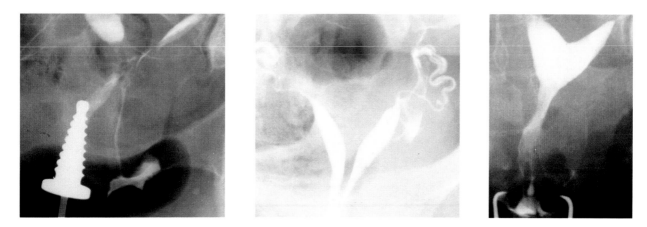

Figure 5 Complete uterine septum, hysterography. Left: before the first step; center: 2 months after the resection of the cervical septum (first step), a normal single cervical canal is seen; right: 2 months after the removal of the uterine septum (second step), hysterography reveals a normal uterine cavity

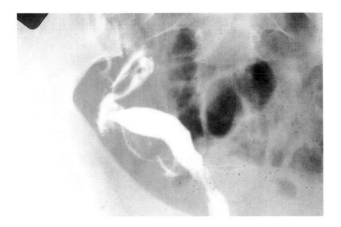

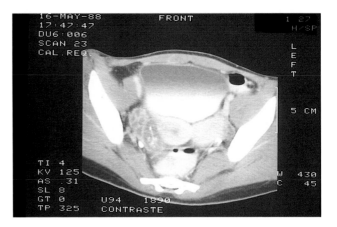

Figure 6 Rudimentary left uterine horn: (a) hystero-graphy: normal right hemi-uterus; (b) computerized tomography: a small uterine horn is seen on the left side; (c) laparoscopic view

Figure 6(b)   *See legend opposite*

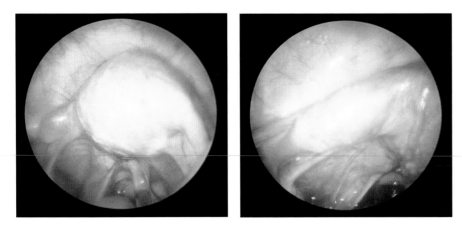

Figure 6(c)   *See legend above*

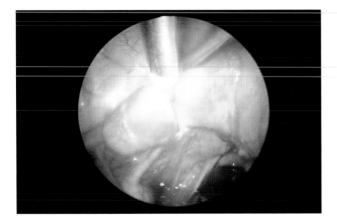

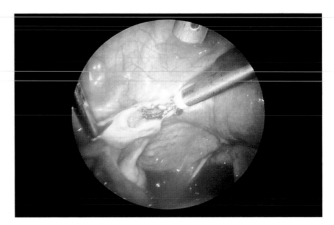

Figure 7 Hemihysterectomy: (a) coagulation of the space between both uterine horns

Figure 7(b)   Section

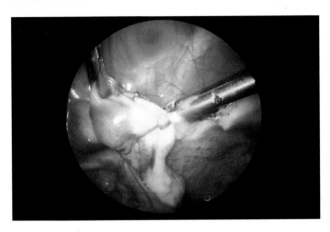

Figure 7(c) and (d) Coagulation and section of the broad ligament and the uterine artery

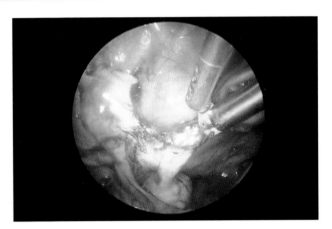

Figure 7(d) *See legend opposite*

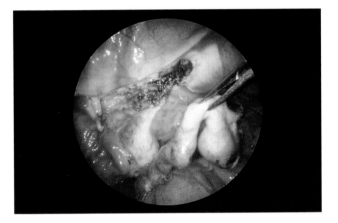

Figure 7(e) Salpingectomy of the affected horn is then carried out

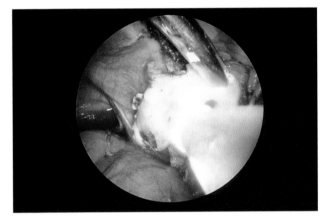

Figure 7(f) Removal of the rudimentary horn through the operating channel or through the trocar

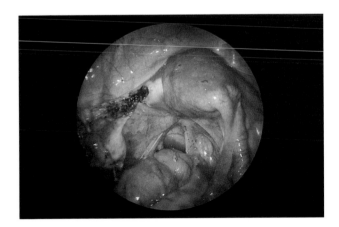

Figure 7(g) Final view

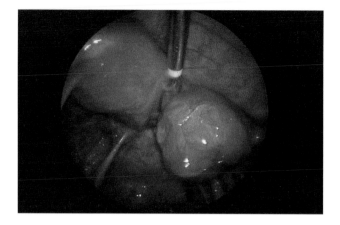

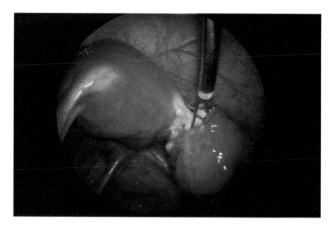

Figure 8(a)–(c)   The same procedure as described in Figure 7 can also be performed if the size of the rudimentary horn is similar to the 'normal' horn

Figure 8(b)   *See legend opposite*

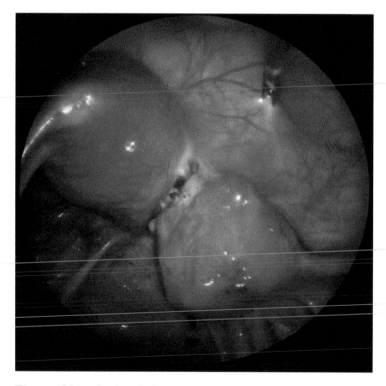

Figure 8(c)   *See legend above*

a term pregnancy rate of 80%. The full-term pregnancy rate reported in various studies[5] ranges from 70 to 80%. Operative hysteroscopy is a safe and effective method of management of uterine septa associated with recurrent pregnancy loss, and makes future vaginal delivery possible.

HEMIHYSTERECTOMY OF THE NON-COMMUNICATING RUDIMENTARY HORNS

Rudimentary pregnancy in a non-communicating horn (Figure 6) is uncommon and usually results in abortion or uterine rupture. Such cases are due to transmigration of sperm into the Fallopian tube of the affected horn. Most of the complictions occur within the first 20 weeks: the most severe are uterine rupture and maternal death. Raman and colleagues[14] recently described a 17-week pregnancy occurring in a rudimentary horn, treated by laparotomy and excision. In order to avoid maternal complications, we systematically perform an excision of the rudimentary horn. A laparoscopic hemihysterectomy (Figure 7) can easily be carried out using the same techniques as for laparoscopic hysterectomy.

Operative technique

A Foley catheter is inserted during surgery to empty the bladder. Four laparoscopic puncture sites including the umbilicus are used: 10 mm umbilical, 5 mm right, 5 mm medial and 5 mm left lower quadrant sites. These are placed just above the pubic hairline and the lateral incisions are made next to the deep epigastric vessels. A cannula is placed in the single cervix for appropriate uterine mobilization. A bipolar forceps is used to compress and desiccate the fibrous tissue between the horns. The tissue is then cut with scissors and with a CO_2 laser. Bipolar coagulation is used to coagulate the pedicle. Scissor division is carried out close to the line of desiccation to ensure that a compressed pedicle remains. The mesosalpinx is then cut. If necessary, the peritoneum of the vesico-uterine space is grasped and elevated with a forceps, while the scissors dissect the vesico-uterine space. Aquadissection may be used to separate the leaves of the broad ligament, distending the vesico-uterine space and defining the tendinous attachments of the bladder in this area, which are coagulated and cut. The tube of the affected horn is then removed. The external tubal vessel is identified and exposed by applying traction to the adnexa with an opposite forceps.

The dissection of the two horns is performed as follows. If there is true separation of the two horns, the fibrous tissue is coagulated with bipolar coagulation and then cut with scissors or with the CO_2 laser.

If there is no external separation of the two horns, the dissection is more difficult (Figure 8); after coagulation, the myometrium must be cut in order to allow the removal of the rudimentary horn. For this purpose, bipolar coagulation and the CO_2 laser or the Nd : YAG laser fiber can be used, permitting coagulation and resection of the myometrium.

The rudimentary horn is removed either through the trocar of the laparoscope (Figure 7), or through a posterior colpotomy in cases of larger rudimentary horns.

The procedure has been successfully performed in our department in more than 10 women. All women who became pregnant had a normal vaginal delivery (> 36 weeks), except one woman in whom Cesarean section was performed for fetal reasons.

REFERENCES

1. Edström, K. and Fernström, I (1970). The diagnostic possibilities of a modified hysteroscopic technique. *Acta Obstet. Gynecol. Scand.*, **49**, 327
2. Chervenak, F.A. and Neuwirth, R.S. (1981). Hysteroscopic resection of the uterine septum. *Am. J. Obstet. Gynecol.*, **141**, 351
3. Valle, R.F. and Sciarra, J.J. (1986). Hysteroscopic resection of the septate uterus. *Obstet. Gynecol.*, **67**, 253
4. Gallinat, A. (1993). Endometrial ablation using the Nd : YAG laser in CO_2 hysteroscopy. In Leuken, R.P. and Gallinat, A. (eds.) *Endoscopic Surgery in Gynecology*, pp.109–16. (Berlin: Demeter Verlag GmbH)
5. DeCherney, A.H., Russel, L.J.B., Graebe, R.A. *et al.* (1986). Resectoscopic management of müllerian defects. *Fertil. Steril.*, **45**, 726
6. Corson, S.L. and Batzer, F.R. (1986). CO_2 uterine distension for hysteroscopic septal incision. *J. Reprod. Med.*, **31**, 710
7. Hamou, J. (1993). Electroresection of fibroids. In Sutton, C. and Diamond, M. (eds.) *Endoscopic Surgery for Gynaecologists*, pp.327–30. (London: Saunders)
8. Daniell, J.F., Osher, S. and Miller, W. (1987). Hysteroscopic resection of uterine septi with visible light laser energy. *Colpos. Gynecol. Laser Surg.*, **3**, 217
9. Loffer, F.D. (1986). Hysteroscopic management of menorrhagia. *Acta Eur. Fertil.*, **17**, 463
10. Donnez, J. and Nisolle, M. (1989). Operative laser hysteroscopy in Mullerian fusion defects and uterine adhesions. In Donnez, J. (ed.) *Laser Operative Laparoscopy and Hysteroscopy*, pp.249–61. (Leuven: Nauwelaerts Printing)
11. Querleu, D., Brasme, T.L. and Parmentier, D. (1990). Ultrasound-guided transcervical metroplasty. *Fertil. Steril.*, **54**, 995–8
12. Rock, J.A., Murphy, A.A. and Cooper, W.H.

(1987). Resectoscopic technique for the lysis of a class V complete uterine septum. *Fertil. Steril.*, **48**, 495

13. Perino, A., Mencaglia, L., Hamou, J. and Cittadini, E. (1987). Hysteroscopy for metroplasty of uterine septa: report of 24 cases. *Fertil. Steril.*, **48,** 321

14. Raman, S., Tai, C. and Neom, H.S. (1993). Noncommunicating rudimentary horn pregnancy. *J. Gynecol. Surg.*, **9**, 59–62

Hysteroscopic lysis of intrauterine adhesions (Asherman's syndrome)

32

J. Donnez and M. Nisolle

Intrauterine adhesions have been related to recurrent abortion, sterility and menstrual disorders. Relief from adhesions has been associated with pregnancy rates of 50% and the disappearance of menstrual disorders in more than 75% of cases.

In 1948, Asherman described 'amenorrhea traumatica' as amenorrhea secondary to intrauterine adhesions, following a curettage for incomplete or missed abortion and postpartum hemorrhage[1]. The term 'Asherman's syndrome' is used to describe this condition.

ETIOPATHOGENESIS

Infection (endometritis) rarely causes adhesions, except in cases of tuberculous endometritis. Most frequently (> 90%) intrauterine adhesions develop after a curettage[2]. The most important factor in the development of intrauterine adhesions is traumatic curettage or manipulation of the endometrium during the post-partum or postabortal period. The denudation of the basalis layer and exposure of the muscularis layer produce adhesions by coaptation between the opposing uterine walls.

DIAGNOSIS AND CLASSIFICATION

Dilatation and curettage are not of diagnostic value for intrauterine adhesions. In amenorrheic women with a biphasic basal body temperature curve, failure of the progesterone challenge test to cause withdrawal bleeding, may suggest the diagnosis, if the patient has a medical history of postpartum or postabortal curettage.

Hysterosalpingography is the most accurate screening method in the diagnosis of intrauterine adhesions[3]. Adhesions are suggested by radiographic filling defects. Hysteroscopy confirms the presence of intrauterine adhesions and allows definitive surgical treatment. Although adhesions can be diagnosed by hysterosalpingography (HSG) or hysteroscopy, both are necessary to confirm their presence and their location.

There are many classifications of adhesions based on histology, hysterography, symptomatology and hysteroscopy. To be able to compare the results of treatment and to determine the therapeutic regimen, the adhesions should be classified from the hysteroscopic and hysterosalpingographic (HSG) findings according to the IUA

classification of the European Society of Hysteroscopy (ESH)[4]. We use our own classification (Table 1)[5], essentially based on the location of the intrauterine adhesions. We consider location to be one of the most important prognostic factors in determining the postoperative pregnancy rate. Degree 1 adhesions are central (Figure 1 and 2) and are classified as thin or filmy adhesions and myofibrous adhesions. Degree 2 adhesions are marginal (Figures 3 and 4). Degree 3 adhesions are revealed by the absence of the uterine cavity at hysterography (Figure 5).

Table 1 Classification according to the location and the aspect of the adhesions[5]

Degree	Location
I	Central adhesions (bridge-like adhesions) (a) thin or filmy adhesions (endometrial adhesions) (b) myofibrous or connective adhesions
II	Marginal adhesions (always myofibrous or connective) (a) ledge-like projections (b) obliteration of one horn
III	Uterine cavity 'absent' on hysterosalpingography (a) occlusion of the internal os (upper cavity normal) (pseudo-Asherman's syndrome) (b) extensive coaptation of the uterine walls (absence of uterine cavity) (true Asherman's syndrome)

Valle and Sciarra[6] classified intrauterine adhesions as mild, moderate and severe, based on the degree of intrauterine involvement on HSG and the extent and type of adhesions found on hysteroscopy. Mild adhesions are defined as filmy adhesions composed of basalis endometrial tissue, producing partial or complete uterine cavity occlusion; moderate adhesions are fibromuscular, characteristically thick and still covered with endometrium: severe adhesions are composed of connective tissue only[7].

The American Fertility Society[8] has proposed a classification of intrauterine adhesions based on the findings at HSG and hysteroscopy and the correlation with menstrual patterns.

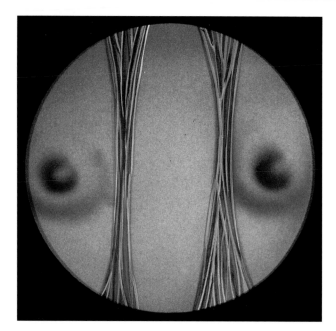

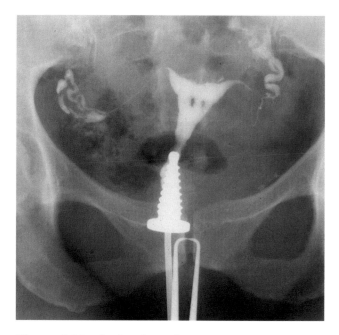

Figure 1(a) and (b) Intrauterine adhesions: degree Ia central adhesions (bridge-like adhesions)

Figure 1(b) *See legend opposite*

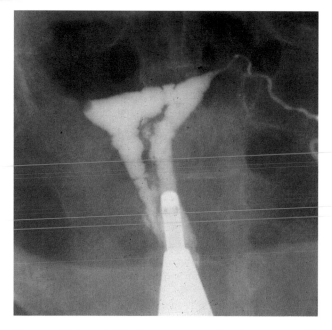

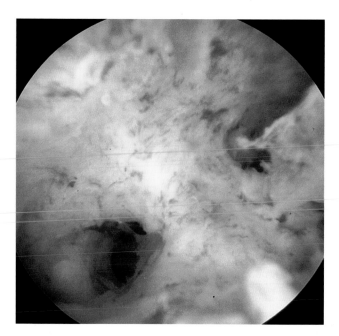

Figure 2(a) and (b) Intrauterine adhesion, degree Ib myofibrous central adhesions

Figure 2(b) *See legend opposite*

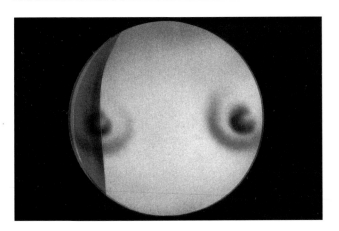

Figure 3(a)–(c) Intrauterine adhesion, degree IIa marginal adhesions (always myofibrous or connective adhesions)

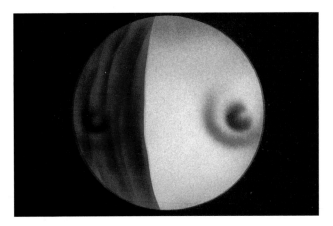

Figure 4(a)–(c) Intrauterine adhesions, degree IIb right marginal adhesion, obliterating the horn

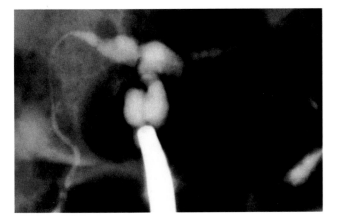

Figure 3(b) *See legend above*

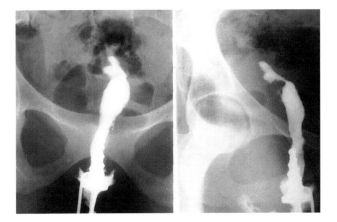

Figure 4(b) *See legend above*

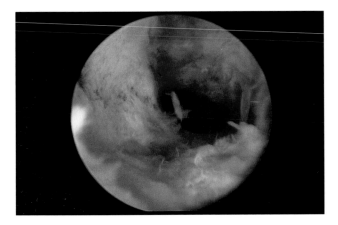

Figure 3(c) *See legend above*

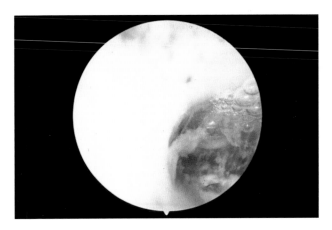

Figure 4(c) *See legend above*

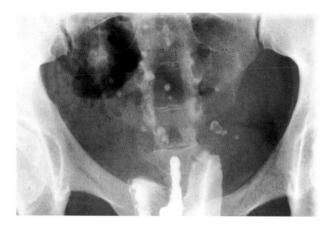

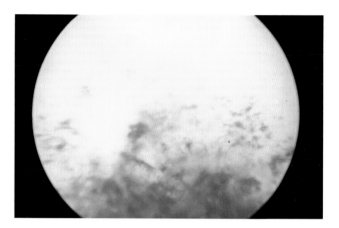

Figure 5(a) and (b)   Intrauterine adhesion, degree III. The cervical canal is visible. The uterine cavity is 'absent'. Only preoperative evaluation permits the differentiation of pseudo-Asherman's from 'true' Asherman's syndrome

Figure 5(b)   *See legend opposite*

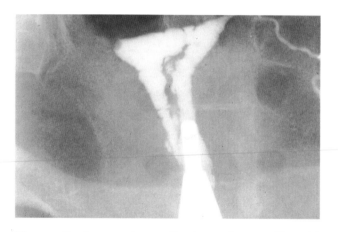

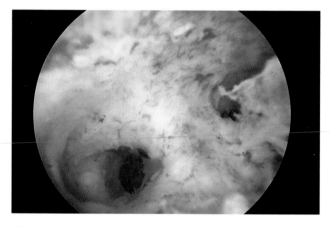

Figure 6   Intrauterine adhesion, degree Ib: (a) hysterosalpingography determines the location

Figure 6(b)   Hysteroscopy determines the type (connective tissue)

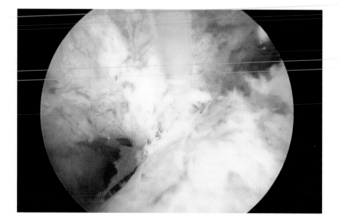

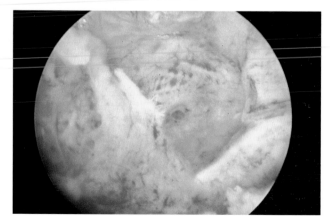

Figure 6(c)   The adhesion is divided with the help of the laser (Nd : YAG) fiber

Figure 6(d)   Final view: the fundus of the uterine cavity (with tubal ostium)

TREATMENT AND RESULTS

Hysterotomies for the division of adhesions and other blind transcervical manipulations are only of historical interest. Blind division of intrauterine adhesions by dilatation does not provide accurate and precise treatment.

Thin or filmy endometrial adhesions are often removed easily by pushing with the tip of the hysteroscopic sheath. Myofibrous or connective adhesions require a synechiotomy. The surgical treatment of intrauterine adhesions thus consists of dividing the adhesions mechanically, or using electrosurgery and/or fiberoptic lasers. The gynecological resectoscope with a modified knife electrode has been used to divide adhesions electrosurgically. Fiberoptic lasers, such as the argon, KTP 532, and Nd:YAG laser with sculptured or extruded fibers, have also been used.

In our series, the Nd:YAG laser was used to remove endometrial adhesions, even when they were multiple and fibrous. Degree 1 and 1b adhesions were easily cut by the laser fiber (Figure 6). Combined laparoscopy and hysteroscopy can be used, if indicated, to decrease the risk of uterine perforation.

The lateral, back and front scattering of KTP and Nd:YAG laser beams may decrease the viability of the surrounding healthy endometrium. When the adhesions partially occlude the uterine cavity (degree Ib), their division is simple: they are divided in the middle, the remaining stumps retract, and the uterine cavity distends, permitting a panoramic view (Figure 6). Marginal or lateral adhesions (degree IIa and b), particularly if they are extensive and fibromuscular or composed of connective tissue, may be difficult to divide (Figure 7). The Nd:YAG laser may not be a good tool for treatment of this type of adhesion. More severe adhesions may even develop, due to the scattering of the laser, decreasing the viability of the surrounding healthy myometrium.

For uterine adhesions of degree III (Figure 8), hysteroscopic observation of the uterine cavity should begin at the internal cervical os: if the adhesions extend to that area, their selective division begins there. As the adhesions are divided and the uterine cavity opens, the hysteroscope is advanced to the fundal area, and both uterotubal ostia are visualized. Sometimes, increased pressure in the uterine cavity, obtained by increasing the inflow pressure, can facilitate the dissection by distending the uterine cavity. Although the plane of dissection is better exposed, this procedure can lead to excessive fluid intravasation if prolonged.

Low viscosity fluids are frequently chosen for operative hysteroscopy because of their ability to remove debris and cleanse the uterine cavity, even in the presence of slight uterine bleeding. Normal saline and Ringer's lactate are excellent media to distend the uterine cavity when treating intrauterine adhesions with hysteroscopic scissors or with the Nd:YAG laser. Care must be taken to avoid solutions containing electrolytes while using electrocoagulation, to control the volume of fluids not accounted for, and to prevent excessive fluid intravasation, particularly when using fluids without electrolytes. Intrauterine adhesions of the moderate and severe type require extensive dissection, increasing the risk of excessive intravasation.

Prophylactic antibiotics are given 1 h prior to hysteroscopic treatment and for 2–3 days postoperatively, when a splint is left in the uterine cavity. We have not found a second hysteroscopy to be of any particular value. A second therapeutic hysteroscopy is performed only if hysterosalpingography demonstrates residual adhesions.

The subsequent insertion of an intrauterine device (IUD) and hormonal treatment have been associated with increasing success rates. In our department, estrogen and progestogen replacement therapy is initiated after surgery for 3 months (ethinylestradiol 100 μg/day and Lynestrenol 10 mg/day for 6 weeks). The doses are doubled for the following 6 weeks.

SUCCESS RATE

In collective series (Table 2), success rates of 74–94% have been obtained[8]. It is very difficult to compare different series because the results have not been evaluated according to the degree of severity. In a recent review[8], the pregnancy rate was 60.5%, and 80% of those pregnancies reached term.

Table 2 Hysteroscopic lysis of intrauterine adhesions

Reference	Patients (n)	Technique	Menses normal n	%	Pregnancy n	%	Term pregnancy n	%
9	27	scissors alongside hysteroscope	20	74	14	51.8	13	48.1
4	36	scissors/biopsy forceps	34	94.4	17	62.9	12	44.4
6	187	flexible/semi-rigid/ rigid scissors	167	89.3	143	76.4	114	79.7

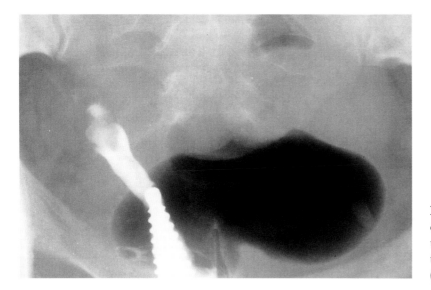

Figure 7 Intrauterine adhesions: (a) degree IIb adhesions in a unicornuate uterus; (b) and (c) the area of connective tissue appears white and fibrotic; (d) and (e) synechiotomy

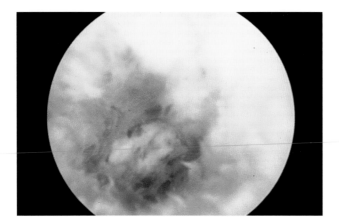

Figure 7(b) *See legend above*

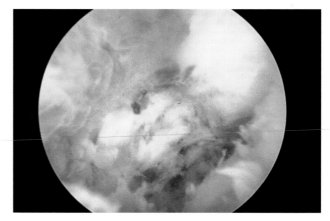

Figure 7(c) *See legend above*

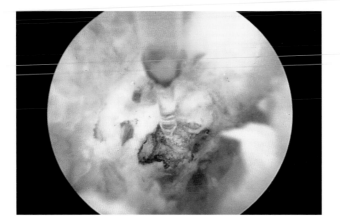

Figure 7(d) *See legend above*

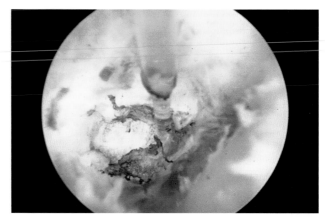

Figure 7(e) *See legend above*

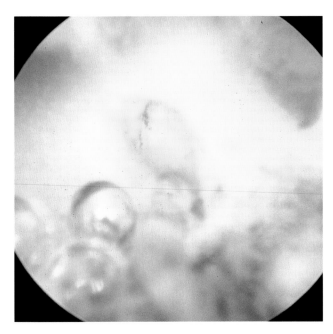

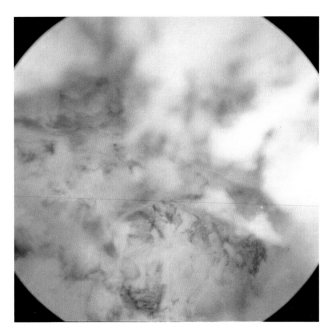

Figure 8 Asherman's syndrome: (a) uterine cavity absent; (b) synechiotomy; (c) rugged aspect of uterine cavity at the end of the procedure

Figure 8(b) *See legend opposite*

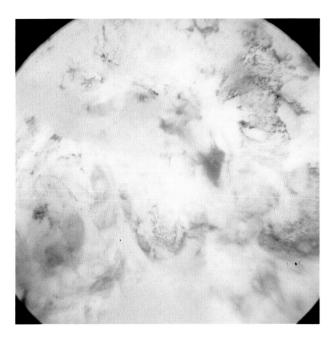

Figure 8(c) *See legend above*

In our series of 74 patients treated for intrauterine synechiae, eight patients were amenorrheic with an absent uterine cavity at hysterography. Four were classified as degree IIIa, and four as degree IIIb. Surgery was successfully performed in group IIIa, with a pregnancy rate of 100%. In group IIIb, however, adhesions recurred; a second-look hysteroscopy showed only a tunnel-shaped uterine cavity with an absence of healthy endometrium. Hysterosalpingography, carried out 3 months after surgery, confirmed the presence of adhesions; some were more severe than the initial adhesions.

CONCLUSION

The hysteroscopic treatment of intrauterine adhesions restored normal menstruation in >80% of treated patients[8]. The results in terms of normal menses and pregnancy rates are excellent for those with adhesions of degrees Ia, Ib, IIa and IIIa. Degree IIb and IIIb adhesions tended to recur and to be more severe in six out of 10 women, and no pregnancy occurred in this group.

Patients treated for moderate or severe adhesions should be considered at risk during delivery. Following delivery, care must be taken to make an early diagnosis of any abnormalities, such as placenta accreta or percreta[6].

REFERENCES

1. Asherman, J.G. (1948). Amenorrhoea traumatica (atretica). *J. Obstet. Gynecol. Br. Empire*, **55**, 23–30
2. Schenker, J.G. and Margalioth, E.J. (1982). Intrauterine adhesions; an updated appraisal. *Fertil. Steril.*, **37**, 593
3. Donnez, J. and Nisolle, M. (1989). Operative laser hysteroscopy in Müllerian fusion defects and uterine adhesions. In Donnez, J. (ed.) *Operative Laser Laparoscopy and Hysteroscopy*, p. 249. (Leuven: Nauwelaerts Printing)
4. Wamsteker, K. (1984). Hysteroscopy in the management of abnormal uterine bleeding in 199 patients. In Siegler, A.M. and Lindemann, H.I. (eds.) *Hysteroscopy, Principles and Practice*, pp. 128–31. (Philadelphia: J. B. Lippincott)
5. Donnez, J. and Nisolle, M. (1989). Operative laser hysteroscopy in Müllerian fusion defects and uterine adhesions. In Donnez, J. (ed.) *Laser Operative Laparoscopy and Hysteroscopy*, pp. 249–61. (Leuven: Nauwelaerts Printing)
6. Valle, R.F. and Sciarra, J.J. (1988). Intrauterine adhesions: hysteroscopic diagnosis classification treatment and reproductive outcome. *Am. J. Obstet. Gynecol.*, **158**, 1459–70
7. Valle, R. (1993). Lysis of intrauterine adhesions (Asherman's syndrome). In Sutton, C. and Diamond, M. (eds.) *Endoscopic Surgery for Gynecologists*, p. 338. (London: Saunders)
8. American Fertility Society (1988). The American Fertility Society classifications of adnexal adhesions, distal tubal occlusion, tubal occlusion secondary to tubal ligation, tubal pregnancies, Müllerian anomalies and intrauterine adhesion. *Fertil Steril.*, **49**, 944–55
9. Neuwirth, R.S., Hussein, A.R., Schiffman, B.M. and Amin, H.K. (1982). Hysteroscopic resection of intrauterine scars using a new technique. *Obstet. Gynecol.*, **60**, 111–13

Endometrial ablation in dysfunctional bleeding: size of the uterine cavity

33

J. Donnez, M. Nisolle, S. Gillerot, F. Clerckx, M. Smets, S. Bassil and V. Anaf

Hysteroscopic surgical techniques, which allow destruction of the endometrium under direct vision, have proved to be successful in the control of menorrhagia[1,2]. Both the electrical current of the resectoscope[3,4] and the energy of the Nd:YAG laser[1,5-7] effectively destroy endometrial tissue to a sufficient depth to avoid regeneration. Patients who are considering this procedure must be aware that further childbearing is impossible, although there is an apparently minimal risk of pregnancy. Laser ablation is not a sterilization procedure, and concomitant sterilization may be proposed. Patients should undergo diagnostic hysteroscopy with endometrial sampling prior to laser ablation. The technique cannot be used for the treatment of patients with abnormal endometrial conditions because some areas of endometrium may not be destroyed.

The aim of the procedure is to decrease the menstrual flow sufficiently to avoid hysterectomy. Indeed, amenorrhea and hypomenorrhea are recognized as sequelae of intrauterine adhesions; the laser ablation procedure is designed to create this condition. Other methods which have been used in an attempt to create endometrial destruction and scarring include cryotherapy, superheated steam, intracavitary radium, rigorous curettage, quinocrine methylcyanoacrylate, oxalic acid, paraformaldehyde and silicone rubber. However, only the neodymium: yttrium-aluminum-garnet (Nd:YAG) laser[1,2,8,9] and the resectoscope[3,4] have produced acceptable results.

The resectoscope has the advantage that it does not require the major capital investment needed for a laser. However, the resectoscope is a unipolar electrical instrument and there is a risk of damaging the bowel or bladder with the current transmitted through the uterine wall or by actual penetration of the uterine wall with the cutting loop. There is also a risk of bleeding if major uterine vessels are transected by cutting too deeply into the uterine wall.

Laser energy, on the other hand, has some advantages in precision of tissue destruction that are not shared by the electrical energy used in the resectoscope. Unlike electricity, laser energy does not travel through tissue; its tissue effect depends on the amount of power used, and its effects are quite reproducible.

There are three reasons favoring the use of the Nd:YAG laser for endometrial ablation:

(1) The use of a flexible quartz fiber;

(2) The ability to transmit laser energy to the tissue surface through a liquid distending medium (saline solution can be used);

(3) The ability to penetrate tissue to a controlled depth.

METHODS

Preoperative therapy

Once the decision to proceed with surgery has been made, the endometrium is brought into a resting phase by treatment with Danazol (400 mg twice daily beginning during the menses)[2] or with a gonadotropin releasing hormone (GnRH) agonist[8]. Administration of GnRH analogs (Zoladex implant; Decapeptyl injection) reduces uterine size and facilitates the surgical procedure[6-8].

In our department, the implant is injected subcutaneously at the end of the luteal phase, to curtail the initial gonadotropin stimulation phase always associated with a rise in estrogens. Significant uterine shrinkage occurs after 8 weeks of therapy. Hysterosalpingography (using the short-line 'multipurpose test system' described by Weibel)[10] revealed an average decrease in the uterine cavity area of 35%[7,8] (range 5-60%). This decrease was greater in patients with a very enlarged uterine cavity (> 10 cm^2) than in those with an initial uterine cavity area of < 10 cm^2 (Figure 1).

The advantages of preoperative therapy are:

(1) Endometrial ablation is easily performed (thin endometrium, small uterine cavity).

(2) The risk of fluid overload is decreased[7,11,12].

Equipment

The quartz fiber used to carry the laser light is 'bare', extending for several millimeters beyond its thin plastic jacket. The fiber is sterilized using gas or alcohol. The laser power is generally set between 60 and 80 W. Several hysteroscopic instruments are suitable for endometrial ablation. The cystoscope designed for the Nd:YAG laser has a deflecting arm, which stabilizes the quartz fiber, and an integrated bundle that screws into a compatible operative port. A hysteroscopic bridge (Storz) is now also available (see Chapter 27).

Constant uterine distension is achieved using a 3000 ml plastic bag of 1.5% glycine solution or 0.9%

saline solution wrapped in a pressure infusion cuff. The tubing is connected to the hysteroscope, with a pressure of 100–150 mmHg. As soon as the bag begins to empty, the nurse gives the surgeon an evaluation of the fluid volume absorbed by the patient; since fluid overload is a reported problem[13], the amount of fluid retained by the patient must be monitored. Unlike dextran, 1.5% glycine solution and 0.9% saline solution do not caramelize when heated.

Endometrial ablation technique

Regional or general anesthesia is recommended, as the use of local anesthesia is accompanied by considerable cramp. All operative hysteroscopies are performed with the uterine cavity well distended (intrauterine pressure exceeding venous pressure), to prevent bleeding from the endometrial surface.

There are three techniques for applying laser energy to the endometrial cavity:

(1) The touch technique[1,14];

(2) The non-touch technique[2]; and

(3) A combination of both techniques.

The original description[14] and most of the cases that have been reported have used the touch technique, in which the quartz laser fiber is in actual contact with the endometrium. This creates furrows in the endometrium, which are clearly visible (Figure 2). The endometrium, and presumably the deeper areas of myometrium (Figure 3), are actually vaporized as the quartz fiber cuts into the tissue. Care must be taken to photocoagulate the endometrium in the uterine horns, close to the tubal ostium (Figure 4). The procedure is performed more easily with a flexible fiber than with the resectoscope.

A considerable amount of debris, including endometrial fragments and bubbles, is created with both the touch and the non-touch techniques. Blood, bubbles and debris can be eliminated by a continuous-flow hysteroscope, as mentioned above. The two different sheaths allow the continued distension of the endometrial cavity, while fluid is drained from the uterine cavity. True aspiration is generally not necessary as the pressure of the distending medium will push debris out through the out-flow sheath. If a large piece of endometrial tissue blocks the entrance, it may be necessary to remove the sheath and the telescope from the uterine cavity.

In the non-touch technique[2], the end of the quartz fiber is brought as near to the lining of the uterus as possible, since power density diminishes when the fiber is at a distance from the surface. The fiber is also directed, as perpendicularly as possible, at the uterine wall to decrease the amount of reflection and increase the amount of absorption. There is a distinct whitening and slight swelling of the endometrium as it is coagulated. Although the end point of endometrial coagulation with the non-touch technique is determinable by the blanching and swelling of tissue, this change is not as easily detectable as the changes observed with the touch technique. When applying the laser beam to the uterine wall, it is helpful to outline small contiguous areas (Figure 5) so that roughly equal amounts of energy can be applied to all areas (Figure 6). As these sections are connected, they advance towards the internal os and eventually cover the anterior uterine wall. The smaller lateral walls are done next, while the posterior wall is treated last, in much the same way as the anterior wall.

Loffer[2] has described a combination of the touch and non-touch techniques. The decision to switch to a touch technique was not made because of dissatisfaction with the non-touch technique, but rather in order to gain experience and to determine whether a higher amenorrhea rate could be obtained. After the endometrial cavity has been completely covered using the non-touch technique as described, the surface is re-treated with the touch technique. The uterine cavity is small, and it is difficult to apply the laser beam perpendicularly to the lower uterine segment using the non-touch technique. The deflecting arm of the hysteroscope can be used, but it is not of particular value, since the interior of the uterine cavity is not large enough to allow the fiber to be flexed at right angles to the uterine wall. Using the touch technique, the fiber can simply be drawn along the lower uterine segment. The procedure aims to decrease the menstrual flow and avoid the need for hysterectomy: amenorrhea and hypomenorrhea are recognised sequelae of endometrial destruction and uterine shrinkage (Figure 7). When only partial endometrial ablation is performed, an area of normal endometrium can be seen at hysterosalpingography (Figure 8).

Selection of patients

In a series of more than 750 patients treated for meno-metrorrhagia by hysteroscopy, we tried to classify the uterine pathology, in order to evaluate the use of endometrial ablation in dysfunctional bleeding. Only women without intrauterine lesions were considered. Two groups of patients were defined according to the size of the uterine cavity ($< 10\ cm^2$; $> 10\ cm^2$) prior to GnRH agonist therapy. The endometrium was brought into a resting phase by subcutaneous injection of a depot GnRH agonist at the end of the luteal phase and then 4 and 8 weeks later[8]. We currently consider the ideal therapy to be preoperative GnRH agonist injection at weeks 0 and 4, followed by hysteroscopic surgery at week 5 or 6. A period of 4–5 weeks of very low estradiol levels is sufficient to reduce the endometrium to a very thin post-menopausal state.

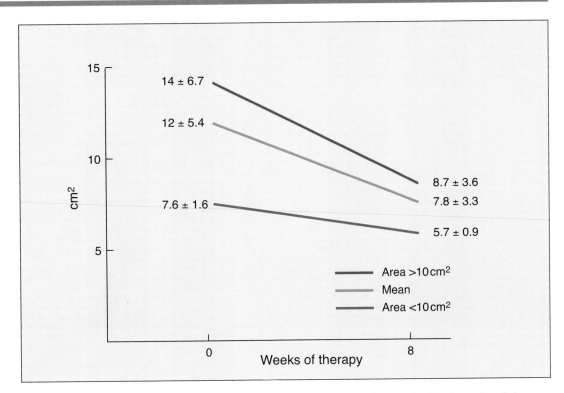

Figure 1 Uterine cavity area as assessed by hysterography before and after 8 weeks of therapy with a gonadotropin releasing hormone agonist

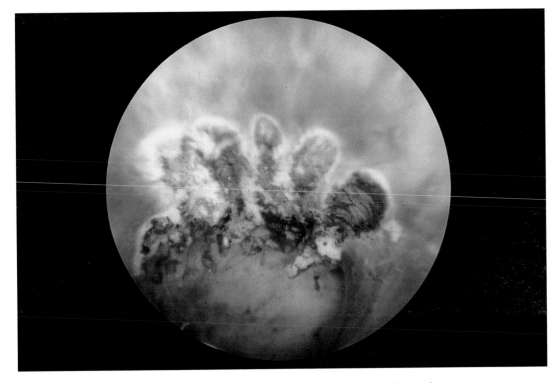

Figure 2 With the touch technique, furrows are created in the endometrium

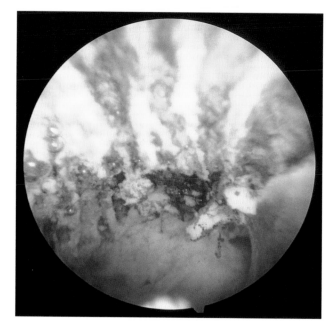

Figure 3 Areas of myometrium are visible proving ablation of the endometrium to a sufficient depth

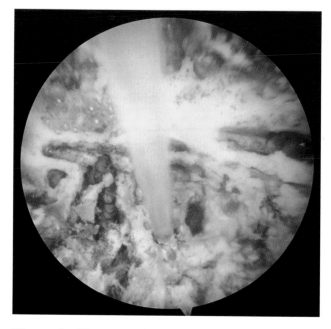

Figure 4 Photocoagulation of the endometrium in the uterine horns and between the horns (fundus of the uterine cavity)

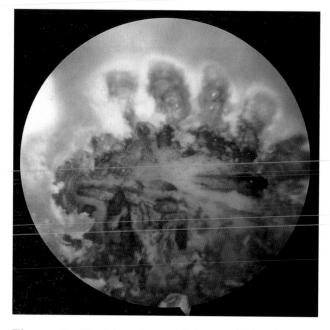

Figure 5 Partial endometrial laser ablation involves leaving area of about 1 cm above the upper part of the cervical canal not photocoagulated

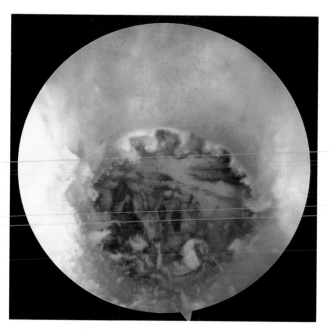

Figure 6 Final view of endometrial ablation

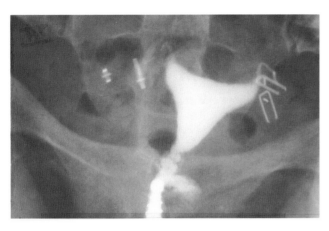

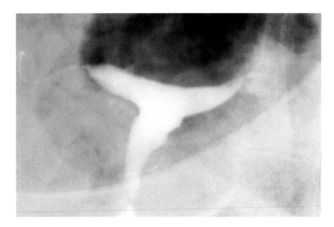

Figure 7 Hysterography (a) before endometrial ablation; (b) 3 months after; and (c) 6 months after the procedure

Figure 8 Hysterography (a) before partial endometrial laser ablation; and (b) 3 months after the procedure. The arrow shows the clear separation between the ablated (above the arrow) and the non-ablated area (beneath the arrow)

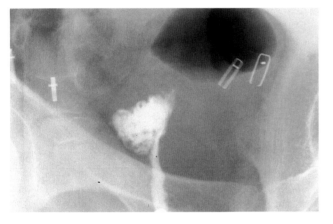

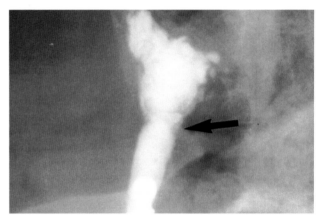

Figure 7(b)   *See legend above*

Figure 8(b)   *See legend above*

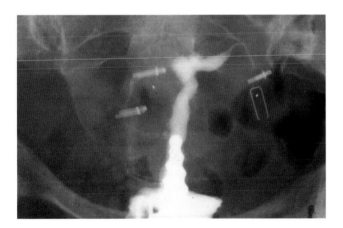

Figure 7(c)   *See legend above*

Table 1 Nd:YAG laser hysteroscopic endometrial ablation in two consecutive series of 50 patients who underwent endometrial laser ablation (ELA) and 270 patients who underwent partial endometrial laser ablation (PELA) for dysfunctional bleeding (myomas excluded)

| | | PELA ($n = 270$) Uterine cavity area | |
Results	ELA ($n = 50$)	$< 10\ cm^2$ ($n = 200$)	$> 10\ cm^2$ ($n = 70$)
Amenorrhea	17 (34%)	3 (1.5%)	1 (1%)
Hypomenorrhea	30 (60%)	189 (94.5%)	59 (84%)
Normal flow	2 (4%)	6 (3%)	6 (9%)
Failed	1 (2%)	2 (1%)	4 (6%)
Recurrence of meno-metrorrhagia (2-year follow-up)	2/50 (4%)	3/146 (2%)	10/49 (20%)
Total failures (at 2 years)	3/50 (6%)	5/146 (3%)	14/49 (28%)

RESULTS

Table 1 shows the results of our patients, treated by the touch technique. In a first series of 50 patients, endometrial ablation was carried out in the entire uterine cavity. Amenorrhea was obtained in 34% of patients. Hypomenorrhea, amounting to little more than several days of spotting, was observed in 60% of patients. Bleeding similar to that experienced before the development of menstrual problems, was observed in 4% of women. Failure of treatment, with no significant decrease in the amount of menstrual flow, was demonstrated in 2% of patients.

In a second series of 270 patients[7], endometrial ablation was carried out in the uterine cavity, except in an area 1 cm above the uterine isthmus. The proposed goal was to obtain hypomenorrhea rather than amenorrhea. This was achieved in 94.5% of women with a uterine cavity of $< 10\ cm^2$. Amenorrhea occurred in 1.5% of these women, and treatment failed in 1% (Table 1). In patients with a uterine cavity $> 10\ cm^2$ the failure rate was higher (4/70; 6%).

The operating time varied from 15 to 25 min. Blood loss was minimal and no uterine perforation occurred.

Patients were followed up for long enough to prove that regeneration of endometrial tissue does not occur after treatment with the touch technique. The decrease in menstrual flow that occurred within the first 3–4 months did not vary over the ensuing years, and hysterosalpingography revealed shrinkage of the uterine cavity (Figures 7, 8). In women with a uterine cavity of $> 10\ cm^2$, the recurrence rate of meno-metrorrhagia was significantly higher (28%; $p < 0.01$) than in women with a uterine cavity of $< 10\ cm^2$ (3%) (Table 1).

The use of GnRH agonist therapy and the continuous flow hysteroscopic system ensured that the fluid overload syndrome did not occur.

COMPLICATIONS

Peroperative complications

Patients should be warned prior to the procedure about the postoperative bloody discharge, lasting 3–4 weeks. The first one or two menses may be rather heavy, but by the third month the results of the treatment should be apparent. Postoperative pain is limited to cramp for which antiprostaglandins and analgesics may be administered.

This procedure is relatively free of complications. The only case of perforation in our series of more than 700 women occurred in a patient exposed to diethylstilbestrol in whom the myometrium of the uterine horn was very thin. Perforation occurred during an attempt at tubal sterilization.

Postoperative bleeding and fluid overload of the first series, leading to pulmonary edema, have occurred in some cases. Fluid overload was originally believed to have been caused by the reabsorption by the peritoneal cavity of large volumes of distending medium that had passed through patent Fallopian tubes. The problem is similar to that described in transurethral resection of the prostate[13]. When a touch technique is used, there is the potential for the quartz fiber to cut into the myometrium and open up vessels anywhere in the uterus. If vessels are either too large, or have not been treated long enough with the laser to become coagulated and provide hemostasis, they can bleed once the pressure of the uterine distending medium is removed. The same mechanism can account for fluid overload and pulmonary edema: vessels open transiently and allow the distending medium, which is under pressure, to infuse into the vascular system. The vessels are later closed by the laser beam or by contraction of the distended uterus and do not cause significant postoperative bleeding.

Loffer has suggested that bleeding and fluid overload do not occur with the non-touch technique because this technique first seals vessels. Using the non-touch technique, Loffer claims to have lost no more than 1000 ml of fluid. This amount had migrated into the peritoneal cavity through the open Fallopian tubes.

In our series of 700 patients, > 1000 ml of fluid was not recovered, yet none of our patients experienced fluid overload. All were carefully monitored for this potential problem. In our first series of 50 patients, three had developed fluid retention (> 2500 ml), and two showed fluid overload syndrome. No fluid overload was observed in the last 700 cases: it does not occur with the systematic administration of GnRH agonist therapy. Another mechanism responsible for fluid absorption may be the thickness of the endometrium and the vascularization of the chorion, parameters which are influenced by GnRH agonist therapy.

Gas embolism occurs when a coaxial quartz fiber carrying a gas is used, rather than a bare fiber. This design was commonly used in gynecology to cool the junction of a sapphire fiber and the quartz fiber. Only a liquid should be used in the uterine cavity if this system is used.

Long-term complications

In our series, some patients complained of cramp and dysmenorrhea, even when they were amenorrheic. In one such patient, echography showed two hypo-echogenic areas (< 1 cm^2) located in the uterine horns (Figure 9). These areas were hematometria.

In one patient, the dysmenorrhea was so severe that a vaginal hysterectomy was required (Figure 10). Histological examination confirmed the presence of residual endometrial tissue in the uterine horns (Figure 11).

The other patients were treated with progestogens for a few months. In two, hysteroscopy was performed in order to cut intrauterine synechia and to eliminate collected blood. Thereafter, an IUD was inserted for several months. No recurrence of hematometria and/or pain was noted.

Obscuring of adenocarcinoma of the endometrium has been suggested as a potential risk but has not been reported. Experimental data[11] suggest that this risk is probably non-existent.

DISCUSSION

Numerous methods have been used in an attempt to create endometrial destruction and scarring. However, only the neodymium: yttrium-aluminum-garnet (Nd:YAG) laser and the resectoscope have had acceptable results.

There are several hysteroscopic lasers suitable for endometrial ablation. An operating channel allows the quartz fiber to be held in place. The double channel system (continuous flow hysteroscopy), which has one sheath for inflow and one sheath for outflow, is used for removing blood, bubbles and debris, which would otherwise obscure vision. True aspiration through the catheter is generally not necessary, as the pressure of the distending medium will push the debris out through the catheter, provided that the outflow channel remains patent. We have never used the rotary pump connected to an integral pressure transducer (Hamou Hysteromat). Intrauterine pressure levels never rise, a clear view of the uterine cavity is achieved and the continuous flow system itself eliminates the risk of excessive fluid absorption[6,8].

There are three techniques for applying laser energy to the endometrial cavity. The touch technique[14], the non-touch technique[2] and a combination of both techniques.

When the overall results are analyzed, it appears that the touch technique, used in the Goldrath series and in our series, increases the chances of the creation of Asherman's syndrome, and hence a greater amenorrhea and hypomenorrhea rate, more often than the non-touch technique of the Loffer series[8].

In the second series of 270 women[7], partial endometrial laser ablation was carried out in order to induce hypomenorrhea rather than amenorrhea. This procedure may be proposed in the future for women in their forties, in order to reduce menstrual flow, even in the absence of dysfunctional bleeding.

Most published studies show a high incidence of immediate good results (Table 2), but few[7] long-term results have been published. Significant differences in outcome have been observed: significant differences in the area of the uterine cavity account for some discrepancies in results.

Postoperative bleeding and fluid overload leading to pulmonary edema never occurred in our second series of patients. Preoperative GnRH agonist therapy and the use of the continuous flow hysteroscopic system help avoid these complications. Care must be taken to photo-coagulate and destroy the endometrium in the uterine horns in order to avoid hematometria and dysmenorrhea.

Table 2 Immediate good results after Nd:YAG laser ablation

Reference	Number of patients	Good results (amenorrhea or hypomenorrhea)
Goldrath[1]	214	209 (96%)
Loffer[2]	55	38 (69%)
Lomano[16]	62	47 (76%)
Baggish et al.[17]	14	10 (71%)
Donnez et al.[5]	50	47 (94%)
Nisolle et al.[7]	270	250 (92%)
Garry et al.[9]	479	288 (60%)
Gallinat[18]	145	136 (94%)

In conclusion, GnRH agonist therapy decreases the total uterine cavity area, facilitating surgical treatment and reducing the risk of fluid overload syndrome. Endometrial laser ablation can be performed quickly by experienced gynecologists. The morbidity rate and hospitalization time are reduced, and hysterectomy can be avoided in young women suffering from abnormal bleeding.

Preoperative evaluation of uterine cavity area can indicate the risk of long-term failure: laparoscopic supra-cervical hysterectomy should be proposed in patients

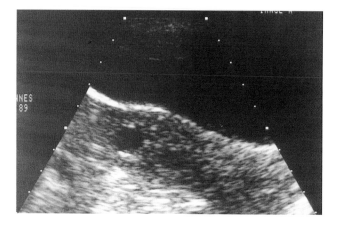

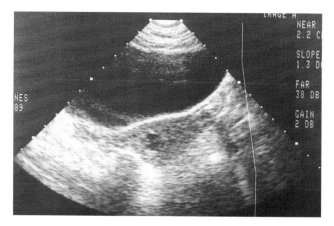

Figure 9(a) and (b)   Echography shows hypoechogenic areas suspected to be hematometria located in the uterine horns

Figure 9(b)   *See legend opposite*

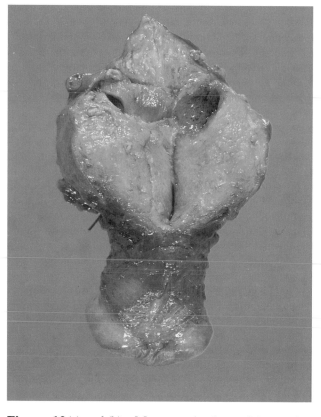

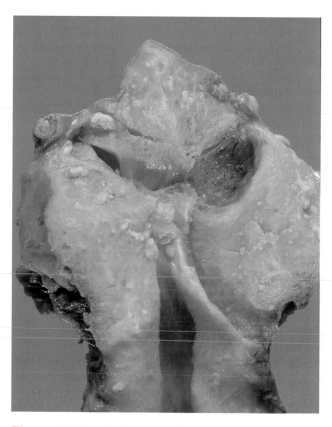

Figure 10(a) and (b)   Macroscopic views of the uterine cavity. Hematometria is visible in the uterine horns

Figure 10(b)   *See legend opposite*

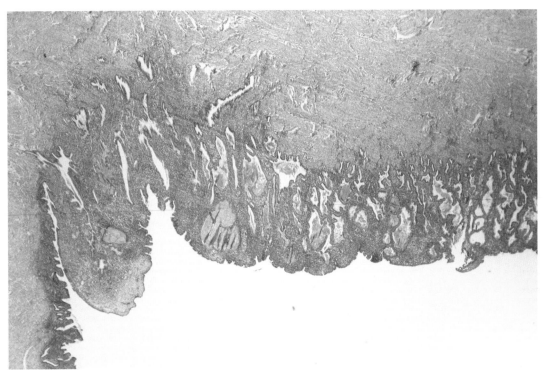

Figure 11 (a) and (b)   Histology shows residual endometrial tissue in the uterine horn. Menstrual bleeding from this non-photocoagulated area was responsible for the hematometria formation

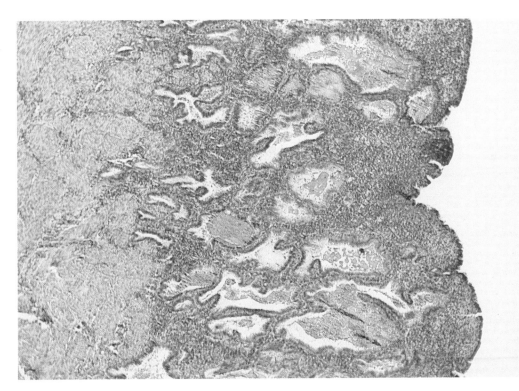

Figure 11 (b)   *See legend above*

with a very large uterus[7,14]. Since 1992, partial endometrial laser ablation has been proposed not only for women suffering from abnormal bleeding but also for women aged over 40 desiring a reduction in menstrual flow.

REFERENCES

1. Goldrath, M.H. (1985). Hysteroscopic laser surgery. In Baggish, M.S. (ed.) *Basic and Advanced Laser Surgery in Gynecology*, p. 357. (Norwalk, CT: Appleton-Century-Crofts)

2. Loffer, F.D. (1988). Laser ablation of the endometrium. *Obstet. Gynecol. Clin. N. Am.*, **15**, 17

3. Van Caillie, T. (1989). Electrocoagulation of the endometrium with the ball-end resectoscope. *Obstet. Gynecol.*, **74**, 425

4. Hamou, J. (1993). Eletroresection of fibroids. In Sutton, C. and Diamond, M. (eds.) *Endoscopic Surgery for Gynecologists*, pp. 327–30. (London: W.B. Saunders)

5. Donnez, J. and Nisolle, M. (1989). Laser hysteroscopy in uterine bleeding: endometrial ablation and polpectomy. In Donnez, J. (ed.) *Laser Operative Laparoscopy and Hysteroscopy*, p. 277. (Louvain: Nauwelaerts)

6. Donnez, J. and Nisolle, M. (1992). Hysteroscopic surgery. *Curr. Opin. Obstet. Gynecol.*, **4**, 439

7. Nisolle, M., Grandjean, P., Gillerot, S. and Donnez, J. (1991). Endometrial ablation with the Nd-YAG laser in dysfunctional bleeding. *Min. Invasive Ther.*, **1**, 35–9

8. Donnez, J., Schrurs, B., Gillerot, S., Sandow, J. and Clerckx, F. (1989). Treatment of uterine fibroids with implants of gonadotropin-releasing hormone agonist: assessment by hysterography. *Fertil. Steril.*, **51**, 947

9. Garry, R., Erian, J. and Grochmal, S. (1991). A multicentre collaborative study into the treatment of menorrhagia by Nd-YAG laser ablation of the endometrium. *Br. J. Obstet. Gynaecol.*, **98**, 357–62

10. Weibel, E.R. (1979). Practical methods for biological morphometry. In Weibel, E.R. (ed.) *Stereological Methods*, Vol.1, p. 101. (Bern: Academic Press)

11. Donnez, J., Gillerot, S., Bourgonjon, D., Clerckx, F. and Nisolle, M. (1990). Neodymium : YAG laser hysteroscopy in large submucous fibroids. *Fertil. Steril.*, **54**, 999

12. Donnez, J., Malvaux, V., Nisolle, M. and Casanas-Roux, F. (1990). Hysteroscopic sterilization with the Nd-YAG laser. *J. Gynecol. Surg.*, **6**, 149

13. Loffer, F.D. (1988). Laser ablation of the endometrium. *Obstet. Gynecol. Clin N. Am.*, **15**, 17

14. Goldrath, M.H., Fuller, T.A. and Segal, S. (1981). Laser photovaporization of endometrium for the treatment of menorrhagia. *Am. J. Obstet. Gynecol.*, **140**, 14

15. Donnez, J. and Nisolle, M. (1993). Laparoscopic supracervical hysterectomy (LASH). *J. Gynecol. Surg.*, **9**, 91–4

16. Lomano, J.M. (1988). Photocoagulation of the endometrium with the Nd-YAG laser for the treatment of menorrhagia. *J. Reprod. Med.*, **31**, 148–50

17. Baggish, M.S. and Baltoyannis, P. (1988). New techniques for laser ablation of the endometrium in high risk patients. *Am. J. Obstet. Gynecol.*, **159**, 287–92

18. Gallinat, A. (1993). Endometrial ablation using the Nd : YAG laser in CO_2 hysteroscopy. In Lueken, R.P and Gallinat, A. (eds.) *Endoscopic Surgery in Gynecology*, p.109. (Demeter Verlag GmbH)

Hysteroscopic myomectomy

34

J. Donnez, M. Nisolle, F. Clerckx, S. Gillerot and P. Saussoy

Laser energy has some advantages in precision of tissue destruction that are not shared by the electrical energy used in the resectoscope[1,2]. Since the most popular laser in gynecology has been the carbon dioxide (CO_2) laser, efforts have been made to adapt this for hysteroscopic use. However, several features of the CO_2 laser make it impractical for hysteroscopic use. The Nd : YAG laser, however, has three specific features, making it readily adaptable for hysteroscopic myomectomy:

(1) Its ability to transmit the beam of energy easily into the uterine cavity by means of a flexible quartz fiber;

(2) Its ability to transmit laser energy to the tissue surface through a liquid distending medium;

(3) Its ability to penetrate tissue to a controlled depth.

The depth at which tissue destruction will occur can be controlled by varying the power used[3,4]: this physical quality can be applied for myomectomy and hysteroscopic myolysis[5,6]. This report describes the different techniques of hysteroscopic myomectomy.

HYSTEROSCOPIC EQUIPMENT

The fiber used to carry the laser light consists of quartz, surrounded by a thin plastic jacket, beyond which the tip of the fiber extends for several millimeters. The fiber is gas-sterilized or wiped with alcohol or cidex prior to use.

The deflecting arm is not of particular value, but allows the fiber to be stabilized. New instruments are now available in which the telescope is inserted into two different sheaths of varying diameter: one for inflow and the other for outflow. This resembles the classic resectoscope[7] and permits the constant cleaning of the uterine cavity. This system has been called the continuous flow hysteroscope (CFH). The author provides constant uterine distension by attaching one 3000 ml plastic bag of 1.5% glycine or saline solution to the blood infusion tubing. The bag is then wrapped in a pressure infusion cuff, similar to that used to infuse blood under pressure. The tubing is connected to the hysteroscope. Since the CFH has been used, overload syndrome has not occurred and this very simple system, which does not require any sophisticated and expensive pumps, allows the surgeon to perform hysteroscopic surgery in optimal conditions.

A Sharplan 2100 apparatus (Sharplan, Tel Aviv, Israel) is used for generating the laser. A power output of 80 W is used.

THE ROLE OF PREOPERATIVE GONADOTROPIN RELEASING HORMONE AGONIST THERAPY

We treated 376 women aged between 23 and 43 years (mean 33 years) with symptomatic submucous uterine fibroids, with a biodegradable gonadotropin releasing hormone (GnRH) agonist (Zoladex implant, ICI; Cambridge, UK). The implant was injected subcutaneously at the end of the luteal phase to curtail the initial gonadotropin stimulation phase always associated with a rise in estrogen. One implant was systematically injected at weeks 0, 4 and 8. Hysteroscopic myomectomy was carried out at 8 weeks. After the initial stimulation of estrogen secretion, GnRH agonist administration produces estrogen levels in the postmenopausal range (15 ± 6 pg/ml). Luteinizing hormone and follicle stimulating hormone levels were significantly suppressed within 2 weeks of treatment. Recovery of ovarian secretion occurred an average of 4–5 weeks after the last injection[6] (Figure 1).

Using the method previously described[5,6], the reduction in area of large submucous fibroids was calculated. When more than one fibroid was present, only the largest was evaluated. In all but four patients the fibroid area decreased by an average of 38%[8] (range 4–95%). The fibroid area was found to decrease significantly ($p < 0.01$), from the baseline area (7.2 ± 4.7 cm^2) to 4.4 ± 3.5 cm^2 after 8 weeks of therapy. Figure 2 shows the mean fibroid area in patients with a pretreatment fibroid area < 5 cm^2 versus those with an area of > 5 cm^2 to < 10 cm^2. In all subgroups, a significant decrease ($p < 0.005$) was noted.

There was no significant difference between the different subgroups, but there was a significant difference (Figure 3) between individual myomas. About 10% of myomas did not appear to respond very well to GnRH agonist treatment (Figure 3).

CLASSIFICATION OF MYOMAS

According to hysterosalpingography data, submucosal fibroids were classified as:

(1) Submucosal fibroids whose greatest diameter was inside the uterine cavity (Figure 4);

(2) Submucosal fibroids whose largest portion was located in the myometrium (Figure 5); and

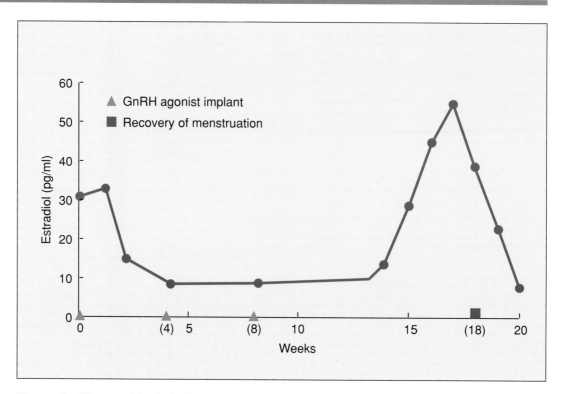

Figure 1 Hormonal levels (17β-estradiol) during gonadotropin releasing hormone agonist therapy. An implant of Zoladex was injected at weeks 0, 4 and 8

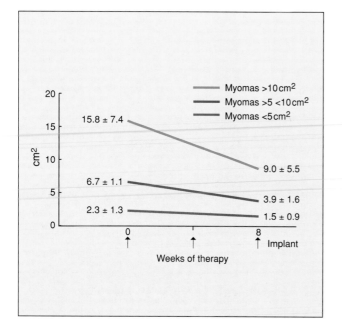

Figure 2 Decrease in fibroid area after 8 weeks of gonadotropin releasing hormone agonist therapy relative to the initial value

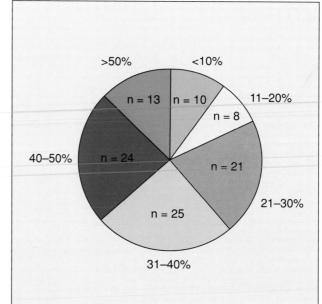

Figure 3 Distribution of the myomas according to their size decrease. Ten per cent of patients were non-responders

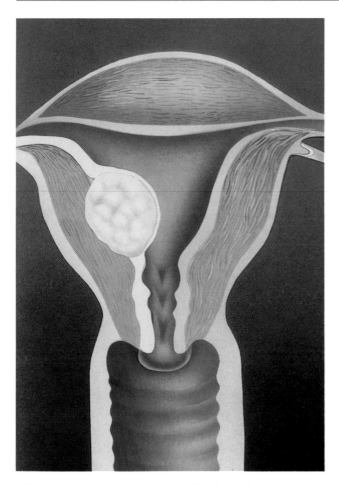

Figure 4(a)–(c) Submucosal fibroids whose greatest diameter was inside the uterine cavity; (d) computerized tomography: intracavitary myoma

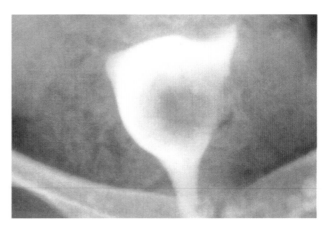

Figure 4(b) Hysterography reveals that the greatest diameter is inside the uterine cavity

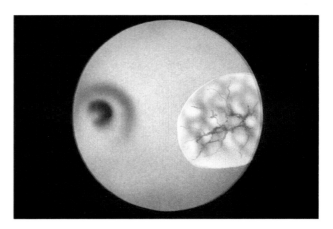

Figure 4(c) *See legend above*

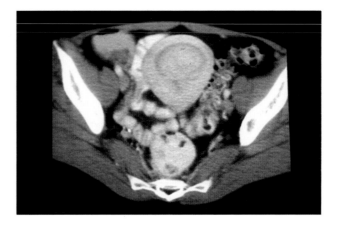

Figure 4(d) *See legend above*

325

(3) Multiple (> 2) submucosal fibroids (myofibromatous uterus with submucosal fibroids and intramural fibroids) diagnosed by hysterography (Figure 6) and echography.

TECHNIQUES

Submucosal fibroids whose greatest diameter was inside the uterine cavity

All patients ($n = 233$) underwent myomectomy by hysteroscopy and Nd:YAG laser. In all but three patients, the operation was easily performed. The myometrium overlying the myoma was less vascular and 'shrinkage' of the uterine cavity may have accounted for the relative ease with which the myomas could be separated from the surrounding myometrium (Figures 7–9).

The myoma was left in the uterine cavity (Figure 10) unless no decrease in size was observed after GnRH agonist therapy – in this case, histological examination was required. No complications such as infection, bleeding or uterine contractions occurred. Hysteroscopy, performed 2–3 months after myomectomy, confirmed the complete disappearance of the myoma, which was probably ejected during the first menstruation after the procedure.

No hormonal therapy was given. The operating time ranged from 10 to 50 min (mean 24 ± 6 min).

Large submucosal fibroids whose largest portion was located in the uterine wall

For large submucous fibroids whose largest portion was not inside the uterine cavity but inside the uterine wall ($n = 78$), a two-step operative hysteroscopy was proposed[6]. After 8 weeks of preoperative GnRH agonist therapy, partial myomectomy was carried out by resecting the protruding portion of the myoma (Figure 11). The laser fiber was then directed, as perpendicularly as possible, at the remaining (intramural) fibroid portion and was introduced into the fibroid to a depth of 5–10 mm (Figure 12). During the application of laser energy, the fiber was slowly removed so that the deeper areas were coagulated. The end-point of fibroid coagulation with this technique was identifiable by the observation of distinct craters with brown borders on all fibroid areas. The depth of the intramural fibroid portion was already known from the results of echographic examination performed the day before surgery. The aim of this procedure was to decrease the size of the remaining myoma by decreasing its vascularity. This technique induces a necrobiosis (Figure 13) and can be called 'transhysteroscopic myolysis'[16].

GnRH agonist therapy was administered for another 8 weeks. At second-look hysteroscopy, the myoma was found to protrude inside the uterine cavity and appeared very white and without any apparent vessels on its surface (Figure 14). The shrinkage of the uterine cavity allowed the residual myoma portion to be easily separated from the surrounding myometrium and dissected off (Figure 15). Myomectomy was then carried out. At the end of the procedure, the myoma could be left in the uterine cavity.

In all but five patients, two-step therapy allowed successful myomectomy. In the five remaining cases, a 'third-look' hysteroscopy was necessary to achieve myomectomy. When removed, the myoma revealed areas of histological necrosis (Figure 13). In some cases, the residual myoma appeared white and necrotic (Figure 16). When performed, hysterography (Figure 17) revealed a normal appearance of the uterine cavity, less than 3 months after the procedure.

Fibromatous uterus

In cases of multiple submucosal fibroids, each myoma was either separated from the surrounding myometrium or totally photocoagulated (Figure 18). When only a small portion of the myoma was visible, the laser fiber was introduced into the intramural portion to a depth depending on the myoma diameter (diagnosed by echography). While firing, the fiber was slowly removed. Each myoma was systematically destroyed. At the end of surgery, endometrial ablation with the Nd:YAG laser was carried out (Figure 18) in order to induce uterine shrinkage only in women older than 35 years who did not wish to become pregnant.

RESULTS

Table 1 shows the long-term results according to the myoma classification of Donnez and Nisolle[9]. Surgery was successful in 230 of 233 patients with large submucous fibroids whose greatest diameter was inside the uterine cavity. In three cases, a stromal tumor was diagnosed. In one of these (Figure 19), dissection of the myoma from the myometrium was impossible because the plane of dissection could not be found. Frozen histology of a biopsy revealed histological characteristics of a stromal tumor (Figure 20). Vaginal hysterectomy was then carried out. The other two cases were diagnosed by histological examination of the removed myomas, which appeared hysteroscopically as benign. The incidence of stromal tumors in apparently benign myomas is thus 1.2% (3/233). All three tumors were observed in patients who did not respond very well (< 10% decrease) to GnRH agonist therapy.

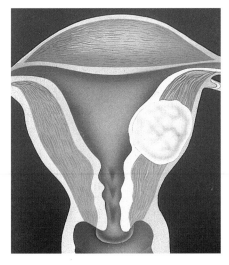

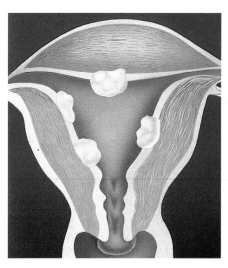

Figure 5(a)–(c) Submucosal fibroids whose largest portion was located in the myometrium

Figure 6(a)–(c) Hysterography reveals the presence of multiple submucosal myomas

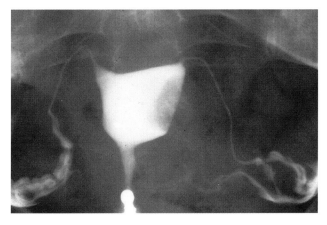

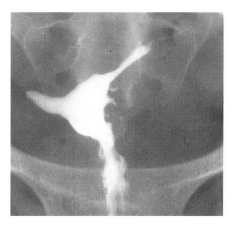

Figure 5(b) *See legend above*

Figure 6(b) *See legend above*

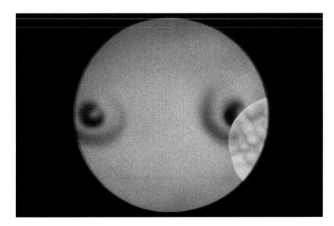

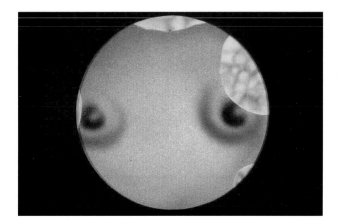

Figure 5(c) *See legend above*

Figure 6(c) *See legend above*

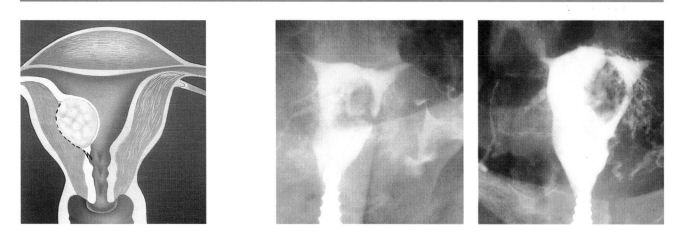

Figure 7 Hysteroscopic myomectomy in cases of submucosal fibroids whose greatest diameter was inside the uterine cavity: (a) illustration of the technique; (b) hysterography; (c) and (d) hysteroscopy

Figure 7(b)   *See legend opposite*

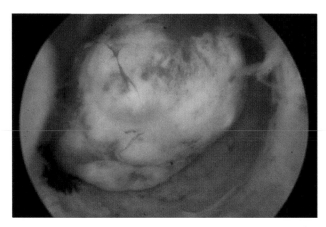

Figure 7(c)   *See legend above*

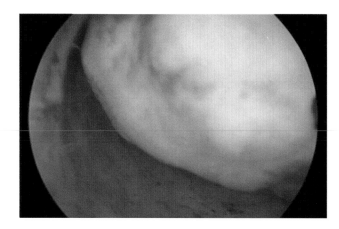

Figure 7(d)   *See legend above*

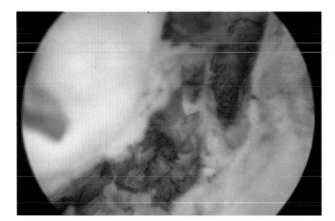

Figure 8 Dissection of the myoma from the surrounding myometrium

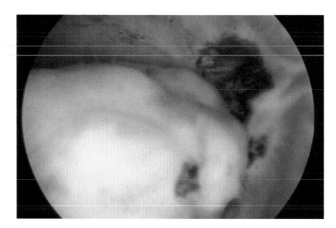

Figure 9 Dissection of the myoma from the surrounding myometrium

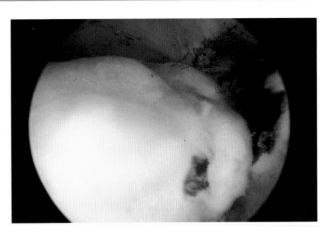

Figure 10 Myoma can be left in the uterine cavity

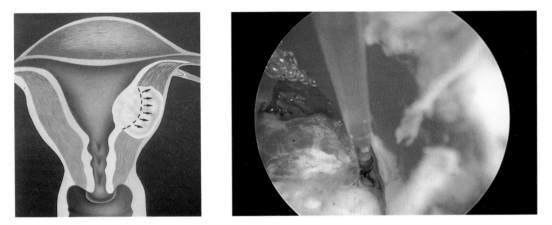

Figure 11 Submucosal fibroid whose largest portion was located in the myometrium. Resection of the protruding portion of the myoma: (a) illustration; (b) hysteroscopic view

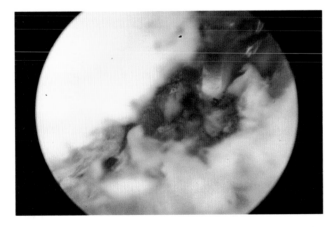

Figure 12 The laser fiber is introduced into the remaining fibroid portion to a depth of 5–10 mm and slowly removed during the application of laser energy

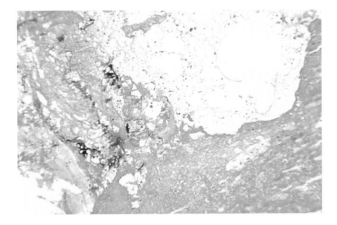

Figure 13 Myoma necrobiosis induced by the Nd : YAG laser (Gomori's trichrome, × 25). Carbonized particles phagocyted by macrophages are clearly seen. In front of them, an area of 'necrobiosis' is visible

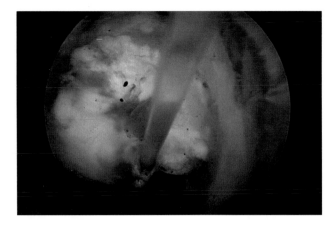

Figure 14 Eight weeks after transhysteroscopic myolysis, the intramural portion of the myoma protrudes inside the uterine cavity

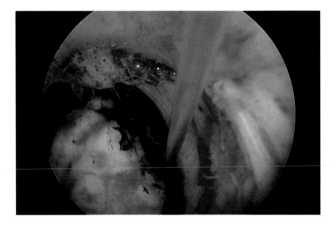

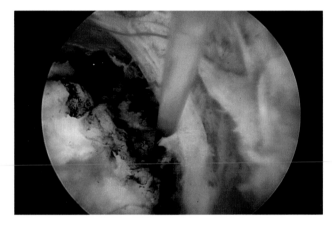

Figure 15(a) and (b) Second-step hysteroscopic procedure. The residual myoma portion is easily separated from the surrounding myometrium and dissected off

Figure 15(b) *See legend opposite*

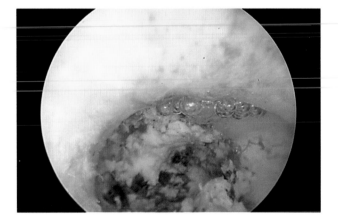

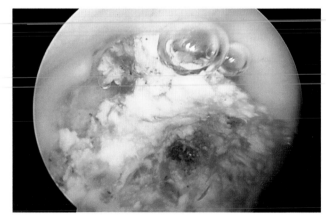

Figure 16(a) and (b) Necrotic appearance of the residual myoma portion, 8 weeks after coagulation with the Nd : YAG laser

Figure 16(b) *See legend opposite*

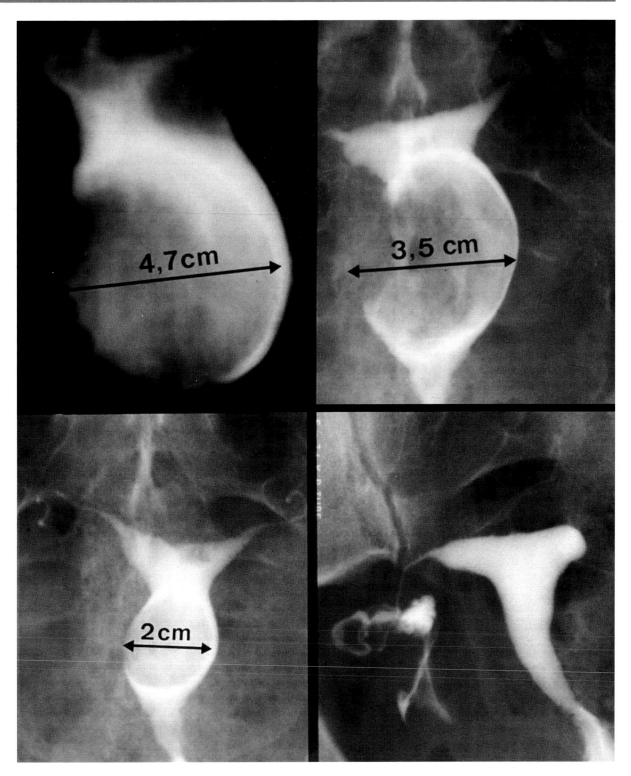

Figure 17 Hysterography. Top left, before GnRH agonist therapy; top right, after GnRH agonist therapy; bottom left, hysterography 8 weeks after partial myomectomy and coagulation. The residual intramural portion was found protruding again in the uterine cavity; bottom right: hysterography 8 weeks after the second hysteroscopic myomectomy

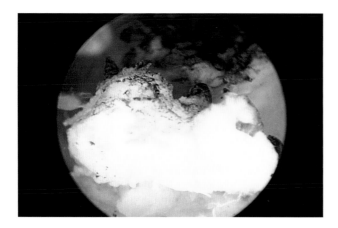

Figure 18(a) Transhysteroscopic multiple myomectomy; (b) multiple myomectomy was associated with endometrial ablation

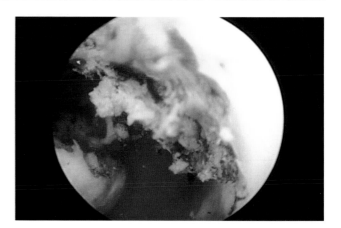

Figure 18(b) *See legend opposite*

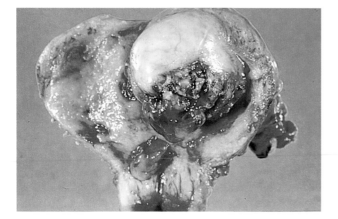

Figure 19(a) and (b) Hysteroscopically, the intrauterine lesion appeared as benign myomas, but no plane of dissection could be found. Histology revealed a stromal tumor invading the myometrium

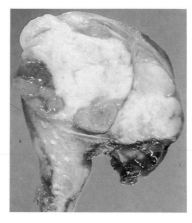

Figure 19(b) *See legend opposite*

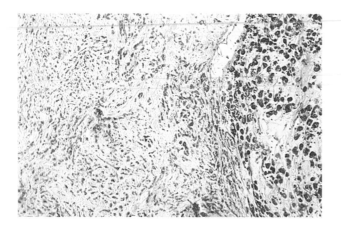

Figure 20(a) Low-grade stromal sarcoma with areas of epithelial differentiation (on the right). In these areas, cells are considerably more atypical than those seen on the left, which resemble the stromal cells of proliferating endometrium

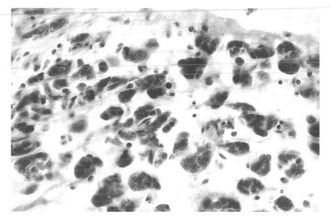

Figure 20(b) Areas of epithelial differentiation (high-power view

Successful myomectomy permits the restoration of normal menstrual flow. Long-term results show that recurrence of menorrhagia occurs more frequently (22%) in patients with multiple submucosal myomas than in those with single submucosal myomas[8]. Recurrence of menorraghia is provoked by the growth of myomas in other sites, as shown by hysterography and hysteroscopy.

Fertility

A first evaluation of a series of 60 women was published in 1990[6]. Twenty-four of 60 treated women wished to become pregnant and had no other infertility factors. Sixteen (66%) of them became pregnant during the first 8 months after the return of menstruation. No miscarriages or premature labor occurred in these women; one Cesarean section was necessary because of fetal distress.

DISCUSSION

Because most leiomyomata return to pretreatment size within 4 months of cessation of GnRH agonist therapy, these agents cannot be used as definitive medical therapy[10–13]. Several reports have demonstrated reductions in uterine and fibroid volumes of 52–77% after 6 months of GnRH agonist therapy, as assessed by ultrasound imaging. In our study, hysterographic imaging documented an average decrease of 35% in uterine cavity size[5,14]. Another study[6] demonstrated reductions in fibroid volume of 38% after 8 weeks of GnRH agonist therapy. The response was variable, however, ranging from 2% to 95%. There was no difference in the extent of the decrease according to the pretreatment fibroid area.

In patients with submucosal uterine fibroids, hysteroscopic myomectomy was carried out if the greatest diameter of the leiomyoma, as assessed by hysterography, was inside the uterine cavity. Hormonal treatment for 8 weeks before hysteroscopic myomectomy was advised since this produced a significant uterine shrinkage.

Peroperative blood loss was minimal, possibly because of the decreased vascularity of the myometrium. This was demonstrated by a significant reduction in the uterine arterial blood flow (Doppler) after treatment with a GnRH agonist[15]. In all patients (except when no decrease in the myoma size was observed), the myoma was left in the uterine cavity and there were no complications. Probably, after a necrotic phase, the myoma was ejected with menstrual blood.

For very large fibroids whose largest diameter was not inside the uterine cavity, myomectomy was carried out in two stages. During the first surgical procedure, the protruding portion was removed and the intramural portion was devascularized by introducing the laser fiber into the myoma, to a depth of 5–10 mm, depending on the depth of the remaining intramural portion (evaluated by echography). The pelvic structures were protected from injury because the distance between the top of the fiber and the external surface of the uterus was never < 1.5 cm. There was no risk of introducing the laser fiber as much as 1 cm into the remaining portion if the diameter of the fibroid was > 3–4 cm.

A very interesting finding was that this intramural portion of the myoma became submucosal and protruded

Table 1 Surgical procedures and long-term results according to the site of myomas

	Greatest diameter inside the uterine cavity	Largest portion located in the uterine wall	Multiple submucosal myomas (myomectomy and endometrial ablation)
Surgical procedures			
Total patients	233	78	55
Successful	230	74	51
Failed	3*	4†	4‡
1-year follow-up			
Total patients	132	42	39
Recurrence of menorrhagia	1 (1%)	1 (2%)	8 (20%)
2-year follow-up			
Total patients	98	24	24
Recurrence of menorrhagia	2 (2%)	1 (4%)	6 (25%)

*, Stromal tumor; †, A third-look hysteroscopy allowed the removal of the myoma; ‡, Myomectomy was not totally successful (in two cases, second-look laser hysteroscopy was successfully performed. In the other two cases, vaginal hysterectomy was proposed and successfully performed)

inside the uterine cavity, possibly because of the GnRH agonist-induced uterine shrinkage. In all cases, the largest diameter of the remaining portion of the myoma was inside the uterine cavity, and myomectomy was easily performed by separating the myoma from the surrounding myometrium with the Nd : YAG laser.

CONCLUSION

Preoperative GnRH agonist treatment reduces tumor size and makes subsequent surgical treatment by hysteroscopy possible. In our series, even when the largest diameter of the myoma was in the myometrium, a two-step hysteroscopic therapy combined with GnRH agonist therapy[6,16] represented ideal management of large submucous myomas, decreasing the need for laparotomy, which is often accompanied by increased operative blood loss and postoperative adhesion formation.

When numerous submucosal and intramural myomas were present a higher risk of recurrence was observed than in patients with only one submucosal myoma[8]. Because of this high rate of recurrence, we prefer to perform a laparoscopic supracervical hysterectomy instead of the hysteroscopic procedure[16,17].

By preventing uterine bleeding, preoperative GnRH agonist therapy restores a normal hemoglobin concentration, and allows for the possibility of a later autologous transfusion[6]. The hormonal endometrial status is one of the factors affecting fluid absorption. Endometrial vascularization may account for liquid resorption, and this was reduced after preoperative GnRH agonist therapy. Less fluid was absorbed if the endometrium was atrophic, reducing the risk of fluid overload. This represents another major advantage of the combined medical and surgical approach to therapy.

The advantages of the preoperative use of a GnRH agonist are:

(1) Reduction of the myoma size;

(2) Decreased risk of fluid overload;

(3) Restoration of normal hemoglobin concentration;

(4) Detection of a stromal tumor.

Like Gallinat and Lueken[18], we believe that, although Nd : YAG laser treatment requires experience and a thorough knowledge of the technique, it nevertheless has the lowest complication rate, when compared to the resectoscope. Nd : YAG laser treatment of large myomas must be considered the safest method in the hysteroscopic surgical treatment of large myomas.

REFERENCES

1. Hallez, J.P., Netter, A. and Cartier, R. (1987). Methodical intrauterine resection. *Am. J. Obstet. Gynecol.*, **156**, 1080

2. Loffer, F.D. (1988). Laser ablation of the endometrium *Obstet. Gynecol. Clin. N. Am.*, **15**, 77

3. Goldrath, M.H., Fuller, T. and Segal, S. (1981). Laser photovaporization of endometrium for the treatment of menorrhagia. *Am. J. Obstet. Gynecol.*, **140**, 14

4. Goldrath, M.H. (1985). Hysteroscopic laser surgery. In Baggish, M.H. (eds.) *Basic and Advanced Laser Surgery in Gynecology*, p. 357. (Norwalk: Appleton-Century-Crofts)

5. Donnez, J., Schrurs, B., Gillerot, S., Sadow, J. and Clerckx, F. (1989). Treatment of uterine fibroids with implants of gonadotropin-releasing hormone agonist: assessment by hysterography. *Fertil. Steril.*, **51**, 947

6. Donnez, J., Gillerot, S., Bourgonjon, D., Clerckx, F. and Nisolle, M. (1990). Neodymium : YAG laser hysteroscopy in large submucous fibroids. *Fertil. Steril.*, **54**, 999

7. Neuwirth, R.S. (1983). Hysteroscopic management of symptomatic submucous fibroids. *Obstet. Gynecol.*, **62**, 509

8. Donnez, J., (1993). Nd - YAG laser hysteroscopic myomectomy. In: Sutton, C. and Diamond, M. (eds.) *Endoscopic Surgery for Gynecologists*, p. 331. (London: W.B. Saunders)

9. Donnez, J. and Nisolle, M. (1993). Nd : YAG laser hysteroscopic surgery: endometrial ablation, partial endometrial ablation and myomectomy. *Reprod. Med. Rev.*, **2**, 63

10. Healy, D.L., Fraser, H.M. and Lawson, S.L. (1984). Shrinkage of a uterine fibroid after subcutaneous infusion of a LH-RH agonist. *Br. Med. J.*, **209**, 267

11. Maheux, R., Guilloteau, C., Lemay, A., Bastide, A. and Fazekas, A.T.A. (1985). Luteinizing hormone-releasing hormone agonist and uterine leiomyoma: pilot study. *Am. J. Obstet. Gynecol.*, **152**, 1034

12. Andreyko, J.L., Blumenfeld, Z., Marschall, L.A., Monroe, S.E., Hricak, H. and Jaffe, R.B. (1988). Use of an agonistic analog of gonadotropin-releasing hormone (nafarelin) to treat leiomyomas: assessment by magnetic resonance imaging. *Am. J. Obstet. Gynecol.*, **158**, 903

13. Friedman, A.J., Barbieri, R.L., Doubilet, P.M., Fine, C. and Schiff, I. (1988). A randomized, double-blind trial of gonadotropin releasing-hormone agonist (leuprolide) with or without medroxyprogesterone acetate in the treatment of leiomyomata uteri. *Fertil. Steril.*, **49**, 404

14. Donnez, J., Clerckx, F., Gillerot, S., Bourgonjon, D. and Nisolle, M. (1989). Traitment des fibromes

utérims per implant d'agoniste de la GnRH: evaluation per hysterographie. *Contrac. Fertil. Sex.*, **17**, 569–73

15. Matta, W.H.M., Stabile, I., Shaw, R.S. and Campbell, S. (1988). Doppler assessment of uterine blood flow changes in patients with fibroids receiving the gonadotropin-releasing hormone agonist Buserelin. *Fertil. Steril.*, **49**, 1083

16. Donnez, J. and Nisolle, M. (1992). Hysteroscopic surgery. *Curr. Opin. Obstet. Gynecol.*, **4**, 439

17. Donnez, J. and Nisolle, M. (1993). Laparoscopic supracervical (subtotal) hysterectomy (LASH). *J. Gynecol. Surg.*, **9**, 91–4

18. Gallinat, A. (1993). Hysteroscopic treatment of submucous fibroids using the Nd:YAG laser and modern electrical equipment. In Leuken, R.P. and Gallinat, A. (eds.) *Endoscopic Surgery in Gynecology*, pp. 72–88. (Berlin: Demeter Verlag GmbH)

Hysteroscopic sterilization

35

J. Donnez, V. Malvaux, M. Nisolle and F. Casanas-Roux

Transcervical approaches to tubal occlusion have been proposed as alternatives to the transabdominal approach and hysteroscopy as an alternative to laparoscopy.

As stated by Thatcher[1], in developing any new sterilization method, which is potentially the ideal contraceptive, an advance should be made in one of the following areas without significantly compromising the positive benefits of the other areas:

(1) Effectiveness, that is, low failure rate;

(2) Safety, or low morbidity of the procedure and its use;

(3) Ease of application and use, namely, short operating time, minimal operative management, and a high level of patient acceptance and tolerance;

(4) Low cost;

(5) Reversibility.

Tubal occlusion performed laparoscopically is the most common technique for elective sterilization. However, it is not without risks.

The development of a reversible method of 'temporary' sterilization is very important; approximately 3–5% of patients, electively sterilized, request reversal.

HYSTEROSCOPIC STERILIZATION: TECHNIQUES

Numerous agents and devices have been used for transcervical tubal occlusion. Often new techniques have not passed animal trials and many have been abandoned after preliminary human trials. The different types of agents and devices have been divided into the following categories:

(1) Hot and cold cauterization;

(2) Chemical agents;

(3) Polymer casts;

(4) Mechanical devices;

(5) Laser ablation.

Hot and cold cauterization

Electrocautery and cryocautery are attractive because of their ease and simplicity, but they are associated with high failure and complication rates. The major

complication involves transluminal cauterization and extension into the peritoneal cavity, with ensuing bowel damage and peritonitis. The high failure rate is due to the regeneration of damaged tubal epithelium.

The results of an international multicenter study of 587 women who were sterilized with electrocautery via the hysteroscope were reported in 1978. Successful occlusion on the first attempt was possible in only 57% of women, and the study reported 25 major complications including one death[2].

Chemical agents

A large variety of chemical agents has been used for tubal occlusion. All of these agents have the same mode of action: they induce inflammation, epithelial destruction and finally luminal fibrosis. These agents also share the same high complication rate and unacceptable failure rate, and their effects are impossible to reverse. The use of quinacrine, an antimalarial drug, capable of tubal destruction with reduced peritoneal toxicity, has also been reported[3].

Polymer plugs

A very promising development is the use of transcervical instillation of silicone that polymerizes in the uterine tube to form an occlusive cast. This method is currently marketed under the trade name Ovabloc[4,5].

Mechanical devices

Surgical nylon loop

Hamou[6] has designed a device made of 1 mm surgical nylon, with a loop at its distal end that can be opened to varying widths to fit the intratubal diameter. The device is inserted in an outpatient procedure, usually without anesthesia, using the Hamou hysteroscope at a magnification of 20×. The device is loaded into a catheter that is passed through the uterotubal junction.

In 144 of 166 patients, the procedure was completed on the first attempt. Reasons for failure were severe uterine retroversion, atretic tubal orifices, and pain. Microhysteroscopy performed 1 month after insertion revealed four expulsions. When the insertion was performed before salpingectomy, as part of unrelated planned surgery, the tubes showed histological changes of mild to moderate inflammation, flattening of the epithelial folds, and, occasionally, fibrinoid necrosis of the epithelial surface.

Hydrogel device

Brundin[7] has proposed a device designed to block the isthmic section of the tube; the hydrogel device is fixed on a nylon skeleton with two small wings to prevent expulsion during the 30 min it takes to form the plug.

Blockage of uterotubal junction

Blockage of the uterotubal junction with a removable device has been pronounced as both effective and the most easily reversible of sterilization techniques. Hosseinian and Morales[8] have developed a 10 mm polyethylene plug with four small metal hooks on the base that anchor the device to the endometrium at the uterotubal junction.

Intramural Nd : YAG laser sterilization

The basic physical properties of the Nd : YAG laser might help us to find a rational explanation for its use. The Nd : YAG laser has the ability to penetrate tissue; it coagulates with self-limiting penetration, at a depth no greater than 7 mm. Surrounding organs are thus theoretically protected from danger, at least in women. In a previous study, Goldrath[9] found that, when firing the laser into a freshly excised hysterectomy specimen, the maximum temperature at 1 cm was 48°C, well below the threshold for enzyme and protein denaturation which occurs, within a short exposure time, at temperatures in excess of 52°C.

EXPERIMENTAL STUDY

The Nd : YAG laser was first used in gynecology a few years ago to treat patients with excessive persistent bleeding. Laser photocoagulation of the endometrium was performed endoscopically as an alternative to hormonal therapy or hysterectomy. This procedure, using a flexible fiber through a malleable fiberscope or a rigid hysteroscope, later allowed the destruction of several types of intrauterine lesions.

In spite of the increasingly frequent applications of the Nd : YAG laser in conservative gynecologic surgery, there was no experimental model in the animal, giving us precise information about the possible damage to the female genital tract induced by this device.

The aim of our study was to provide such a model in the female rabbit, in order to permit an analysis of the histological changes produced by the application of Nd : YAG laser energy to the uterine horn.

The right uterine horn was opened through a 2 cm longitudinal incision in its middle portion using microscissors with the laser as a coagulating tool. Photovaporization of both the uterine horn endometrium and the isthmic Fallopian tube was performed under direct vision and with continuous cooling using 0.9% sterile saline solution. Careful inspection through an OPMI Zeiss microscope allowed control of penetration of the quartz fiber through the isthmic portion. A power output of 60 W was used. The mean total energy applied was about 5400 J.

To apply the laser energy, the touch technique was used with the quartz fiber coming into contact with the endometrium during the application of laser energy. Biopsies were taken in order to evaluate the effects of the laser on tissue and the degree of obstruction.

Results

When the laser beam was fired onto the endometrial surface of the uterine horn, the pink-red color of the endometrium changed to white as the tissue temperature rose, and then to brown-black because of carbonization of the underlying myometrium. The smooth, velvety surface of the untreated area disappeared, leaving small holes and channels. The coagulated tissue shrank and appeared fragile and non-vascularized.

Macroscopic evaluation 3 weeks after the procedure

In all the rabbits, macroscopic examination revealed the presence of a 2 cm fibrous streak in the portion of the horn where photocoagulation had occurred. There were no adhesions with the adjacent peritoneum in any of the cases nor did surrounding tissue show any evidence of thermal damage. The genital tract did not present any major deformity. In some cases, the coagulated area had completely disappeared, leaving only the 7/0 suture. The broad ligament was intact and no adhesions with adjacent organs were found.

Microscopic evaluation

Serial sections from the photocoagulated area were examined. Histological evaluation revealed that the tubal epithelium and endometrium were completely destroyed. Neither endometrial glands nor tubal epithelium survived, the cytogenetic stroma was sparse or absent and the myometrium appeared normal. The tubal lumen and virtual cavity of the uterine horn were

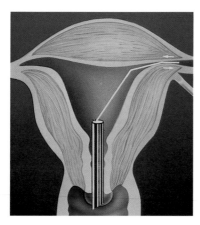

Figure 1(a)–(c) Nd : YAG laser sterilization. The fiber is introduced into the intramural Fallopian tube

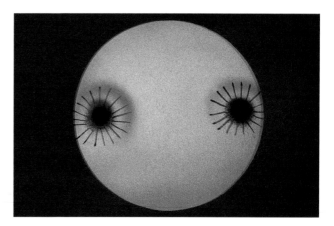

Figure 1(b) *See legend opposite*

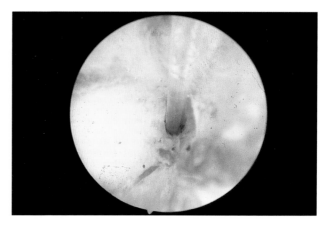

Figure 1(c) *See legend above*

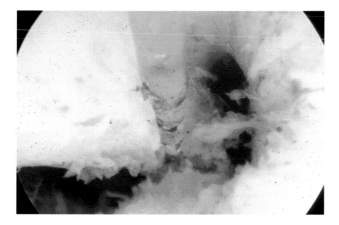

Figure 2(a) and (b) Nd : YAG laser sterilization. The touch technique is used to apply laser energy to the uterine cavity, close to the tubal ostium

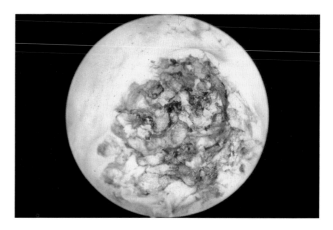

Figure 2(b) *See legend opposite*

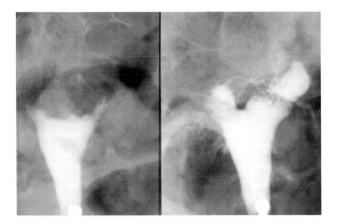

Figure 3 The hysterosalpingography confirms the tubal occlusion

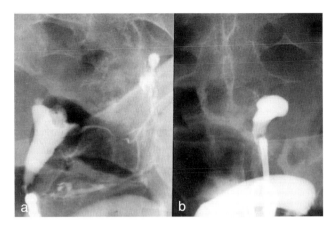

Figure 4(a) Hysterography shows a patent tube on the left side; (b) after 6 months, fibrosis and shrinkage of the uterine horn induced a complete stenosis

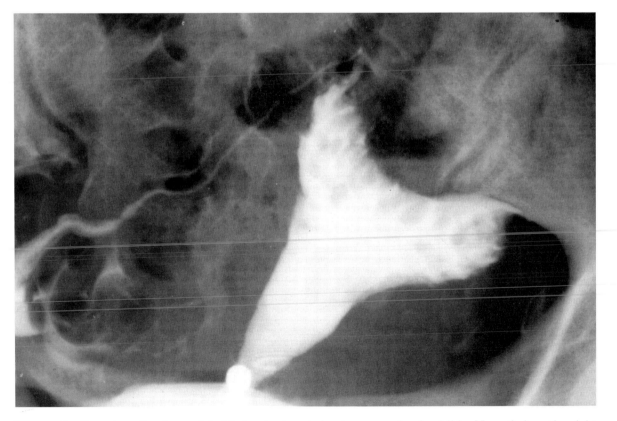

Figure 5 Sequelae of endometrial ablation in the uterine horn are clearly visible. Nevertheless, the right tube was found to be patent

completely obstructed. Neovascularization and fibro-blastic proliferation occurred, replacing the normal endometrium and its stroma with connective tissue and newly formed capillaries. There was almost no inflammatory reaction; polymorphonuclear neutrophils were rare, while many foreign body giant cells surrounding carbon particles attracted attention.

Our experimental model fulfils the goal of provoking adhesion of the tubal folds of the uterine horn walls to one another and, thus, complete obstruction of the cavity. Histologic evaluation of serial sections proved that tubal endometrial photocoagulation was complete in all cases. Indeed, no viable tissue, not even the smallest gland was ever found.

Another interesting observation, similar to that made in women and in mice, concerns the absence of inflammation. Besides the numerous foreign body giant cells observed around carbon particles in each biopsy, only very rare polymorphonuclear neutrophils were seen. The tissue replacing the tubal epithelium and the endometrium and its stroma is a connective tissue; this suggests that the occlusion is not only complete but that it will also be permanent.

FEMALE Nd : YAG LASER STERILIZATION

The author uses the touch technique. The quartz fiber is introduced about 1 cm into the intramural portion of the Fallopian tube. In order to apply the laser energy, the fiber is slowly removed while firing. The same procedure is repeated five times. The power used is 80 W and the total energy applied is about 5000–8000 J. The touch technique is then used to apply the laser energy to the uterine cavity, close to the tubal ostium (Figure 1). By allowing the quartz fiber to be in contact with the endometrium during the application of laser energy, the endometrium and the deeper areas of myometrium (1 cm around the tubal ostium) are coagulated (Figure 2).

Hysterosalpingography must be performed to confirm tubal occlusion (Figure 3). In a series of 80 cases, tubal occlusion was proved in all cases, except two. In one case, the left tube was found patent after 3 months and occluded after 6 months (Figure 4). In the other case, one tube was patent. A second procedure was successfully carried out (Figure 5).

In conclusion, this hysteroscopic approach to tubal occlusion could be feasible in women aged over 40 years who undergo a hysteroscopy for another reason. This technique is not the procedure of choice for young women, because of its very low degree of reversibility.

REFERENCES

1. Thatcher, S.S. (1988). Hysteroscopic sterilization. Obstet. Gynecol. Clin. N. Am., **15**, 51
2. Darabi, K.F., Roy, K. and Richart, R.M. (1978). Collaborative study on hysteroscopic sterilization procedures: final report. In Sciarra, J.J., Zatuchni, G.I. and Speidel, J.J. (eds.) Risks, Benefits, and Controversies in Fertility Control, p. 81. (Hagerstown: Harper & Row Publishers)
3. Richart, R.M. (1981). Female sterilization using chemical agents. In Zatuchni, G.I. (ed.) Research Frontiers and Fertility Regulation, Vol. 5, No.1, p.1. (Chicago: Program for Applied Research on Fertility Regulation)
4. Erb, R.A. (1983). Hysteroscopic tubal occlusion procedure with formed-in-place silicon plugs: instruments and technique. In Zatuchni, G.I., Shelton, J.D., Goldsmith, A. et al. (eds.) Female Transcervical Sterilization, p. 245. (Philadelphia: Harper & Row Publishers)
5. Loffer, F.D. (1984). Hysteroscopic sterilization with use of formed-in-place silicone plugs. Am. J. Obstet. Gynecol., **149**, 261
6. Hamou, J., Gasparri, F., Scarselli, G.F. et al. (1984). Hysteroscopic reversible tubal sterilization. Acta Eur. Fertil., **15**, 123
7. Brundin, J. (1983). Hydrogel tubal blocking device: P-block. In Zatuchni, G.I., Shelton, J.D., Goldsmith, A. et al. (eds.) Female Transcervical Sterilization, p. 240. (Philadelphia: Harper & Row Publishers)
8. Hosseinian, A.H. and Morales, W.A. (1983). Clinical application of hysteroscopic sterilization using uterotubal junction blocking devices. In Zatuchni, G.I., Shelton J.D., Goldsmith, A. et al. (eds.) Female Transcervical Sterilization, p. 234. (Philadelphia: Harper & Row Publishers)
9. Goldrath, M.H., Fuller, T. and Segal, S. (1981). Laser photovaporization of endometrium for the treatment of menorrhagia. Am J. Obstet. Gynecol., **140**, 14–19

Complications of hysteroscopic surgery in gynecology

36

S. Bassil, M. Nisolle and J. Donnez

INTRODUCTION

Hysteroscopic surgery has developed from a diagnostic tool into an effective surgical technique. It is now a standard investigational and therapeutic tool in gynecology which, when performed properly for the right indications in patients with no contraindications, has practically no complications. In a recent survey[1], the overall complication rate for almost 14 000 hysteroscopic procedures performed in 1988 was reported as 2%, with major complications occurring in less than 1% of procedures. Although complications are infrequent, their description helps us understand their causes and thus take steps to avoid them. There are five groups of complications of operative hysteroscopy: traumatic, hemorrhagic, distension-medium hazard, infection, and thermal surgery damage.

Our purpose is to describe the diagnosis, management and prevention of such complications. Complications of anesthesia, and treatment failures will not be described.

TRAUMATIC COMPLICATIONS OF HYSTEROSCOPY

Traumatic complications of diagnostic hysteroscopy have been well documented. Hysteroscopic surgery, however, also involves some blind manipulation. Dilating the cervix to accommodate wide-caliber operating instruments may cause cervical laceration and/or uterine perforation, with or without hemorrhage. The frequency of these complications is unknown, and has been estimated as 1–9%[2–4].

Diagnosis

Cervical lacerations are diagnosed only if cervical bleeding occurs. Uterine perforation is suspected if the depth of passage of the sound or the dilator is greater than the apparent size of the uterus. Very rapid flow of liquid or very low distension pressure with CO_2 at the time of insertion of the hysteroscope should raise this suspicion. Diagnosis is sometimes made by the visualization of the bowel. Any hemorrhage before the beginning of the surgical procedure is highly suggestive of traumatic damage.

Management

Cervical laceration is of little consequence, although sutures are occasionally required to prevent or to stop cervical bleeding. Uterine perforation does not usually need surgical repair. If perforation is diagnosed before the surgical procedure, surgery must be delayed and the patient observed for 24h. If perforation is diagnosed intraoperatively or after the surgical procedure, a diagnostic laparoscopy is recommended to ensure that no damage has been caused to adherent or adjacent structures and that there is no unsuspected laceration of the large blood vessels.

Prevention

To prevent such complications, careful placement of the tenaculum and gentle dilatation of the cervix are recommended. Advancement of the hysteroscope must always be performed under visual control, accommodating the instrument axis to the direction of the cervical canal and to the position of the uterus. The use of laminaria tents is favored by some hysteroscopists, but avoided by others, because of the possible risk of overdilatation, resulting in loss of distension medium and intrauterine pressure, and causing poor visualization.

HEMORRHAGIC COMPLICATIONS OF HYSTEROSCOPY

Intraoperative bleeding, other than that due to cervical laceration or uterine perforation, is usually the result of inadvertent or intentional trauma to the uterine wall. The reported rate of bleeding requiring surgery or uterine tamponade ranges from 0 to 22.4%[5–8]. This wide variation is attributed to the gynecologist's experience, and to the pathology treated. Hemorrhage can occur from false passages, with or without perforation, created during either the dilatation or the insertion of the hysteroscope. Bleeding can also occur after operative procedures, especially when penetration of healthy myometrium is too deep. This can occur after the use of scissors or thermal energy (laser, resectoscope).

Diagnosis

Heavy and continuous vaginal bleeding during or after surgery must be investigated, in order to determine if it is intrauterine or cervical bleeding. Management should be effected according to the origin of the hemorrhage.

Management

Intraoperatively, rapid bleeding can be controlled by coagulation, using either the tip of the laser fiber or the electrical loop. Postoperative and uncontrolled intra-operative bleeding may sometimes require intrauterine tamponade. A Foley catheter is introduced into the uterine cavity and the balloon is inflated with 15 ml of liquid. After approximately 3 h, one half of the liquid is removed; if no bleeding recurs over the next hour, the catheter is removed and the patient is usually discharged. If active bleeding recurs, the balloon is reinflated and left in place overnight.

Prevention

Recommendations for avoiding trauma also apply to hemorrhagic complications. In addition, the entire surgical procedure must be carried out under strict visualization of the dissection plane. If large submucosal myomas or dense intrauterine synechiae are present, performing the procedure in two parts decreases the risk of such complications. The use of intracervical vasopressin has been described to decrease the risk of bleeding[6]. This drug must be used with consideration of its systemic effects. The use of preoperative medical therapy (gonadotropin releasing hormone agonists, danazol, progestins) has been reported to decrease postoperative bleeding. Such therapy decreases the thickness and vascularity of the endometrium and shrinks myomas[3,5,9,10] and may be helpful in avoiding this type of complication.

DISTENSION MEDIUM COMPLICATIONS

Complications specifically related to distension media occur in 4% of procedures[1] and vary according to the medium used.

Carbon dioxide

Venous gas embolism is the most feared complication of using CO_2 gas as a distension medium. This risk is low when using adequate hysteroflators. Most reports of fatal CO_2 embolism during operative hysteroscopy are the result of using inadequate or faulty insufflators[11–14].

High molecular weight dextran

The major complication feared from the use of dextran 70 (Hyskon) is anaphylactic shock. This can be prevented by performing an intravenous injection test with a small amount of dextran 15% 2 min before using dextran 70. This distension medium also induces ascites and intravascular overload if a substantial volume is retained in the patient.

Low viscosity liquid complications

These fluids (mainly sorbitol, glycine and dextrose in water) are used primarily during electrosurgical intrauterine procedures. When retained by the patient they may cause hyponatremia and fluid overload. Glycine has toxic effects on the central nervous system[15].

Diagnosis

Venous air embolism and anaphylactic shock are easily recognized. Manifestations of fluid overload are treacherous and can occur any time postoperatively. The monitoring of intake and output of liquids during and after the procedure is mandatory to assess the fluid balance. A discrepancy of 800 ml requires an assessment of serum electrolytes to permit the diagnosis.

Management

Venous air embolism and anaphylactic shock are acute complications. Admission to the intensive care unit and hyperbaric oxygen therapy are required for embolism[16], corticosteroids and cardiotonics are administered for anaphylactic shock. Fluid overload with abnormal serum electrolytes is managed with diuretics and fluid restriction. The patient is usually able to void the excess fluid and the problem is thus solved.

Prevention

The first rule for hysteroscopy with CO_2 is the use of adequate insufflators. The insufflation pressure must not exceed 100 mmHg. Faulty routes, especially submuscosal passages, increase the risk of embolism. Repeated introduction of the hysteroscope in such cases must be avoided, as must the use of CO_2 for cooling laser tips. During hysteroscopy with liquid medium, monitoring of the inflow and outflow volumes is essential to prevent the retention of too much distension medium by the patient. An infusion pressure of more than 150 mmHg increases the risk of fluid absorption, but intravasation of the fluid often occurs, through open uterine venous channels or in the presence of unrecognized perforation with normal infusion pressure[17]. If uterine perforation and/or fluid balance discrepancy of over 800 ml is detected the procedure must be stopped.

INFECTIOUS COMPLICATIONS

Infection is rare, with a frequency of 0.25–1%[6,18,19]. Usually, the infection follows prolonged operative procedures, especially when repeated insertion and removal of the hysteroscope through the cervical canal has been necessary. It occurs about 72 h postoperatively and manifests with fever, vaginal discharge and pelvic pain. It can be treated successfully with broad-spectrum oral antibiotics. Hospitalization is rarely required. To prevent this complication, the use of prophylactic antibiotics is recommended.

THERMAL ENERGY COMPLICATIONS

There is little information in the gynecological literature regarding the occurrence and management of injury to viscera during hysteroscopy. Such injuries could be caused directly by the electrical current or by the thermal diffusion of energy.

Improvements in instrument design and in energy generators have eliminated the risk of electrical shock to the patient from the body of the resectoscope. Such injuries often occur in the presence of uterine perforation. They can be induced by the prolonged application of strong electrical or laser energy to the uterine wall, especially in the area of tubal ostia.

Diagnosis

The diagnosis is missed intraoperatively in the majority of cases. Postoperative symptoms include fever, abdominal pain, leukocytosis and signs of peritonitis. Laparoscopy is helpful in suspicious cases, but this may be insufficient to fully evaluate the bowel, and laparotomy is then required[20].

Management

Guidelines described in Chapter 25 for vessel injuries or bowel burns with laparoscopy apply to such injuries.

Prevention

The success of prevention depends on respecting the technical conditions of surgical hysteroscopy. If uterine perforation occurs, the procedure must be delayed for the patient's safety. In addition, the energy source must always be activated with a completely clear visualization of the tip of the laser fiber or the resectoscope loop.

DISCUSSION

Operative hysteroscopy has provided new possibilities for the conservative treatment of gynecological pathologies. Although complications are not frequent, some serious problems do occur. Besides the common complications described above, rupture of the tubes, rupture of the diaphragm with the patient's death, rupture of the uterine wall, trauma to pelvic vessels and rupture of the uterus in twin pregnancy after hysteroscopic perforation have been reported[6,21]. Most of the complications described are induced by traumatic injuries. The safety of the procedure depends on the experience of the surgeon, and the increasing number of gynecologists performing operative hysteroscopy will increase the potential risk of complications. Understanding the risks inherent in the use of the instruments and media selected will minimize the chances of complications and enhance the chances of good surgical results.

REFERENCES

1. Peterson, H.B., Hulka, J.F. and Phillips, J.M. (1990). American Association of Gynecologic Laparoscopist's 1988 membership survey on operative hysteroscopy. *J. Reprod. Med.*, **35**, 590
2. Lindemann, H.J. and Mohr, J. (1976). CO_2 hysteroscopy: diagnosis and treatment. *Am. J. Obstet. Gynecol.*, **124,** 129
3. Donnez, J. and Nisolle, M. (1992). Hysteroscopic surgery. *Curr. Opin. Obstet. Gynecol.*, **4,** 439
4. Cooper, J.M. (1992). Hysteroscopic sterilization. *Clin. Obstet. Gynecol.*, **35**, 282
5. Brooks, P.G., Serden, S.P. and Davos I. (1991). Hormonal inhibition of the endometrium for resectoscope endometrial ablation. *Am. J. Obstet. Gynecol.*, **164,** 1601
6. Brooks, P.G. (1992). Complications of operative hysteroscopy: how safe is it? *Clin. Obstet. Gynecol.*, **35** 256
7. De Cherney A.H., Diamond, M.D., Lavy, G. and Polan, M. L. (1987). Endometrial ablation for intractable uterine bleeding: hysteroscopic resection. *Obstet. Gynecol.*, **70,** 668
8. Donnez, J., Gillerot, S., Bourgonjon, D., Clerckx, F. and Nisolle, M. (1990). Neodymium : Yag laser hysteroscopy in large submucous fibroids. *Fertil. Steril.*, **54**, 999
9. Siegler, A.M., Valle, R.F., Lindemann, H.J. and Mencaglia, L. (1990). *Therapeutic Hysteroscopy, Indications and Techniques.* (St Louis: CV Mosby)
10. Donnez, J., Schrurs, B., Gillerot, S., Sandow, J. and Clerckx-Braun, F. (1989). Treatment of uterine fibroïds with implants of gonadotropin releasing hormone agonist: assessment by hysterography. *Fertil. Steril.*, **51**, 947

11. Perry, P.M. and Baughman, V.L. (1990). A complication of hysteroscopy: air embolism. *Anesthesiology*, **73**, 546

12. Challener, R.C. and Kaufman, B. (1990) Fatal venous air embolism following sequential unsheathed (bare) and sheathed quartz fiber Nd : YAG laser endometrial ablation. *Anesthesiology*, **73**, 551

13. Food and Drug Administration. (1990). Gas/air embolism associated with intrauterine laser surgery. *FDA Bull.*, **19**, May 11

14. Baggish, M.S. and Daniell, J.F. (1989). Death caused by air embolism associated with neodymium : yttrium-aluminium-garnet laser surgery and artificial sapphire tips. *Am. J. Obstet. Gynecol.*, **161**, 877

15. Hoekstra, P.T., Kahnoski, R., McCamish, M.A., Bergen, W. and Heetderks, D.W. (1983). Transurethral prostatic resection syndrome: a new perspective: encephalopathy with associated hyperammonemia. *J. Urol.*, **130**, 704

16. Tur-Kaspa, I. (1990). Hyperbaric oxygen therapy for air embolism complicating operative hysteroscopy. *Am J. Obstet. Gynecol.*, **163**, 680

17. Vulgaropulos, S.P., Haley, L.C. and Hulka, J.F. (1992). Intrauterine pressure and fluid absorption during continuous flow hysteroscopy. *Am. J. Obstet. Gynecol.*, **167**, 386

18. Taylor, P.J. and Hamou, J.E. (1983). Hysteroscopy. *J. Reprod. Med.*, **28**, 359

19. Mergui, J.L., Raossanaly, K. and Salat-Baroux, J. (1990). Place de l'hystéroscopie opératoire en 1990. *Lett. Gynécol.* **132**, 21

20. Sullivan, B., Kenney, P. and Seibel, M. (1992). Hysteroscopic resection of fibroïd with thermal injury to sigmoïd. *Obstet. Gynecol.*, **80**, 546

21. Creinin, M. and Chen, M. (1992). Uterine defect in a twin pregnancy with a history of hysteroscopic fundal perforation. *Obstet. Gynecol.*, **79**, 879

Hysteroscopic surgery: the anesthetist's point of view

M.J. Van Boven, P.E. Pendeville and F.J. Singelyn

Endoscopic intrauterine hysteroscopic surgery is only possible by distension of the uterine cavity. Distension of the uterus and separation of its walls require a pressure of approximately $10 \, cmH_2O$. When the intrauterine pressure exceeds $50 \, cmH_2O$, fluid refluxes through the patent Fallopian tubes and accumulates in the cul-de-sac of Douglas[1].

Both gas and liquid can be used as a distension medium, but gas is no longer used for operative hysteroscopy because of its potential for causing gas embolism. The use of liquid distension medium causes concern due to its possible resorption.

LIQUID DISTENSION MEDIA

The main qualities of a distension medium are as follows. The solution should be isotonic, non-hemolytic, non-electrolytic, non-toxic when absorbed, and not metabolized. It should not influence the osmolarity of blood, should be rapidly excreted and should be an osmotic diuretic[2]. Moreover, it must give the surgeon perfect vision during the procedure.

Several media may be used to distend the cavity: water, 0.9% sodium chloride, 5% dextrose in water, 5% dextrose in Ringer lactate, Ringer lactate, dextran solutions and glycine solution.

During the procedure, the high pressure required to distend the poorly compliant uterine cavity, forces fluid into the open veins, resulting in a potential volume overload. Significant fluid overload in patients with a compromised cardiovascular status can lead to pulmonary edema and congestive heart failure[3-5].

Fluid overload is essentially due to poor monitoring of fluid administration rather than to the inherent properties of any particular solution. Overload with colloids is much more difficult to treat than is overload with crystalloids[6]. In order to prevent fluid overload in patients with cardiovascular diseases, the monitoring of central venous pressure has been suggested[4,7].

The absorption of a large volume of electrolyte-free solution may also lead to the dilution of blood components.

Several factors may contribute to resorption of the distending medium (Table 1). First, because of the low compliance of the uterine cavity, the infusion pressure rises well above the normal venous pressure. It has also been suggested that there is a retrograde flow into damaged arteries due to the high pressure in the uterine cavity[8]. Second, the solution may pass through the permeable Fallopian tubes into the peritoneal cavity. Formerly, tubal closure was recommended in order to reduce the amount of fluid which is present in the abdominal cavity and which is absorbed[9]. In our experience, only a small amount of liquid can be reaspirated by culdosynthesis from the peritoneal cavity when an associated laparoscopy is performed. This suggests that the distension medium is mainly absorbed by the open blood vessels and that the extent of resection is of more significance than the duration of the resection.

Table 1 Factors affecting fluid absorption

Infusion pressure
Permeability of the Fallopian tubes
Open blood vessels
Resection area
Resection time
Surgical technique
Hormonal endometrial status

A study by Loffer[9] indicates that the surgical technique used for endometrial ablation is important with regard to fluid resorption. In a comparison of the dragging and blanching techniques, he showed that less liquid was resorbed with the latter[9].

During the second phase of the menstrual cycle, the endometrium is well developed and there is a high degree of vascularization; this may well account for the greater liquid resorption. This high vascularization can be reduced by gonadotropin releasing hormone treatment[5]. Matta studied uterine blood flow by Doppler ultrasound in eight patients treated with a gonadrotopin releasing hormone agonist. At the end of the treatment, a reduction in the uterine volume was associated with a significant reduction in uterine blood flow[10].

Specific problems related to dextran solutions

Hyskon (32% dextran 70 in 10% dextrose) is an optically clear electrolyte-free, viscid, sterile, non-pyrogenic, non-conductive, biodegradable mixture which is immiscible with blood. Several complications may occur during its use (Table 2). Many cases of anaphylactic reactions to dextran have been described after its intravenous injection[11]. Data collected from 208 dextran-induced

Table 2 Specific problems related to dextran solutions

Dextran-induced anaphylactoid reactions
Fluid overload
Pulmonary capillary toxicity
Blood clotting disturbances
Renal failure

anaphylactoid reactions (DIAR) in Germany, revealed that DIAR commonly occurs in the early phase of the infusion [12,13]. Symptoms range from mild (flush, urticaria) to gastrointestinal, respiratory and cardiovascular problems.

DIARs are mediated by dextran reactive antibodies (IgG immunoglobulins) formed in response to dextran polysaccharides and resulting from exposure to dextran contaminants in sugar, dextran in dental plaque and from cross-reactivity with bacteria. Dextran reactive antibodies are present in the general population and this places many patients at risk of a reaction to dextran.

However, by prior administration of a hapten, a substance able to combine with immunoglobulins without producing a reaction, the immunoglobulin reactive sites are occupied and unable to react to the antigen. Intravenous injection of 20 ml dextran 1 (Promit®, Promiten® – a low molecular weight dextran) before the infusion of dextran has been shown to be a very effective and safe method of prophylaxis against severe DIAR [12-16]; however, one case of a severe reaction has been published [16].

Moreover, after an infusion of more than 20 ml/kg/24 h, dextran 70 may interfere with normal blood clotting, leading to disturbances in blood cross-matching and to bleeding diathesis. These clotting defects are due to reduced platelet adhesiveness secondary to an antithrombin effect.

Renal failure has been reported in several patients following the administration of dextran 40 in amounts exceeding 20 ml/kg.

Intravascular absorption of 32% dextran 70 may have a direct toxic effect upon the pulmonary capillaries, resulting in extravasation and interstitial pulmonary edema. This mechanism may be similar to the drug-induced non-cardiogenic pulmonary edema reported with Ritodrine and dextran 40 [11]. During Nd : YAG laser procedures, dextran 70 in 10% dextrose produces large bubbles and, as a result of heating, caramelizes around the laser fiber. Because of its high molecular weight, dextran solution may lead to a dramatic intravenous fluid overload.

Specific problems related to 1.5% glycine solution (Table 3)

Glycine solution has excellent optical and non-hemolytic properties during hysteroscopic surgery [5]. This electrolyte-free solution is widely used by urologists during transurethral resections [17]. Glycine is a non-essential amino acid which exists naturally in the body. Its normal plasma level is 120–155 μmol/l, and it readily crosses the blood–brain barrier. Glycine functions as an inhibitory transmitter in the spinal cord and in the brainstem and retina. The toxicity of intravenously administered glycine has been demonstrated in dogs and in humans (Table 3). Symptoms include nausea, vomiting, fixed and dilated pupils, weakness and muscular incoordination [18-21].

Degradation of glycine in the body takes place in several ways. The main route of metabolism is by reversible oxidative cleavage to carbon dioxide, ammonia and N5,N10-methylene-tetrahydrofolate by glycine synthetase. Glycine may also be converted to serine by serine hydroxymethyltransferase with pyridoxal phosphate as coenzyme [2]. Glycine is also metabolized to oxalate.

During the surgical procedure, very large quantities of glycine solution may be resorbed into the intravascular and extravascular space, leading to the well-documented transurethral resection (TUR) syndrome. This is commonly considered to be basically water intoxication with hypervolemia and hemodilution. The symptoms that usually appear during surgery performed under regional anesthesia include apprehension, nausea, blurred vision or even temporary blindness, and eventually convulsions, coma and vascular collapse [17,22]. Cardiac symptoms may be predominant in the early phase. Early signs of water intoxication include an increase in arterial and central venous pressure, bradycardia, cardiac arrhythmias and electrocardiographic changes, including a widening and increased amplitude of the QRS complex and T-wave inversion. Complete recovery within 24–48 h is the rule, although severe reactions can occur. Other important factors are the decrease in serum osmolarity and the rapid drop in the serum sodium level.

Table 3 Specific problems related to 1.5% glycine solution

Fluid overload
Electrolyte dilution
Hyperglycinemia and ammonia toxicity

There are reasons to believe that an overload of glycine will, in some patients, result in a marked elevation of blood ammonium levels and encephalopathy. The effect of hyperglycinemia in the presence of a low serum sodium level also has to be considered. It has been suggested that glycine or its metabolites may be a cause of visual disturbances and encephalopathy, independent of changes in serum sodium levels or osmolarity [19,20,23-25].

Recent observations suggest that ammonium toxicity may be an important, and in some instances, the sole

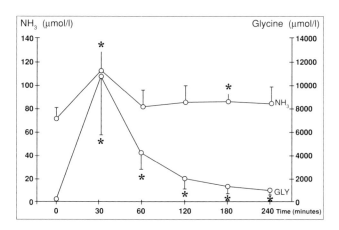

Figure 1 Concentrations of glycine and ammonia measured in serum of seven artificially menopausal patients undergoing Nd : YAG laser endoscopic procedures

cause of encephalopathy in patients showing signs of water intoxication during or following transurethral resection using glycine as the irrigant solution[25]. Such a possibility should be considered when large quantities of glycine solution are absorbed during uterine endoscopic surgery. Since oxalate is one of the metabolic products of glycine, a high absorption of the amino acid might lead to hyperoxaliuria, possibly accompanied by elevated urinary glycolate[26].

In order to study the metabolism of glycine after endoscopic uterine surgery, serum concentrations of the amino acid and its metabolites were measured in seven artificially menopausal patients scheduled for Nd : YAG laser endoscopic procedures. Fluid balance was determined by a volumetric method (comparison of the volume of injected irrigating fluid and the volume of fluid collected during the procedure). The mean irrigant absorption was 1128 ± 673 ml. A significant increase in glycine concentration during and after the procedure (up to 100 times the normal value) was correlated with a rise in serum ammonia levels (Figure 1). Recovery was uneventful in all cases. Serum sodium levels and osmolarity remained normal during and after surgery and there was no increased oxaliuria[27].

Table 4 Precautions in operative hysteroscopic surgery when a liquid distending medium is used

Monitor in-and-out fluid balance
Restrict intravenous fluid
(Monitor central venous pressure)
(Favor regional anesthesia)
(Monitor electrolyte serum concentration)
When dextran is used, prevent dextran-induced
  anaphylactoid reaction (DIAR) by using low molecular
  weight dextran

Other liquid distension media (low viscosity liquids)

Ringer lactate, sodium chloride and 5% or 10% dextrose were employed as distension media. These solutions are very miscible with blood rendering surgery more difficult. Moreover, they may lead to fluid overload and water intoxication if they are electrolyte free. Hyperglycemia has been reported after the use of dextrose-containing solutions.

CONCLUSION

Besides anaphylactoid reactions (dextran-containing solutions), water intoxication (electrolyte-free solutions), hyperglycemia and hyperglycinemia, fluid overload is certainly the most important problem related to the use of a liquid distending medium. As only a small amount of liquid can be re-aspirated by culdosynthesis after the procedure, it seems that the distension medium is mainly resorbed by open blood vessels, and that the extent of the resection could be of more significance than the resection time.

General anesthesia masks the early signs of fluid overload, as well as of water intoxication and transurethral resection syndrome. As recommended by many authors, regional anesthesia must be the procedure of choice both for transurethral resections as well as for hysteroscopic laser surgery[18,19,25]. Unfortunately, when additional laparoscopy has to be performed, general anesthesia seems inevitable. When an extensive procedure is planned, fluid load and central venous pressure should be carefully monitored. In patients with a history of heart failure, the insertion of a Swan-Ganz catheter should be considered. Although hysteroscopic surgery has been proposed in high-risk patients as an alternative to hysterectomy[3,28], the potential danger of fluid overload should be considered carefully when choosing the surgical technique (Table 4).

REFERENCES

1. Lavy, G., Diamond, M.P., Shapiro, B. and Decherney, A.H. (1987). A new device to facilitate intrauterine instillation of dextran 70 for hysteroscopy. *Obstet. Gynecol.*, **70**, 955–7
2. Norlen, H., Allgen, L.G., Vinnars, E. and Bedrelidou-Classon, G. (1986). Glycine solution as an irrigating agent during transurethral prostatic resection. *Scand. J. Urol. Nephrol.*, **20**, 19–26
3. Baggish, M.S. and Baltoyannis, P. (1988). New techniques for laser ablation of the endometrium in high-risk patients. *Am. J. Obstet. Gynecol.*, **159**, 287–93
4. Osborne, D.A., Rudkin, G.E and Moran, P.

(1991). Fluid uptake in laser endometrial ablation. *Anaesth. Intensive Care*, **19**, 217-9

5. Donnez, J. and Nisolle, M. (1989). Laser hysteroscopy in uterine bleeding. Endometrial ablation and polypectomy. In Donnez, J. (ed.) *Laser Operative Laparoscopy and Hysteroscopy*. p. 277. (Leuven: Nauwelaerts)

6. Ibister, J.P. and Fisher, M. (1987). Adverse effects of plasma volume expanders. *Anaesth. Intensive Care*, **8**, 145-51

7. Morrison, L.M.M., Davis, J. and Summer, D. (1989). Absorption of irrigating fluid during laser photocoagulation of the endometrium in the treatment of menorrhagia. *Br. J. Obstet. Gynaecol.*, **96**, 346-52

8. Garry, R. (1990). Safety of hysteroscopic surgery. *Lancet*, **336**, 1013-4

9. Loffer, F.R. (1987). Hysteroscopic endometrial ablation with the Nd:YAG laser using a non-touch technique. *Obstet. Gynecol.*, **69**, 679-82

10. Matta, W.H.M., Stabile, I., Shaw, R.W. and Campbell, S. (1988). Doppler assessment of uterine blood flow changes in patients with fibroids receiving the gonadotropin releasing hormone agonist Buserelin. *Fertil. Steril.*, **49**, 1083-5

11. Leake, J.F., Murphy, A.A. and Zacur, H.A. (1987). Noncardiogenic pulmonary edema: a complication of operative hysteroscopy. *Fertil. Steril.*, **48**, 497-9

12. Ring, J. (1984). Colloids. *Clin. Anesthesiol.*, **2**, 619-41

13. Hedin, H., Richter, W., Messmer, K., Renck, H., Ljungström, K.G. and Laubenthal, H. (1981). Incidence, pathomechanism and prevention of dextran-induced anaphylactoid/anaphylactic reactions in man. *Dev. Biol. Stand.*, **48**, 179-89

14. Ljungström, K.G., Renck, H., Strandberg, K., Hedin, H., Richter, W. and Widerlöv, E. (1983). Adverse reaction to dextran in Sweden 1970-1983. *Acta Chir. Scand.*, **149**, 253-62

15. Renck, H. Ljunström, K.G., Rosberg, B., Dhuner, K.G. and Dahl, S. (1983). Prevention of dextran-induced anaphylactic reactions by hapten inhibition. *Acta Chir. Scand.*, **149**, 349-53

16. Berstein, R.L., Rosenberg, A.D., Iada, E.Y. and Jaffe, F.F. (1987). A severe reaction to dextran despite hapten inhibition. *Anesthesiology*, **67**, 567-9

17. Charlton, A.J. (1980). Cardiac arrest during transurethral prostatectomy after absorption of 1.5% glycine. *Anaesthesia*, **35**, 804-6

18. Bowman, T.M., Rein, P. and Keenan, R. (1986). Glycine-induced ammonia toxicity following transurethral resection of the prostate. *Anesthesiol. Rev.* **13**, 39-42

19. Ovassapian, A., Joshi, C.W. and Brunner, E.A. (1982). Visual disturbance: an unusual symptom of transurethral surgery. *Anesthesiology*, **57**, 332-4

20. Vila, R., Salvadores, M., Puig, R. and Inturbe, F. (1987). Résection endoscopique sous irrigation de glycine. *Ann. Fr. Anesth. Réanim.*, **6**, 48-9

21. Casey, W.F., Hannon, V., Cunningham, A. and Heany, J. (1988). Visual evoked potential and changes in serum glycine concentration during transurethral resection of the prostate. *Br. J. Anaesth.*, **60**, 525-9

22. Bready, L.L., Hoff, B.H., Boyd, R.C., Wilson, M.A. and Ritter, R.R. (1985). Acute hyponatremia associated with transurethral surgery. *Anesthesiol. Rev.*, **12**, 37-41

23. Zucker, J.R. and Buff, A.P. (1984). Independent plasma levels of sodium and glycine during transurethral resection of the prostate. *Can. Anaesth. Soc. J.*, **31**, 307-13

24. Mei-Li Wang, J., Wong, K.C., Creel, D.J., Clark, W.M. and Shahangian, S. (1985). Effects of glycine on hemodynamic responses and visual evoked potentials in the dog. *Anesth. Analg.*, **64**, 1071-7

25. Roesh, R.P., Stoelting, R.K., Lingeman, J.E., Kahnosky, R.J., Backes, D.J. and Gephardt, S.A. (1983). Ammonia toxicity resulting from glycine absorption during a transurethral resection of the prostate. *Anesthesiology*, **58**, 577-9

26. Fitzpatrick, J.M., Kasidas, G.P. and Rose, G.A. (1981). Hyperoxaliuria following glycine irrigation for transurethral prostatectomy. *Br. J. Urol.*, **53**, 250-2

27. Van Boven, M., Pendeville, P.E. and Singelyn, F.J. (1993). Glycine and its metabolites during and after intrauterine YAG laser surgery. *Br. J. Anaesthesia*. **70**, (Suppl. 1), A87

28. DeCherney, A., Diamond, M.P., Lavy, G. and Polan, M.L. (1987). Endometrial ablation for intractable uterine. *Obstet. Gynecol.*, **70**, 668-70

Section III

The future

Nd : YAG laser ITT multifiber device (the Donnez device): endometrial ablation by interstitial hyperthermia

38

J. Donnez, R. Polet, P.-E. Mathieu, E. Konwitz, M. Nisolle and F. Casanas-Roux

INTRODUCTION

Dysfunctional uterine bleeding has been treated using numerous non-surgical intracavitary procedures with varying degrees of success. The techniques of endometrial resection and transhysteroscopic photocoagulation by Nd : YAG laser have been mastered and are extremely effective in experienced hands[1-5].

The recent development of new Nd : YAG optic fibers with lateral diffusion (ITT fibers, E. Konwitz, personal communication), with the aim of simplifying the technical performance, has given rise to the idea of a multifiber Nd : YAG device (the Donnez device), conceptually close to the intrauterine device (IUD). These new fibers act rather like an interstitial hyperthermic modality.

Before embarking on clinical trials with this device, an initial study of the thermometric measurement on hysterectomy specimens was conducted, in order to determine the appropriate power intensity and duration of treatment. As a second step, the device was tested on a first series of four patients.

MATERIALS AND METHODS

This new multifiber device (the Donnez device, DD) is composed of three prototype ITT fibers designed for lateral diffusion (Figure 1); the two lateral segments have a diffusion length of 3 cm while the central segment measures 4 cm. The whole piece is contained inside a system of sliding sheaths. The ends of each fiber are cuffed by a semi-supple Teflon bridge, giving the assembly some degree of rigidity. The device was developed in collaboration with Sharplan Laser Industry (Tel Aviv, Israel). Once the device has been inserted into the uterus, the removal of the first sheath exposes the active segment of the fibers; pushing the two lateral fibers together gives the system an inverted triangular configuration, which conforms to the shape of the uterine cavity.

In order to ensure a homogeneous distribution of power between the three fibers, the apparatus is equipped with an intermediate fiber fixed to a mirrored coupler to which the three fibers are connected (Figure 2).

In vitro thermometric study on hysterectomy specimens

Eight uteri of normal volume were obtained from patients undergoing vaginal hysterectomy for benign pathologies.

The specimens were opened by a right lateral incision using a scalpel in order to allow the insertion of the device into the cavity; the edges of the incision were then closed using stitches.

Five thermocouples were inserted at the following sites: right uterine horn, fundus, left uterine horn, anterior wall and the isthmus (Figure 3). After immersion of the specimens in a thermostatic solution, an echo-guided technique was used for the precise measurement of the distance between the thermocouples and the fibers.

The laser beam was then switched on for a total duration of 600 s, using a power of 30 W in continuous mode, with the specimens immersed in a thermostatic 37°C saline solution. Temperatures were noted every minute and recorded on a graph.

Clinical thermometric study

The device was used in four patients scheduled for various surgical procedures: two were to undergo a routine hysteroscopic endometrial photocoagulation ablation for menorrhagia, with a normal intracavitary investigation (hysterosalpingogram and outpatient hysteroscopy), together with a diagnostic laparoscopy for chronic pelvic pain; the procedure was preceded by injection of one subcutaneous implant of a gonadotropin releasing hormone agonist 4 weeks earlier. The other two patients were to have their uterus removed (one laparoscopy-assisted supracervical hysterectomy (LASH) and one vaginal hysterectomy (VH) for uterine prolapse), providing pathological data immediately following the interstitial hyperthermy procedure.

There was good access in all cases, allowing the translaparoscopic insertion of the thermocouples into the serosa at the following locations: right uterine horn, fundus, left uterine horn, anterior uterine wall, anterior supraisthmus and posterior supraisthmus. The transvaginal insertion of thermocouples into the cervico-vesical space and the rectovaginal space was also carried out. The uteri were of normal size.

Under general anesthesia and endotracheal intubation, the cervix was first dilated with Hegar probes up to no.10. The thermocouples were then fixed, either translaparoscopically or transvaginally. The device was finally inserted and opened, exposing the fibers. A power output of 30 W for a total duration of 5 min was selected. During the energy emission, the serosal temperatures were prospectively recorded and

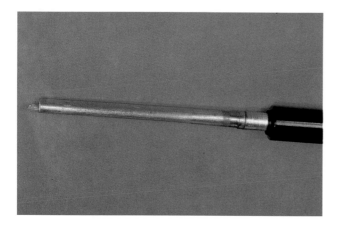

Figure 1 View of the device: (a) and (b) the three fibers are contained in a system of sliding sheaths; (c) the inverted triangular configuration is obtained after pushing the two lateral fibers. This configuration conforms to the shape of the uterine cavity

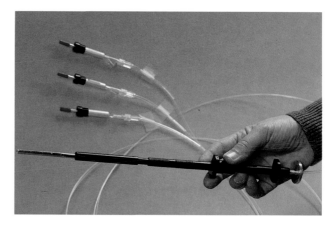

Figure 2 Construction of the system: the three fibers are connected to a mirrored coupler in order to ensure a homogeneous distribution of power between the three fibers

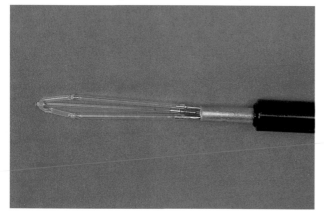

Figure 1(b)   *See legend above*

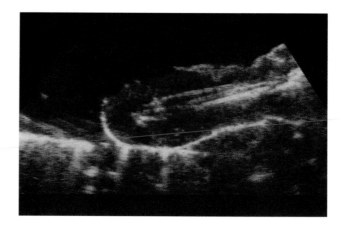

Figure 3 Technique of echoguided insertion of the thermocouples: (a) the location of the fibers is checked precisely

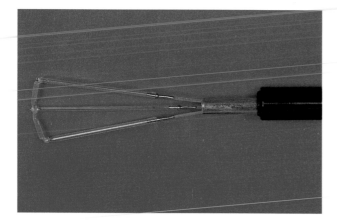

Figure 1(c)   *See legend above*

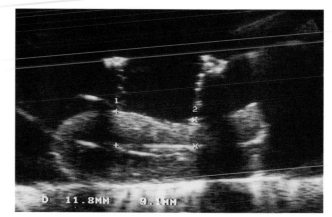

Figure 3(b) The thermocouples are inserted; the distance between the intrauterine device and the thermocouples is carefully evaluated

macroscopic changes were noted; if suspect temperatures had been observed or suspicious serosal blanching had appeared, indicating a possible uncontrolled localized hyperthermia, the procedure would have been immediately discontinued. After 5 min, the device was removed, the intracavitary temperature was measured and a glycine medium hysteroscopy was performed.

Hysterectomy specimens were examined carefully to evaluate the histological changes and, if possible, the depth of the thermal effect.

One patient undergoing endometrial ablation required vaginal hysterectomy 6 weeks later.

RESULTS

In vitro thermometric study

Figures 4 and 5 show the changes in temperature at different sites in one uterus with deeply inserted thermocouples, and in one with thermocouples inserted in the serosa. Because the depth of insertion varied between specimens, an average temperature elevation curve could not be calculated properly.

After some minutes, a specific temperature gradient, corresponding to each insertion site, could be observed within the tissue. The gradients obtained in the distal sites were almost the same; conversely, the gradients

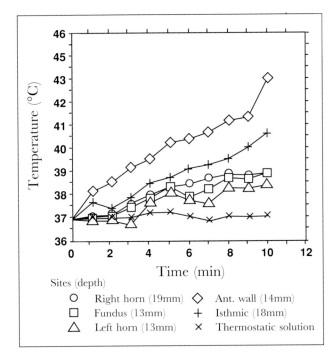

Figure 5 Temperature elevation curve (thermocouples inserted in serosa)

were more marked on the anterior wall and the isthmus (Figures 6 and 7).

The temperature inside the cavity reached 102–103°C after 4–5 min; at a distance of 7 mm, it never exceeded 60°C within 10 min of laser emission.

Macroscopically, at the opening of the treated uterus, a homogeneous and diffuse whitening of the endometrium was seen. Fine superficial traces of carbonization were sometimes observed laterally on the supraisthmic portion, corresponding to pressure sites of the fibers on

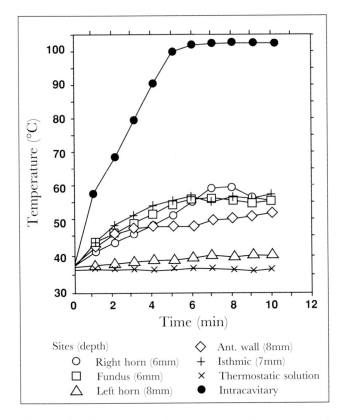

Figure 4 Temperature elevation curve (deeply inserted thermocouples)

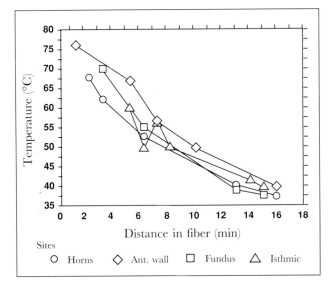

Figure 6 Temperature–distance curves after 5 minutes of emission

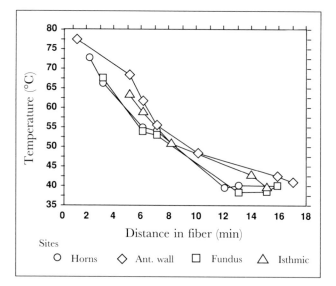

Figure 7 Temperature–distance curves after 10 minutes of emission

the tissue. On section, there was a tough 3 mm-deep white layer, beyond which the myometrium appeared softer and whitish at a depth of 4–5 mm. These features were related to an intense coagulation phenomenon.

Clinical thermometric study

Figure 8 shows the typical temperature changes of the different serosal sites in one of the patients. Serosal temperatures never exceeded 41°C; the temperature elevation curves evoked a saturation effect as initial temperatures rose quickly and soon stabilized. The intracavitary temperature, immediately following discontinuation of laser emission, was 68°C.

A glycine control hysteroscopy performed after photocoagulation showed a homogeneously and uniformly whitened cavity (Figure 9). The supraisthmic portion showed, in two cases, fine traces of superficial carbonization.

Immediate histology was available on two hysterectomy specimens (Figure 10): in both, the endocervical canal showed congestion 2 mm in width, probably related to traumatic dilatation with Hegar probes. On the isthmic portion, the epithelium disappeared and an underlying 2 mm wide edematous zone was observed. At the cavity level, only the superficial layer of the endometrium was strikingly and diffusely ablated following treatment, with no serious damage to the myometrium.

One patient underwent a vaginal hysterectomy 6 weeks after the procedure, as a punch biopsy of the cervix, performed on the day of surgery, revealed a microinvasive carcinoma. On macroscopic observation, the cavity appeared almost completely obliterated, leaving a 1.7 cm-long portion (Figure 11). Microsco-

pically, complete disappearance of the endometrium was noted, together with myometrial damage, estimated at about 4 mm in depth (Figure 12). Postoperative recovery was uneventful.

DISCUSSION

Nd:YAG fibers, routinely used for endometrial photocoagulation, are of the 'bare' type; they diffuse the laser beam axially, forward, and precisely. For this reason, they need to be dragged along the cavity wall, using hysteroscopic control and glycine distending medium, according to a technique requiring prior training [1,2,4].

The advent of new optic fibers, characterized by their ability to diffuse laterally along an active segment of 3–4 cm, has initiated the idea of a multifiber device, inserted and retrieved as simply as an IUD, requiring no distending medium, no hysteroscopic control, no learning curve for the operator and possibly, ultimately, no general or loco-regional anesthesia.

The physical principle of this new technique is very different from the usual transhysteroscopic Nd:YAG fiber dragging technique. In the latter, photocoagulation of the tissue is obtained by a very short application of a very high power density beam; however, the new fibers need to be in contact with the tissue for a long period and then proceed rather like an interstitial hyperthermic modality.

The Nd:YAG laser delivers its energy to tissue in the form of heat through a mechanism of cellular protein absorption. When in contact with the tissue, the beam scatters and covers a vaguely hemispheric territory,

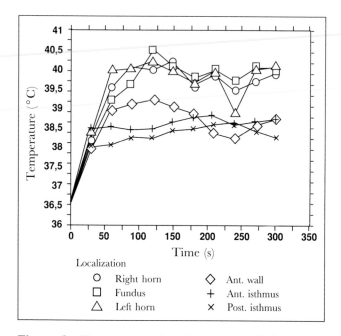

Figure 8 Temperature elevation curve in clinical set-up

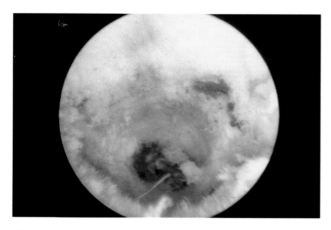

Figure 9 Hysteroscopic view, immediately following the procedure: (a) general view of the cavity, homogeneously whitened

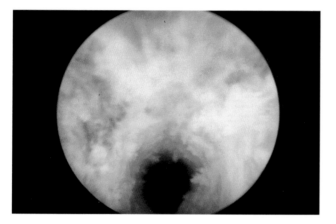

Figure 9(b) A clearcut limit between the photocoagulated cavity and the intact endocervical canal is clearly seen

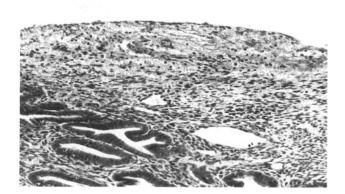

Figure 10 Histological view of hysterectomy specimen (HES × 25). After laser emission, the endometrium was found to be quite normal, except the superficial layers (±300μ), which showed some areas of destruction)

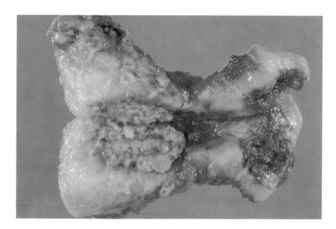

Figure 11 Macroscopic aspect of the endometrial cavity 6 weeks after endometrial ablation by interstitial hyperthermia procedure. A wide surface of the endometrial cavity is obliterated, leaving a supraisthmic portion of the cavity of less than 2 cm

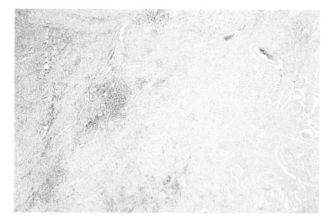

Figure 12 Histological view of uterine wall, 6 weeks after the procedure (HES × 25). The endometrium has virtually disappeared. The myometrium shows signs of fibrosis on a depth of about 4 mm

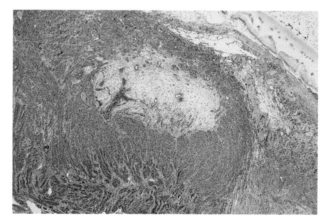

Figure 13 Histological cornual occlusion in the rabbit observed 4 weeks after intracornual laser emission with a third generation ITT fiber–2700 J (Gomori's trichrome, × 25)

measuring 4–6 mm in radius. This measurement can be considered as the optic field of the laser. Beyond this limit, heat diffuses essentially by a simple gradient effect through the myometrium, a tissue of known poor thermal conductivity.

Cellular survival and macroscopic changes associated with short duration hyperthermia are well-known[6]. When tissue temperature reaches 60°C, it suffers irreversible damage. Exposed to lower temperatures, its thermotolerance is time- and temperature-dependent[7,9]: a living tissue is expected to withstand 1 h at 43°C, a limit beyond which the resistance is halved for every degree increase. *In vivo* animal studies[8] have, to some extent, confirmed this. When clinical application of hyperthermic sources is considered in a patient, this principle must be borne in mind.

Interstitial hyperthermia is a therapeutic concept used in oncology to treat primary and secondary malignant tumors[9–11]; its effect is mediated by cytoskeletal and enzymatic protein denaturation. Nd:YAG laser is delivered alone, or in combination with other treatments.

Prior to experimentation with the multifiber device, three successive generations of individual fibers were tested in order to determine the most suitable prototypes (J. Donnez, P.E. Mathieu, personal communication). In laparotomized rabbits, where individual fibers inserted into uterine horns were tested under various energy protocols (ranging from 540 to 3600 J, 10 W for 54–360 s), macroscopic changes observed at the time of the operation and 4 weeks later were noted. Histological examination was also performed in search of tubal occlusion, a condition compatible with an adequate and homogeneous lateral diffusion effect. This feature was found in 80% of cornuas irradiated with third generation fibers only, at energy levels of at least 2700 J, together with a homogeneously stenotic cornua. It was concluded that third generation fibers are the most homogeneous, the most capable of lateral diffusion and, consequently, the most suitable for clinical use. These results were particularly reproducible from experiment to experiment (Figure 13).

In our *in vitro* specimen study, the highest temperatures were reached at the isthmic portion and on the anterior wall, respectively. These localizations both take advantage of a greater 'thermic concentration', related to the geometric positioning of the fibers: the power density would be expected to be higher in sites where the fibers are closer to each other. The close proximity of the bladder and the rectum at the level of the isthmus must be a constant consideration.

Strikingly, *in vitro* temperature elevation and temperature gradients were consistently lower in the left horn. Various factors could account for this, including diffusion heterogeneity linked to the fiber itself, distribution heterogeneity at the level of mirrored coupler, and the overlapping effect of the fibers related to a certain lack of rigidity of the system. It can also be

regarded as an experimental artifact: the uterus opened on its right side may favor accumulation of air in the left horn and this can interfere with an accurate transmission of the beam to the tissue. Because this was not observed during our clinical trials, the latter explanation is probably correct.

The risk of fiber breakage exists. In clinical use, this accident might be detected ultrasonographically by visualizing either the fiber discontinuity, or the abnormally rapid formation of an echographic thermal damage zone[12].

Our system is a completely new delivery system which uses laser emission to induce an endometrial ablation by interstitial hyperthermia. It does not require hysteroscopy and could be used under local anesthesia.

Recent publications confirm a growing interest in new modalities of endometrial ablation in order to make the procedure simpler and less hazardous. Phipps reported a series of menorrhagic patients treated by a microwave probe, on whom a thermometric study was also conducted[13,14].

In vitro, the multifiber device elevated the temperatures in the cavity rapidly up to 102°C; at 6 mm, temperatures of 55°C and 60°C (58–67°C according to the site) were found after 5 and 10 min, respectively, of laser emission. *In vivo*, the intracavitary temperature was 68°C and serosal temperatures never exceeded 41°C at any location after 5 min of laser emission. The discrepancy between *in vitro* and *in vivo* data is related to the cooling effect induced by the uterine arterial flow.

We conclude that the multifiber Donnez device is an extremely simple modality based on interstitial hyperthermy, used to perform endometrial ablation without a hysteroscope. The procedure can be performed under echographic control. Thermometric studies have shown correct temperature distribution, and early clinical experiments indicate good expectations regarding the efficacy according to the first data collected. While improvements are constantly being made with regard to the solidity of the system, further clinical investigations are actively being conducted.

REFERENCES

1. Donnez, J. and Nisolle, M. (1989). Laser hysteroscopy in uterine bleeding: endometrial ablation and polypectomy. In Donnez, J. (ed.) *Laser Operative Laparoscopy and Hysteroscopy*, pp.277–88. (Leuven: Nauwelaerts)
2. Goldrath, M.H., Fuller, T.A. and Segal, S. (1981). Laser photovaporization of endometrium for the treatment of menorrhagia. *Am. J. Obstet. Gynecol.*, **140**, 14–19
3. DeCherney, A. and Polan, M.L. (1983). Hysteroscopic management of intrauterine lesions and intractable uterine bleeding. *Obstet. Gynecol.*, **61**, 392
4. Loffer, F.D. (1988). Laser ablation of the

endometrium. *Obstet. Gyneol. Clin. N. Am.*, **15**, 77

5. Hamou, J. and Salat-Baroux, J. (1984). Advanced hysteroscopy and microhysteroscopy: our experience with 1000 cases. In Siegler, A.P. and Linderman, H.J. (eds.) *Hysteroscopy: Principles and Practice*, p.63. (Philadelphia: JB Lippincott)

6. Hunter, J.G. and Dixon, J.A. (1985). Lasers in cardiovascular surgery – current status. *West. J. Med.*, **142**, 506–10

7. Hall, E.J. and Roizin-Towle, L. (1984). Biological effect of heat. *Cancer Res.*, **44** (Suppl.), 4708s–35s

8. Fajardo, L.F. (1984). Pathological efects of hyperthermia in normal tissues. *Cancer Res.*, **44** (Suppl.), 4826s–35s

9. Hahn, G.M. (1982). *Hyperthermia and Cancer*. (New York: Plenum Press)

10. Masters, A., Steger, A.C., Lees, W.R., Walmsley, K.M. and Bown, S.G. (1992). Interstitial laser hyperthermia: a new approach for treating liver metastases. *Br. J. Cancer*, **66**, 518–22

11. Steger, A.C., Lees, W.R., Walmsley, K.M. and Bown, S.G. (1989). Interstitial laser hyperthermia: a new approach to local destruction of tumors. *Br. Med. J.*, **299**, 362–5

12. Steger, A.C., Shorvon, P., Walmsley, K., Chisholm, R., Bonn, S.G. and Lees, W.R. (1992). Ultrasound features of low power interstitial laser hyperthermia. *Clin. Radiol.*, **46**, 88–93

13. Phipps, J.H., Lewis, B.V., Roberts, T., Prior, M.V., Hand, J.W., Elder, M. and Field, S.B. (1990). Treatment of functional menorrhagia by radio-frequency-induced thermal endometrial ablation. *Lancet*, **335**, 374–6

14. Phipps, J.H., Lewis, B.V., Prior, M.V. and Roberts, T. (1990). Experimental and clinical studies with radiofrequency-induced thermal endometrial ablation for functional menorrhagia. *Obstet. Gynecol.*, **76**, 876–81

Endometrial photosensitization: experimental models

39

Y. Tadir, B. Tromberg, T. Krasieva, R. Steiner, J. Chapman and M.W. Berns

Photodynamic therapy is an experimental technique used in the treatment of certain tumors[1]. The process typically involves intravenous administration of a photosensitizing drug that is retained longer in certain malignant and vascularized tissues. When light of sufficient energy and appropriate wavelength interacts with the sensitizer, highly reactive oxygen intermediates are generated. These intermediates, primarily singlet molecular oxygen, irreversibly oxidize essential cellular components. The resulting photodestruction of crucial cell organelles and vasculature ultimately causes tissue necrosis[2]. In addition to their therapeutic effect, the characteristic red fluorescence exhibited by photosensitizers can be used in tissue diagnosis. By recording the spatial and spectral distribution of drug fluorescence and tissue autofluorescence, high-contrast images of malignancies can be obtained. Endometrial tissue (*in situ* or ectopic, i.e. endometrium, adenomyosis and endometriosis) may well serve as both an experimental model and a target tissue for photodynamic therapy. It is a highly vascular, neoproliferative tissue with selective sensitivity to hormonal stimulation. Schneider and colleagues[3] studied the potential use of photodynamic therapy for selective endometrial ablation in rat uteri. The same group further evaluated the influence of estrogen on the uptake and localization of dihematoporphyrine ether (DHE) in the uterus of ovariectomized rats[4]. The photosensitizer was concentrated in the endometrial tissue and estrogen treatment significantly increased the uterine uptake but had no effect on other organs. Endometrial ablation by means of photodynamic therapy with Photofrin in the rabbit was described recently[5]. The drug was injected intravenously (1, 2, 5 and 10 mg/kg) and 24 h later, intrauterine laser illumination at 630 nm was administered. The authors concluded that endometrial ablation can be achieved effectively in rabbits by means of photodynamic therapy.

The potential of photodynamic therapy for the treatment of endometriosis was evaluated by Manyak and co-workers[6]. The authors induced endometriosis surgically by transplantation of endometrial tissue in female rabbits. The animals were injected intravenously with DHE and 24 h later, transplants were exposed to 630-nm light. Complete and selective epithelial destruction was seen in 60–81% of the animals with a direct relationship to the light dose. Endometrial implants were also surgically induced for photodynamic therapy by Petrucco and associates[7]. Gold vapor laser irradiation (operating at 627.8 nm) of the transplanted area,

pretreated with hematoporphyrin derivative (HPD), produced necrosis of the endometriotic lesions, leaving surrounding tissue healthy.

In a different study, Manyak and colleagues[8] prepared a rabbit model for early-stage endometriosis by intraperitoneal injection of monodispersed viable endometrial cells. They found that DHE fluorescence facilitates detection of endometrial tissue.

Kennedy[9] studied the fluorescence following systemic administration of a different photosensitizer, 5-aminolevulinic acid (ALA), in the mouse uterus. The endometrium became strongly fluorescent, whereas the myometrium did not. Yang and colleagues[10] in a recent study has clearly demonstrated that intrauterine injection of ALA followed by light exposure caused persistent and specific photodynamic ablation of rat endometrium. In a recent presentation, Judd and co-workers[11] have studied fluorescence of the uterine layers following intravenous injection of ALA and phthalocyanine. The endometrium showed a peak fluorescence at 2 and 3 h with ALA and phthalocyanine, respectively. When using the ALA, the endometrial layer showed fluorescence levels five times higher than the myometrium.

The response of human endometrial carcinoma (HEC-1-A cell line) and ovarian carcinoma (OvCar-3) to photodynamic therapy *in vitro* was studied by Raab and colleagues[12]. Both cell lines did not survive photodynamic therapy. Complete ovarian cell death was observed after application of irradiation doses in the range of 5–20 J/cm² combined with drug concentrations of 2.5–10 μg/ml at a fixed incubation of 48 h. The endometrial cells did not survive photodynamic therapy with 10 J/cm² after incubation in 5 μg/ml for 48 h.

In order to better understand the determinants of selective uptake and retention of various photosensitizers in uterine tissue, we have systematically investigated this topic in rat models (phases I and II)[13]. The main questions we addressed in phase I of these studies were: What is the preferred mode of drug application? and What is the influence of estradiol (as an endometrial proliferation stimulator) on the selectivity and duration of drug uptake?

Since Photofrin is currently the most commonly used photosensitizer, this compound was the main drug employed. Initially, we evaluated the relative merits of intravenous, intraperitoneal, and intrauterine administration methods in medically or surgically castrated rats. Extraction of Photofrin from uterine tissue was

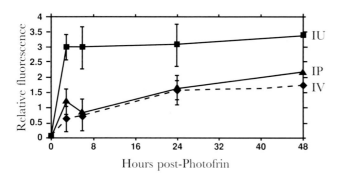

Figure 1 Surface endometrial (columnar epithelium) fluorescence following various application modes of Photofrin: intrauterine (IU, 0.7 mg/kg), intravenous (IV) and intraperitoneal (IP, 7 mg/kg). (Reprinted from reference 13, with permission)

conducted according to a modified porphyrin fecal extraction technique[14]. Frozen sections were analyzed by fluorescence microscopy in order to characterize the distribution of drug fluorescence in uterine layers. Histological specimens were fixed in 10% buffered formalin at room temperature for 24 h and then washed in phosphate buffer, dehydrated in graded alcohol, cleared in histoclear and embedded in paraffin. Using a histomatic tissue processor, 7-μm sections were cut, deparaffined and stained with hematoxylin and eosin.

Intraperitoneal Photofrin administration resulted in a definite pattern of uptake and redistribution within the uterus, as well as a higher overall uptake than with the intravenous approach. This trend suggested that initially there was a high concentration of Photofrin in the serosa; however as time elapsed the drug moved towards the endometrium. Again, myometrial uptake and retention persisted up to 48 h, although it was not significantly higher than with intravenous delivery. It is not clear whether this redistribution was due to diffusion or absorption into the vascular system and subsequent redistribution.

Intrauterine delivery of the photosensitizer appeared to allow more selective retention within the surface endometrial cells (over all time intervals) and minimized myometrial uptake (Figure 1). On the basis of fluorescence intensity, it was determined that the drug remained within the surface endometrial glands with limited diffusion into the deeper stromal layers. Uptake by the endometrial stroma was not significantly different at 48 h as compared to intravenous administration. However, the relative distribution favored uptake within the endometrium with limited uptake by the myometrium. The elevated mitotic activity and increased protein production within the surface endometrial cells and deeper stromal cells may have increased the concentration and retention of the drug in these two layers. Finally, despite a tenfold reduction in dose, intrauterine application yielded a significant increase in extracted

Photofrin, lending support to the hypothesis that site-specific delivery of the photosensitizer can result in selective retention of the drug at a much reduced dose.

In a subsequent experiment[13], all rats were administered the photosensitizer by intrauterine application. The main question focused on the effect of estrogen on uptake and retention of the photosensitizer within the uterine layers and other control organs. Serum estradiol levels were determined by direct radioimmunoassay (the minimum detectable estradiol concentration was 10 pg/ml). Fluorescence activity within the surface of endometrial glands was most prominent in the estradiol-stimulated rats. There was some fluorescence in the deeper stromal cells, with all groups showing some pockets of bright fluorescence. Photofrin, however, tended to be excluded from the myometrial layer, especially following estrogen stimulation. This appeared to be due to the presence of an active, thicker endometrial layer. There are possible explanations for the prolonged retention of Photofrin within the epithelium. As a relatively hydrophobic compound, once it is inside the epithelial cellular lining, it binds to the metabolically active components within the cytosol. If the endometrium has been recently stimulated by estradiol, stromal cells and endometrial glands will exhibit prolonged binding of the Photofrin. The distribution pattern of fluorescence within the endometrial stroma may reflect products from the breakdown of Photofrin within the surface endometrial cells that diffuse into the stroma, while still retaining their fluorescent and photodynamic properties.

Although estradiol stimulation yielded equivocal increases in fluorescence in the endometrial layer (columnar epithelium and stroma), it substantially increased the overall amount of porphyrins extracted from the uterus. Thus, estradiol stimulation appears to result in greater photosensitizer uptake. There were no significant estradiol-induced changes in the uptake of the drug in control organs (spleen and thigh muscle).

Our preliminary studies combined with the limited information available in the literature encouraged further investigation of this approach. Although the intrauterine application of drug appeared promising, drawbacks to these studies included the relatively high Photofrin concentration in the columnar epithelium and the absence of data correlating our drug distribution and studies with photodynamic efficacy. A penetration-enhancing agent, Azone (1-dodecylazacycloheptane-2-one) was added to Photofrin, and a similar rat model was used to compare fluorescence distribution in uterine layers following topical application of Photofrin to Photofrin with Azone. Preliminary data suggest that Photofrin with Azone penetrates much faster than Photofrin alone to the deeper endometrial layers.

A summary of endometrial photosensitization studies can be found in Table 1. Further studies are under way to define the optimal conditions for selective

Table 1 Summary of endometrial photosensitization studies

Author	Model	Photosensitizer	Dose (mg/kg)	Laser wavelength (nm)	Aim
Schneider (1988)[3]	rat endometrium	DHE (IV)	7	630	endometrial ablation
Schneider (1988)[4]	rat endometrium	DHE (IV)	7	630	effect of estrogen
Manyak (1989)[6]	rabbit (surg. induced endometriosis)	DHE (IV)	10	630	endometriosis treatment; laser parameters
Petrucco (1990)[7]	rabbit (surg. induced endometriosis)	HPD (IV)	50	629.7	endometriosis treatment; tissue fluorescence
Manyak (1990)[8]	rabbit (endometrial cell dispersion)	DHE (IV)	10	366 (fluorescence)	endometriosis diagnosis and treatment
Raab (1990)[12]	human endometrial cancer*	porphyrin (in vitro)	0–10 µg/ml medium	630	*in vitro response of endometrial cancer to PDT
Bhatta (1992)[5]	rabbit endometrium	porphyrin	1, 2, 5, 10	630	endometrial ablation
Judd (1992)[11]	rabbit endometrium	ALA (IV)	200	—	compare tissue fluorescence uptake
Kennedy (1992)[9]	mouse uterus	ALA (IV)	N/A	—	compare tissue fluorescence uptake
Yang[10]	rat endometrium	ALA (IU)	4, 6, 16 (mg/0.1 ml)	(non-laser red light)	endometrial ablation
Chapman (1993)[13] Ph. I	rat endometrium	DHE (IV,IP,IU)	7, 7 and 0.7, respectively	—	pharmacokinetics: fluorescence study of various applications
Chapman (1993)[13] Ph. II	rat endometrium	DHE (IU)	0.7	—	pharmacokinetics: fluorescence study; influence of estradiol
Steiner (unpublished) Ph. III	rat endometrium	DHE (IU) DHE Azone (IU)	0.7, 0.7	—	pharmacokinetics: fluorescence study
Steiner (unpublished) Ph. III	rat endometrium	DHE (IU) DHE + Azone (IU)	0.7, 0.7	630	histology following PDT

IV = intravenous; IU = intrauterine; IP = intraperitoneal; DHE = dihematoporphyrine ether; HPD = hematoporphyrin derivative; ALA = 5-aminolevulinic acid; PDT = photodynamic therapy; N/A = not applicable

endometrial ablation. It is expected that photodynamic destruction of endometrial tissue may in future replace surgical procedures that require general anesthesia and hospitalization. Photodynamic therapy has the potential to improve the conventional management of endometrial disease and minimize the cost and invasiveness of treatment.

REFERENCES

1. Dougherty, T.J. (1984). Photodynamic therapy (PDT) of malignant tumors. *CRC Crit. Rev. Oncol. Hematol.*, **2**, 83–116

2. Dougherty, T.J. (1987). Photosensitizers: therapy and detection of malignant tumors. *Photochem. Photobiol.*, **45**, 879–89

3. Schneider, D., Schellhas, H.F., Wessler, T.A. *et al.* (1988). Endometrial ablation by DHE photoradiation therapy in estrogen treated ovariectomized rats. *Colposc. Gynecol. Laser Surg.*, **4**, 73–7

4. Schneider, D., Schellhas, H.F., Wessler, T.A. *et al.* (1988). Hematoporphyrin derivative uptake *in uteri* of estrogen treated ovariectomized rats. *Colposc. Gynecol. Laser Surg.*, **4**, 67–71

5. Bhatta, N., Anderson, R., Flotte, T., Schiff, I., Hasan, T. and Nishioka, N.S. (1992). Endometrial ablation by means of photodynamic therapy with Photofrin II. *Am. J. Obstet. Gynecol.*, **167**, 1856–63

6. Manyak, M.J., Nelson, L.M. and Solomon, D. (1989). Photodynamic therapy of rabbit endometrium transplants: a model for treatment of endometriosis. *Fertil. Steril.*, **52**, 140–5

7. Petrucco, O.M., Sathananden, M., Petrucco, M.F., Knowles, S., McKenzie, L., Forbes, I.J., Cowled, P.A. and Keye, W.E. (1990). Ablation of endometriotic implants in rabbits by hematoporphyrin derivative photoradiation therapy using the gold vapor laser. *Lasers Surg. Med.*, **10**, 344–8

8. Manyak, M.J., Nelson, L.M., Solomon, D., DeGraff, W., Stillman, R.J. and Russo, A. (1990). Fluorescent detection of rabbit endometrial implants

from monodispersed viable cell suspension. *Fertil. Steril.*, **54**, 356–9

9. Kennedy, J.C. and Pottier, R.H., (1992). Endogenous protoporphyrin IX, a clinically useful photosensitizer for photodynamic therapy. *J. Photochem. Photobiol. B. Biol.*, **14**, 275–92

10. Yang, J.Z., Van Vugt, D.A., Kennedy, J.C. and Reid, R.L. (1993). Evidence of lasting functional destruction of the rat endometrium following 5-aminolevulinic acid induced photodynamic ablation: prevention of implantation. *Am. J. Obstet. Gynecol.*, **168**, 995–1001

11. Judd, M.D., Bedwell, J. and MacRobert, A.J. (1992). Comparison of the distribution of phthalocyanine and ALA-induced porphyrin sensitizers within the rabbit uterus. *Lasers Med. Sci.*, **7**, 203

12. Raab, G. H., Schneider, A.F., Eirmann, W., Gottschalk-Deponte, H., Baumgartner, R. and Beyer, W. (1990). Response of human endometrium and ovarian carcinoma cell-lines to photodynamic therapy. *Arch. Gynecol. Obstet.*, **248**, 13–20

13. Chapman, J.A., Tadir, Y., Tromberg, B.J., Yu, K., Manetta, A., Sun, C.H. and Berns, M.W. (1993). Effect of administration route and estrogen manipulation on endometrial uptake of Photofrin. *Am. J. Obstet. Gynecol.*, **168**, 685–92

14. Rossi, E. and Curnow, D. (1986). Porphyrins. In Lim, C.L. (ed.) *HPLC of Small Molecules. A Practical Approach*, pp.266–7. (Oxford: IRL Press)

The future of micromanipulation techniques in reproductive medicine

40

S. Gordts

The rapid development of technologies for investigation and treatment in reproductive medicine, and the use of micromanipulation techniques in assisted reproduction have created new possibilities for couples with fertility problems. These techniques offer new possibilities for the manipulation of gametes and embryos, which will be beneficial for couples with male subfertility, as well as for couples with a high risk of genetic disease.

MALE SUBFERTILITY

Although many couples with fertility problems can be helped by *in vitro* fertilization, the treatment outcome in those with semen subfertility remains poor, because of failure of sperm-oocyte fusion. While the complex mechanism of this fusion process is not fully understood, fertilization rates will be low and it will be difficult to predict the outcome for individual couples. Oocyte-sperm fusion problems can, however, be bypassed, using micromanipulation techniques.

The zona pellucida may be bypassed by *partial zona dissection (PZD)* (Figure 1). In this technique, a gap in the zona pellucida is created chemically or mechanically, permitting the 'best' sperm to pass through and to fuse more easily with the oocyte. Chemicals such as Thyrode acid partially digest the zona pellucida but damage the oocyte, resulting in low fertilization rates and poor quality of the developing embryos, with low or zero pregnancy rates[1,2]. Mechanical disruption of the zona pellucida leads to higher fertilization rates and better embryo quality[3]. The results are still controversial, however, because of varying polyspermia rates.

Differences in polyspermia rates found by different authors can be explained, first and foremost, by the

Table 1 Comparison of fertilization rates after normal insemination and after subzonal injection of sperm (SUZI) in sibling oocytes from couples with male subfertility. PN, pronuclei

	Number of oocytes	2PN (%)	3PN (%)	Total fertilization (%)
Normal insemination	928*	9	—	9
SUZI	1661*	17	9	27

* If fewer than four oocytes were retrieved only SUZI was performed

Table 2 Correlation between the number of subzonally inserted sperm and fertilization and polyspermia rates. PN, pronuclei

Number of injected sperm	2PN (%)	3PN (%)
1– 5	8.5	1.5
5–10	14.5	8
10–15	23.5	9
15–20	22	17.5

Table 3 Influence of morphology on polyspermia rates in normally inseminated and subzonally injected oocytes

	2PN (%)		3PN (%)	
Morphology	Normal	SUZI	Normal	SUZI
< 14%	9	19	0	7
> 14%	11	20	0	22

subjective interpretation of semen parameters, especially of sperm morphology. It is, furthermore, technically impossible to slit the zona pellucida in a standardized and uniform way, to enable fewer or more spermatozoa to enter the perivitelline space[4], depending on the size of the gap, and thus directly influencing the fertilization and polyspermia rate. Third, there is no proof that the gap will remain patent in all the treated oocytes. Obstruction can be caused by sperm crowding, zona elasticity or obstruction by remaining corona cells.

The zona pellucida is completely bypassed by *subzonal insertion of sperm* (SUZI) (Figure 2). In this technique, a few randomly chosen spermatozoa are inserted directly into the perivitelline space. In our own experience, as well as studies of other investigators[5,6] this technique results in a statistically higher fertilization rate (2 pronuclei (PN)) compared to the outcome in normally inseminated sibling oocytes (Table 1). The implantation rate, however, reaches only 13%. This may be an indication of lower embryo quality, related to sperm quality and/or to the micromanipulation procedure, in spite of the microscopically normal aspect of the embryo and a normal cleavage rate. In our own experience, training influenced the outcome of the micromanipulation procedure in terms of fertilization rate, cleavage rate and pregnancy rate (Figure 3). The mean polyspermia rate in our study was 7%, but this was clearly influenced by the number of subzonally injected sperm, and even more, by the morphology of the semen (Tables 2 and 3).

The *intracytoplasmatic injection technique* (ICSI) (Figure 1) bypasses all obstacles as a randomly chosen single sperm is injected into the cytoplasm of the oocyte. This technique seems to offer promising results in terms of fertilization rate[7] reaching a 2PN fertilization rate of 44% and a pregnancy rate per embryo transfer of 18%. The implantation rate per embryo is, however, severely impaired in cases of extreme teratozoospermia. Caution is recommended, because until now, only a few babies have been born from this procedure and there are still too few data available to exclude an increased risk of fetal malformation.

PREIMPLANTATION DIAGNOSIS

The micromanipulation techniques mentioned above are also used for the purpose of preimplantation genetic studies. For couples at high genetic risk, a biopsy of a single cell in the preconceptional stage can be performed by removal and examination of the first polar body[8], or at the embryonic stage, by removal of one or two blastomeres at the eight-cell stage, or by biopsying trophectoderm cells from an embryo in the blastocyst stage[9,10]. Polymerase chain reaction (PCR) or fluorescent *in situ* hybridization (FISH) techniques enable single cells to be analyzed and screened for genetic disorder[11]. If only unaffected embryos are transferred, couples with a known high risk of genetic disease can be offered the possibility of normal offspring, thus avoiding the decisions and risks associated with terminating a pregnancy[8-10].

All of these micromanipulation techniques are mechanical, using holding and injection pipettes. As mentioned above, training is an important factor and influences substantially the final fertilization and pregnancy rates. Although experienced laboratory technicians can easily learn to make different kinds of pipettes, the procedure remains a time-consuming business.

THE FUTURE

The introduction of the laser may offer new perspectives in the evolution of assisted fertilization techniques.

As suggested by Tadir *et al.*[12-15], the laser can be used not only for microinsemination procedures, but also for the destruction of an extra pronucleus, for optical trapping of spermatozoa, or for inducing chromosome movement. So far, however, most experiments have focused on using the laser for microinsemination procedures, mostly for partial zona dissection. For this purpose, different wavelengths have been used, ranging from the infrared (800 nm) to the ultra-violet spectrum at 217 nm. When choosing a laser system, different criteria have to be kept in mind. First, since cells, and particularly oocytes and embryos, contain a high proportion of water, the laser system must be characterized by a high absorption coefficient in water. Second, thermal damage to the oocyte or embryo must be avoided. This is in contrast to the laser systems used for endoscopic surgery, where most of the energy is converted into heat. Even the culture medium may impair the quality of the embryo[16]. For example, when using the same 248 nm krypton fluoride excimer laser, the rise in temperature at the embryo is 16 times higher in human tubal fluid (HTF) medium than in phosphate buffered saline (PBS) medium. Third, operating laser systems employing a non-touch technique would simplify the micromanipulation technique itself, avoiding the time-consuming business of pipette making and offering the possibility of directing the laser beam tangentially at the egg sphere. Lastly, damage to DNA must be prevented. Some experimental investigations have shown a higher incidence of chromosomal abnormalities after irradiation with a 308 nm excimer laser, although these alterations were minor[17]. Some investigators prefer wavelengths with a high absorption coefficient in water, such as the 193 nm radiation laser[18,19] producing laserpulses through micropipettes or using glass-fibers, such as the 2.94 μm Erbium : YAG laser[20]. The 2.94 μm Erbium : YAG laser and the 1064 nm Nd : YAG laser are both in the infrared spectrum. The Nd : YAG laser was used successfully to transect the zona pellucida of hamster oocytes, but the functional incapacity of the treated oocytes to bind sperm and the absence of penetration of the ooplasm with decondensation of the sperm head indicates that the thermal mode of action of this laser induced some alterations in the subcellular structure of the oocyte[21]. Normal embryonic development occurred after treatment of mouse embryos with the Erbium : YAG laser, and in humans, an ongoing pregnancy was achieved[20,22]. The excimer lasers are all in the ultra-violet range of the electromagnetic spectrum. These laser pulses are based on the principle of photoablation, in which an excitation of the organic molecules is induced through the absorption of a UV photon. When the molecules reach a sufficiently excited state, bond-breaking of the molecules occurs, with disruption and the onset of a chemical reaction.

A 308 nm XeCl excimer laser was used to slit the zona pellucida of mouse oocytes, using a non-touch technique. The fertilization rate was improved to 31.5%, compared with only 6% in control oocytes, using sperm from vasectomized males. The incidence of blastocyst formation was 72%. Because the oocytes were put in fresh culture medium following laser exposure, no attention was paid to the possible toxic effect of ablation by-products. This issue was investigated in the study of Blanchet *et al.*[16]. Using a 248 nm krypton fluoride

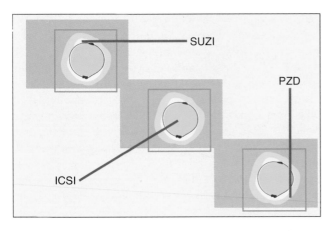

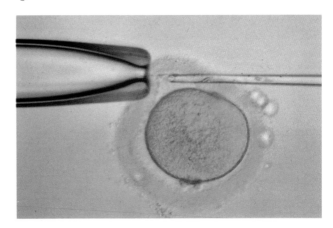

Figure 1 Different techniques of micromanipulation: in PZD an opening in the zona pellucida is made, allowing the sperm to pass the barrier of the zona pellucida. In SUZI several spermatozoa are directly injected in the perivitelline space. ICSI involves injection of one sperm into the cytoplasm of the oocyte

Figure 2 The oocyte is fixed with the holding pipette, while the injection pipette is inserted subzonally, waiting for 5–10 spermatozoa to swim out into the perivitelline space

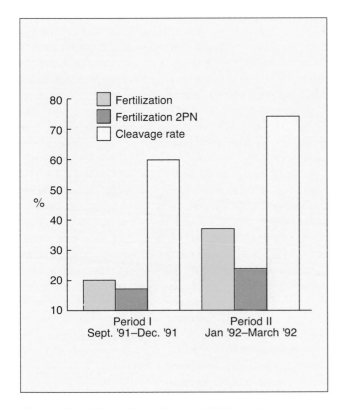

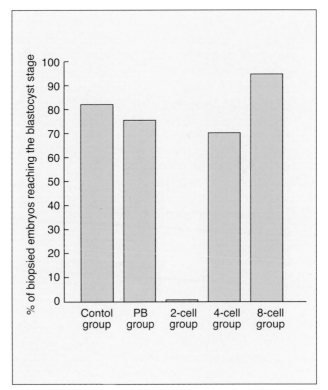

Figure 3 Effect of training on SUZI results

Figure 4 Evolution of mouse embryos to blastocyst stage after removal of the polar body and of one blastomere in different cleavage stages

excimer laser on the zona pellucida of mouse embryos, they found not only a significant difference in blastocyst formation, depending on whether the mouse embryos were cultured in HTF medium or PBS medium (7.4% versus 24%, respectively), but they also observed that this rate of blastocyst formation was lower than in the control group in both media (87% and 92.8%). Ablation by-products were responsible for the inhibition of the embryo development, correlating directly with the time of exposure. The blastocyst formation rate improved to 66% when embryos were immediately transferred to fresh medium after laser exposure.

For drilling of the zona pellucida with the 193 nm argon fluoride excimer laser, micropipettes filled with air were used in contact with the zona[19], because the very high absorption of this laser beam by water makes delivery through liquid interfaces impossible. After a gap in the zona pellucida had been made with minimal damage to the surrounding area, the authors reported a higher fertilization rate compared with the non-treated oocytes, and a higher incidence of hatched blastocysts.

Polyspermia is a possible complication of human *in vitro* fertilization; the mean incidence of 4–6% increases to 25% after micromanipulation[4]. As the male pronuclei can be distinguished by their larger size and the presence of an associated sperm tail, it is possible to remove the supernumerary male pronuclei when this occurs. After the zygote has been fixed using the holding pipette, the smaller handling pipette is pierced through the zona pellucida and then pushed through the plasma membrane near the spot of the male pronucleus. Using light suction, the male pronucleus is aspirated and the micropipette slowly withdrawn. Cellular damage caused by introducing the micropipette into the cytoplasm and by aspirating some of the cytoplasm surrounding the aspirated pronucleus is, however, inevitable.

An XeCl excimer laser can be focused at the desired target within the zona or the cytoplasma and may be used to selectively destroy supernumerary male pronuclei[24,25] without opening or damaging the zona pellucida or plasma membrane. Further research must be carried out on the possible adverse effects of this technique, and normal embryo development has to be evaluated.

It is possible for optical sperm trapping[13,24] to be used for tracking sperm in different micromanipulation procedures. By allowing measurement of the relative force of normal and abnormal sperm, it can give us a better understanding of sperm physiology.

For preimplantation diagnosis at the embryonic stage, a blastomere biopsy is mostly performed at the eight-cell stage[9,10] taking into consideration on the one hand, the implantation window and, on the other hand, the time that is required for genetic analysis of the single cells. The earlier the biopsy, the more time there is for genetic analysis. Our own experiments on mouse embryos have shown no difference in blastocyst formation, compared with the controls, when biopsies were performed at the eight-cell stage. Developmental arrest was observed when the embryo was biopsied at the two-cell stage (Figure 4), probably because of the relatively greater reduction in cellular mass than in later stages.

At the blastocyst stage, the embryonic cells differentiate into an outer epithelial layer and an inner cell mass, responsible for the formation of the fetus. The number of cells removed makes genetic analysis easier and more accurate. Biopsy of the trophectoderm cells has the advantage that the cells upon which the further development of the fetus depends do not have to be removed. Extrusion of trophectoderm cells can be achieved by making a slit in the zona pellucida of the embryo. This may be performed by a tangentially directed laser beam, as previously described. The extruded trophectoderm cells can then be cut from the blastocyst, using the laser beam in a non-touch manner. Until now, however, the formation of blastocysts of human embryos has been limited and only 40–50% of the embryos reach this stage, thus reducing the number of embryos available for biopsy.

CONCLUSIONS

The development of different kinds of laser with low energy output will offer perspectives for the further development of micromanipulation procedures. Although some clinical pregnancies have already been described following the use of laser techniques for micromanipulation procedures, a lot of experimental work still has to be done. Different questions remain unanswered and technical problems are unsolved. The use of lasers in the field of micromanipulation is now at the same point as it was in gynecological endoscopic procedures at the beginning of the 1980s. Wave lengths range between 217 nm and 800 nm. In contrast to endoscopic surgery, energy is delivered not in continuous mode but with ultra-short pulses of 10–14 ns, using a spot size of 1–5 μm. Application has mostly been focused on partial zona dissection. Although an increased fertilization rate is seen using this technique, its importance has not yet been well defined and other micromanipulation techniques such as SUZI and ICSI will probably do better. Application of laser for PZD makes it possible to reproduce gaps of the same size, which is technically impossible with mechanical micromanipulation techniques. This makes a comparison of results possible and helps to determine the right indications for this technique. In order to be clinically interesting and economically feasible, the chosen laser system must be suitable not only for PZD, but also for all other applications.

The toxic effect of photoablation by-products, as described by Blanchet *et al.*[16] has to be further investigated for different types of laser and different kinds of culture medium.

It has been demonstrated that certain wavelengths induce some, albeit minor, chromosomal aberrations. Further studies still have to be carried out to exclude laser-induced chromosomal alterations.

In developing laser systems for micromanipulation, the non-touch technique is preferable, because it will simplify the procedure and there will be no further need for the preparation of injecting or holding pipettes. Furthermore, the non-touch technique offers the possibility of directing the laser beam tangentially at the egg sphere.

Many new possibilities are at our disposal in the field of reproductive medicine. Different new techniques are now being used to assist fertilization, especially in couples with male subfertility. All of these techniques are still under development and the results have to be evaluated in due course. It is certain, however that the introduction of laser techniques in this field will contribute greatly to the further development of all the possibilities.

REFERENCES

1. Gordon, J.W., Grunfeld, L., Garrezi, G.J., Talansky, B.E., Richards, C. and Laufer, M. (1988). Fertilization of human oocytes by sperm from infertile males after zona pellucida drilling. *Fertil. Steril.*, **50**, 68–73

2. Depypere, H.T., McLaughlin, K.J., Seamark, R.F., Warnes, G.M. and Mattheus, C.D. (1988). Comparison of zona cutting and zona drilling as techniques for assisted fertilization in the mouse. *J. Reprod. Fertil.*, **84**, 205–11

3. Garrisi, G.J., Talansky, B.E., Grunfeld, L., Sapira, V., Navot, D. and Gordon, J.W. (1990). Clinical evaluation of three approaches to micromanipulation assisted fertilization. *Fertil. Steril.*, **54**, 671–7

4. Levron, J., Stein, D.W., Brandes, J.M. and Itskovitz-Eldor, J. (1993). Presence of sperm in the perivitelline space predicts fertilization rate after partial zona dissection. *Fertil. Steril.*, **59**, 820–5

5. Gordts, S., Garcia, G., Vercruyssen, M., Roziers, P., Campo, R. and Swinnen, K. (1993). Subzonal insemination: a prospective randomized study in patients with abnormal sperm morphology. *Fertil. Steril.*, **60**, 307–13

6. Fishel, S., Jackson, P., Antinori, S., Johnson, J., Grossi, S. and Versaci, C. (1990). Subzonal insemination for the alleviation of infertility. *Fertil. Steril.*, **54**, 828–35

7. Palermo, P., Hubert, J., Derde, M.P., Camus, M., Devroey, P. and Van Steirteghem, A. (1993). Sperm characteristics and outcome of human assisted fertilization by subzonal insemination and intracytoplasmatic sperm injection. *Fertil. Steril.*, **59**, 826–35

8. Verlinsky, Y., Ginsberg, N., Lifeher, A., Valle, J., Moise, I. and Stram, C.M. (1990). Analysis of the first polar body: preconception genetic diagnosis. *Hum. Reprod.*, **5**, 826–9

9. Handyside, A.H. (1993). Diagnosis of inherited disease before implantation. *Reprod. Med. Rev.*, **2**, 51–61

10. Handyside, A.H., Kontogianni, E.H., Hardy, K. and Winston, R.M.L. (1990). Pregnancies from biopsied human preimplantation embryos sexed by Y-specific DNA amplification. *Nature (London)*, **344**, 768–70

11. Wu, R., Cuppens, H., Hilliker, C., Buyse, I., Decorte, R., Marynen, P., Gordts, S. and Cassiman, J.J. (1993). Coamplification of the cystic fibrosis F508 mutation with the HLADQA1 and 3-color fluorescent *in situ* hybridization for chromosomes X, Y and 18 in single cells: an *in vitro* test for a potentially successful strategy in preimplantation diagnosis. *Prenatal Diagn.*, (in press)

12. Tadir, Y., Wright, W.H., Vafa, O., Liaw, L.H., Asch, R. and Berns, M.W. (19XX). Micromanipulation of gametes using laser microbeams. *Hum. Reprod.*, **6**, 1011–6

13. Tadir, Y., Wright, W.H., Vafa, O., Ord, T., Asch, R. and Berns, M.W. (1989). Micromanipulation of sperm by a laser generated optical trap. *Fertil. Steril.*, **52**, 870–3

14. Tadir, Y., Wright, W.H., Vafa, O., Ord, T., Asch, R. and Berns, M.W. (1990). Force generated by human sperm correlated to velocity and determined using a laser generated trap. *Fertil. Steril.*, **53**, 944–7

15. Neev, J., Tadir, Y., Ho, P., Berns, M.W., Asch, R.H. and Ord, T. (1992). Microscope-delivered ultraviolet laser zona dissection: principles and practices. *J. Assist. Reprod. Genet.*, **9**, 513–23

16. Blanchet, G.B., Russell, J.B., Fincher, C.R. and Portmann, M. (1992). Laser micromanipulation in the mouse embryo: a novel approach to zona drilling. *Fertil. Steril.*, **57**, 1337–41

17. Virsick-Peuckert, R.P., Hillrichs, G., Jahn, R., Jungbluth, K.H. and Neu, W. (1992). Art und Häufigkeit von Chromosomenschädigungen nach Zellbestrahlungen mit einem 308 nm-Excimerlaser. *Lasermedizin*, **8**, 182–7

18. Palanker, D., Ohad, S., Lewis, A., Simon, A., Shenkar, J., Penchas, S. and Laufer, N. (1991). Technique for cellular microsurgery using the 193-nm excimer laser. *Laser Surg. Med.*, **11**, 580–6

19. Laufer, N., Palanker, D., Shufaro, Y., Safran, A., Simon, A. and Lewis, A.(1993). The efficacy and safety of zona pellucida drilling by a 193-nm excimer laser. *Fertil. Steril.*, **59**, 889–95

20. Strohmer, H. and Feichtinger, W. (1992). Successful clinical application of laser for micromanipulation in an *in vitro* fertilization program. *Fertil. Steril.*, **58**, 212–4

21. Coddington, C.C., Veeck, L.L., Swanson, R.J.,

Kaufmann, R.A., Lin, J., Simonetti, S. and Bocca, S. (1992). The yag laser used in micromanipulation to transect the zona pellucida. *J. Assist. Reprod. Genet.*, **9**, 557–63

22. Feichtinger, W., Strohmer, H., Fuhrberg, P., Radivojevic, K., Antinori, S., Pepe, P. and Versaci, C. (1992). Photoablation of oocyte zona pellucida by erbium : Yag laser for *in vitro* fertilization in severe male infertility. *Lancet*, **339**, 811

23. El-Danasouri, I., Westphal, L.M., Neev, Y., Gebhardt, J., Louie, D. and Berns, M.W. (1993).

Zona opening with 308 nm XeCl excimer laser improves fertilization by spermatozoa from long-term vasectomized mice. *Hum. Reprod.*, **8**, 464–6

24. Tadir, Y., Neev, J. and Berns, M.W. (1993). Laser microsurgery and manipulation of single cells. In Sutton, C. and Diamond, M. (eds.) *Endoscopic Surgery for Gynecologists*, pp. 379–86. (London: Saunders)

25. Rawlins, R.G., Binor, Z., Radwanska, E. and Dmowski, W.P. (1988). Microsurgical enucleation of tripronuclear human zygotes. *Fertil. Steril.*, **50**, 266–72

Index